# CASE STUDIES IN CANADIAN HEALTH POLICY AND MANAGEMENT

## Second Edition

*Edited by Raisa B. Deber with Catherine L. Mah*

Covering a wide range of issues, *Case Studies in Canadian Health Policy and Management* is an exceptional resource for bringing real-life policy questions into the classroom. The twenty-two case studies have been developed with input from mid-career professionals with strong field experience, and have been extensively tested in Raisa B. Deber's graduate case study seminar at the University of Toronto. Each case features both a substantive health policy issue and a selection of key concepts and methods appropriate to examining public policy, public health, and health care management issues.

The contributors provide a summary of each case and the related policy issues, a description of events, questions for discussion, supporting information and references, and suggestions for further reading. Suitable for graduate and undergraduate classrooms in programs in a variety of fields, *Case Studies in Canadian Health Policy and Management* is an exceptional educational resource.

This second edition features all new cases, as well as a new introductory chapter that provides a framework and tools for health policy analysis in Canada.

RAISA B. DEBER is a professor at the Institute of Health Policy, Management and Evaluation at the University of Toronto.

CATHERINE L. MAH is an assistant professor in the Division of Public Health Policy at the Dalla Lana School of Public Health at the University of Toronto.

The Teaching Notes for this book are available on a tab on the book's University of Toronto Press webpage: http://www.utppublishing .com/Case-Studies-in-Canadian-Health-Policy-and-Management-Second-Edition.html

EDITED BY RAISA B. DEBER
WITH CATHERINE L. MAH

# Case Studies in Canadian Health Policy and Management

## Second Edition

UNIVERSITY OF TORONTO PRESS
Toronto Buffalo London

© University of Toronto Press 2014
Toronto Buffalo London
www.utppublishing.com
Printed in Canada

ISBN 978-1-4426-4022-1 (cloth)
ISBN 978-1-4426-0996-9 (paper)

Printed on acid-free, 100% post-consumer recycled paper with vegetable-based inks.

A cataloguing record for this publication is available from Library and Archives Canada.

University of Toronto Press acknowledges the financial assistance to its publishing program of the Canada Council for the Arts and the Ontario Arts Council.

 Canada Council  Conseil des Arts
for the Arts  du Canada

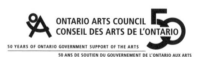

University of Toronto Press acknowledges the financial support of the Government of Canada through the Canada Book Fund for its publishing activities.

*This book is dedicated to all of the students who took and contributed to Raisa B. Deber's case studies course.*

# Contents

# Acknowledgments

Writing this case book has been a complex exercise, spanning many years. We would like to express our appreciation for the many people who helped.

First, we would like to thank the many students who took Case Studies in Canadian Health Policy over the years, and helped write, edit, and clarify what was necessary to make these cases work in a classroom setting. Locating the many contributors to these cases was an interesting challenge. In addition to Google and LinkedIn, we would like to thank Mariana Vardaei, Christina Lopez, Tina Smith, Sue VanderBent, and the Society of Graduates in Health Policy, Management and Evaluation; we also thank the few students we could not locate who had contributed to early versions of some cases, but were not involved in writing the final revised versions.

In their roles as valuable colleagues and friends, Wendy Armstrong, Jan Barnsley, Andrea Baumann, Ahmed Bayoumi, John Blake, Ivy Bourgeault, Adalsteinn Brown, Tamara Brown, Mike Carter, Tony Culyer, Frieda Daniels, Gail Donner, Rick Fisher, Virginia Flintoft, Paul Froese, Brenda Gamble, Vivek Goel, Jillian Clare Kohler, Audrey Laporte, Chris Longo, Fiona Miller, Barbara Mintzes, Bill Ness-Jack, Dorothy Pringle, Michael Rachlis, Brad Sinclair, Cyra Sethna, John Stager, Yves Talbot, Ross Upshur, Michael Villeneuve, Frank Wagner, and Paul Williams also provided superb insight into those cases they were kind enough to review. Kanecy Onate, Christine Day, and Tim Walker provided essential support in editing and formatting cases, locating bibliographic items, and otherwise helping make these cases coherent. We also appreciate the help of Eric Carlson, Doug Richmond, Virgil Duff, and the staff at the University of Toronto Press.

In addition to their roles as loving family members, Charles Deber, Jonathan Deber and Karen Dawson, and Guy Schnitzler provided editorial assistance and unflinching support.

Raisa B. Deber and Catherine L. Mah, Toronto

# Introduction

The cases in this book are products of a popular graduate seminar in health policy at the University of Toronto taught by Raisa B. Deber. All of the cases, and their accompanying teaching notes in the companion volume, have been developed through repeated use in the classroom setting, and the best are included here. Each case has been extensively tested and revised to ensure it can be easily applied in the classroom setting by individuals other than the case writer. This intensive degree of student feedback from individuals with strong field experience is rare among case collections in health and public policy. As can be seen from the brief biographies in the "About the Contributors" section, many of our students and graduates play pivotal roles in health care and public policymaking in Canada and on the international stage. The Canadian Hospital Association Press published the original edition of this case studies book in 1992; this second edition has all new cases.

This book is intended primarily for faculty and students in policy/administration classes with a health policy component. We have found that students at all levels of study (senior undergraduates, graduate students, health care professional students, and health care professionals/executives returning to school) have been able to use the cases and teaching notes readily and successfully. The cases can be used in undergraduate or graduate courses, in a variety of programs, including those directed towards health professional education (including health administration, medicine, public health, nursing, social work, rehabilitation, and health law), as well as in political science/management departments. Students in other disciplines working with public policy issues, and policymakers and health care stakeholders seeking case-based material for professional education seminars should also find the book useful. The cases cover a wide variety of topics, including (but not restricted to) public health, health human resources, resource allocation, and ethics; they deal with a broad array of subsectors (including insurance, primary care, hospitals, long-term care, and pharmaceuticals), and can be used to teach a variety of policy tools (including economic analysis, queuing theory, and screening).

Because the University of Toronto program in which this course is offered takes midcareer students from a variety of professional backgrounds, the case material has been able to draw upon a wide range of expertise. Another unusual (and perhaps unique) feature of the book is that many of the students who took this course have contributed to the generation and refinement of these cases, and are accordingly listed as co-authors when their contributions so warranted; this included reviewing the revised versions of their case, and suggesting revisions and modifications as needed. Rarely, contributors to earlier versions could not be located and hence could not be involved in contributing to this published version; we nonetheless thank them, as well as the other students whose contributions to class discussions also influenced the revisions.

All of the cases in this book are based on real-world issues and situations in health and public policy, but have applicability beyond each specific example. This book contains two pairs of "companion cases" (Chapters 3 and 4, and Chapters 19 and 20) that are linked, but can also be taught separately, as well as several cases (Chapters 15, 16, and 20) that can be taught as role play exercises. Real names are used in the cases when they were already in the public domain; otherwise, names are invented (and at times may make reference to individuals involved in developing the cases). These cases have intentionally been designed to be "rich," in that they can be focused in a number of different ways, depending on what the instructor would like to emphasize. All are two-track, presenting both a substantive health policy issue (e.g., how to manage wait times for cancer treatment) and key concepts and methods for public policy/public administration (e.g., the roles of the bureaucracy vs. the politicians; how to use queuing theory). Instructors may vary as to which of these they wish to emphasize. In addition, although the specific cases have emerged in a Canadian (often Ontario) setting, we have attempted to ensure that the issues and concepts discussed will be applicable to public policymaking and management in other jurisdictions, not only in Canada but also internationally. To reduce duplication, Chapter 1 (Concepts for the Policy Analyst) summarizes a variety of health policy and health care system concepts that we have found give helpful background information and/or recur in multiple cases; cross references to the most relevant Chapter 1 material are noted in the case, and are listed at the end of the teaching notes for that case (teaching notes are available for free download from http://www.utp publishing.com/Case-Studies-in-Canadian-Health-Policy-and-Man agement-Second-Edition.html).

Each case is designed to allow class participants to identify the problems that must be resolved, analyze them, and suggest solutions. We have been particularly cognizant that even incomplete cases may work in the classroom if enough tacit knowledge is present, but that a published case book cannot (and should not) rely on this. We have accordingly tried to ensure that enough information is given to allow these cases to work even when the class members (and perhaps the presenter) are not yet experts in the topics being covered. We have tried to ensure that the cases are up to date and accurate, without becoming bogged down in detail, and that the references properly acknowledge our sources without listing too many.

Each case consists of the following components:

- Short introduction, summarizing the case and the policy issues that might be addressed;
- List of appendices;
- Description of the events in the case, culminating in a decision point;
- Suggested questions for discussion;
- Supporting appendices; and
- References cited and further readings, including websites where appropriate.

In the companion teaching notes, we describe for each case:

- The outcome;
- Points that could be made in discussion, with brief comments on each (linked to the suggested questions from Volume 1);
- A listing of the particularly relevant topics from Chapter 1; and
- References cited and further readings.

The teaching notes can be used in two ways. They can be used as a conventional instructor's manual. Alternatively, as in Deber's graduate course at the University of Toronto, students can be asked to select a case (alone, or in a small group), and to prepare and facilitate a seminar-length discussion on the case, working through the theoretical foci and policy options. We give the presenting student(s) the teaching notes for that case to assist them in preparing for the class. We subsequently distribute those teaching notes to all students in the class, but only after that case has been discussed; students have found the notes to be a helpful review of the material discussed. More detail on how teaching notes can be used is given in Chapter 1 of the teaching notes.

We believe you will find this volume of cases interesting and helpful. If you have any comments or suggestions, please contact Raisa B. Deber (raisa.deber@utoronto.ca).

# 1 Concepts for the Policy Analyst

*RAISA B. DEBER*

In analyzing these case studies, a number of concepts may be helpful. To avoid undue repetition, this chapter briefly describes key concepts that recur in multiple cases. Although it could be read as a unified work, it is primarily designed to allow the reader to dip into these "theory bits." Accordingly, we have not only cross-referenced concepts within Chapter 1, but also sought to cross-reference concepts between Chapter 1 and the cases by noting in each case the sections of Chapter 1 that might be particularly applicable. Chapter 1 in the Teaching Notes also includes a listing of which cases (designated by chapter number) particularly focus on each of the specific theory bits.

For those wishing for a fuller treatment of these concepts, one good starting point is a basic political science / policy analysis text. Here are some texts we have found helpful; this is not intended to be an exhaustive list (Brooks, 2009; Brooks & Miljan, 2003; Courtney & Smith, 2010; Doern & Phidd, 1992; Howlett et al., 2009; MacLean & Wood, 2010; McLean & McMillan, 2003).

## 1. What Is Policy?

*Politics* has been defined as the "authoritative allocation of resources," or, more simply, as "who gets what, when and how" (Lasswell, 1958). Clearly, politics occurs everywhere, not just within government (hence the term "office politics").

There are multiple definitions of *policy*. One definition we have found useful is that of Jenkins: "A set of interrelated decisions taken by a political actor or group of actors concerning the selection of goals and the means of achieving them within a specified situation where these decisions should, in principle, be within the power of these actors to achieve" (Jenkins, 1978). Implications of using this definition include the following:

- As is true for politics, policy occurs everywhere, not just within government. This is particularly important for health policy, where many decisions are made by non-governmental actors.
- Policy is not always written down. (This differs from another way the term "policy" is often used within organizations, in the sense of a "policy and procedures" manual.)
- Policy may involve deciding to do nothing, which Bachrach and Baratz have termed "non-decisions" (Bachrach & Baratz, 1962, 1963). Indeed, some of the deepest held values or assumptions are often revealed in decisions that are never made explicitly, including the acceptance of certain options without question. Comparing policies across jurisdictions often helps highlight when such underlying assumptions have been operative in a particular jurisdiction and/or policy subfield. As one example, Canada has never even considered using primary health care models where patients are assigned to physicians rather than being able to select the provider of their choice, although Canadian school boards do use similar models where elementary and high school students are assigned to schools and teachers.
- Policy involves intentions rather than results; it may not always succeed in achieving its goals. As noted US political scientist Aaron Wildavsky observed, when one is dealing with difficult policy decisions, one rarely solves them (Wildavsky, 1979). Instead, one will often replace one set of problems with a new set of problems; if one is successful, one prefers the new problems to the old ones.

There are also multiple ways political scientists conceptualize policymaking. Some stress the distinction between the *structures* that influence policymaking, the *processes* used, and the policy *outcomes*. Others focus on such policy elements as *ideas*, *institutions*, and *interests*. We will borrow from them all, plus others. We will begin with the institutions/structures that help decide how policies are made, and by whom.

## 2. Institutions/Structures

The term *institutions* can be used to refer not only to the structures that human groups develop to make decisions about economic and social

activities, but also to the rules (or sets of rules) that structure social inter-
actions by shaping and constraining actors' behaviour. Note that these
rules can be both formal and informal. Some are carried out by government, and some by other bodies. Political scientists often speak of
government as "the state," which can be defined as "a specialized type
of political organization characterized by a full-time, specialized, professional work force of tax-collectors, soldiers, policemen, bureaucrats
and the like that exercises supreme political authority over a defined
territory with a permanent population, independent from any endur-
ing external political control and possessing a local predominance of
coercive power (always supplemented with moral and remunerative
incentives as well) great enough to maintain general obedience to its
laws or commands within its territorial borders" (Johnson, 2005).

One useful starting point is to see how the various functions of government are carried out.

## 2.1 Functions: Legislative, Executive, Judiciary

Any political system must perform certain key functions. Note that
these functions can be structured in a number of ways, and can be
handled by a variety of actors (including governments, voluntary organizations, and/or for-profit businesses), and through a variety of mechanisms (including regulation and markets); the approach taken may
vary, depending on both the issue and the jurisdiction. One commonly
used categorization is to distinguish among the *legislative*, *executive*, and
*judicial* functions. The legislative function involves making laws, while
the executive implements them, and the judiciary interprets them.

The *legislative* branch is made up of elected representatives, who are
usually members of political parties. In most systems, legislators will
be elected to represent a particular geographical constituency. Elec-
toral systems vary in how votes are translated into seats. Many models
(particularly those based on English/American models, which include
Canadian legislatures) employ what is called first-past-the-post, where
the candidate with the most votes wins the seat, regardless of the actual
percentage of the vote obtained. Other systems employ variations that
attempt to ensure that the winning candidate has a majority, not just a
plurality, of the vote. These may include proportional representation
(where there is an effort to link the percentage of the vote won to percentage of the seats awarded), run-off elections, and/or preferential
ballots (where the voter can indicate a rank ordering of candidates; if no
candidate wins a majority, the second place votes of the lowest-ranking

candidates are then reallocated, and so on, until a clear winner is determined). Different voting systems have different implications. For example, first-past-the-post strongly favours parties with geographically concentrated support, and works best when there is a two-party system. (When there are multiple parties, they are more likely to split the vote, and give a majority of the seats to parties that may not represent a majority of the electorate.) However, proportional representation systems are not usually compatible with geographically based constituencies electing a single representative; they also encourage a proliferation of parties and hence often lead to coalition governments. No model appears ideal; all have advantages and disadvantages.

The *executive* branch of government contains both political and bureaucratic elements. In democracies, the political element is headed by an elected leader / chief executive (who may have such titles as president, prime minister, premier, governor, or mayor, depending on the jurisdiction). The bureaucratic element is often called the *civil service*, and is responsible for carrying out the day-to-day business of government and implementing its policies.

Depending on the size of the government, the executive branch is often divided on functional lines into a series of units, commonly referred to as departments and/or ministries. (In Canada, the usual term is ministry.) In turn, these ministries are usually subdivided into smaller units, often called branches or divisions. Commonly, each of the departments/ministries will have both a political and a civil service head. In many countries, including Canada and the United Kingdom, the political heads are often called the minister of their branch or portfolio (e.g., Minister of Health); in the United States, they are often called secretary (e.g., Secretary of State). Collectively, these political heads form a council (often called the Cabinet). Depending on the system, Cabinet members either must or must not be members of the legislature (see section 2.1.1, Presidential vs. Parliamentary Models); in presidential models, the Cabinet members cannot be legislators and are more likely to be picked for their subject expertise. In all models, the Cabinet members are appointed by the leader of the executive branch, and serve at his/her pleasure. Ministers can be moved, added, or dropped, in what is usually called a Cabinet shuffle. Note that there is often a perceived hierarchy of portfolios, such that ministers can be deemed to be promoted or demoted if they change portfolios. In Canada, there is a tendency not to leave ministers in particular portfolios for a long time, which in turn affects the balance of power/expertise between the political and bureaucratic heads. Regardless of how they are selected, Cabinets change when governments change (although if governments are re-elected, ministers can be reappointed). The civil service head (in Canada usually called the Deputy Minister) will be a member of the bureaucracy, and may or may not change when the government does. Note that in some systems, including Canada, the Deputy Minister is also appointed by the leader of the executive branch (rather than by the minister for that portfolio), and also serves at his/her pleasure. In Canada, there has also been a tendency for Deputy Ministers to have relatively short tenures in particular ministries, although they can be (and often are) shifted to other portfolios.

The civil servants employed by the executive branch are, in theory, nonpartisan, and are responsible for carrying out the ongoing work of government. They have been described as "nameless and blameless." In general, most civil servants will remain in their jobs even when governments change, particularly those working at more junior levels. (As noted above, the most senior members of the civil service usually serve "at the pleasure" of the government of the day.)

The *judicial* branch is composed of judges; these may be elected or appointed, but are expected to impartially enforce the law.

As noted above, one key distinction when analyzing the structure of political systems is to distinguish between *presidential* and *parliamentary* models.

### 2.1.1 PRESIDENTIAL VS. PARLIAMENTARY MODELS

In *presidential* models, the executive, legislative, and judiciary functions are separated; this is sometimes referred to as a "separation of powers" model. For example, in the United States, people vote separately for the chief executive (president, governor, etc.) and the legislature. All voters in the jurisdiction cast votes for the office of chief executive, in addition to voting for legislative representative(s) for their district. Cabinet members are then appointed by the elected chief executive after he/she takes office; Cabinet members are not allowed to serve in the legislative branch. Indeed, when an elected individual is appointed to Cabinet, he/she must first resign their elected seat. In contrast, a parliamentary system fuses the executive and legislative functions, including the requirement that all members of the Cabinet *must* be members of the legislature.

Canada uses a parliamentary system at the federal and provincial/territorial levels, which also retains elements of the British tradition.

Officially, the head of state is the Crown (i.e., the Queen/King of England). She/he is represented by an appointed Governor General (federally) or Lieutenant Governor (provincially). All legislation must be passed by the legislature, and approved by the Crown. In practice, the Crown does not lead the government, but takes advice from a Privy Council. Appointments to this advisory body are for life, but in practice, all decisions are made by its active committee, the Cabinet, all of whom must be serving members of the legislature. Although in theory legislators are selected/elected as individuals, in practice, as noted above, they are associated with political parties. In parliamentary models, the head of the legislature (the Prime Minister, or Premier) is one of these elected members; he or she is on the ballot only within his/her constituency, but is selected by his/her party as their leader. If that leader does not succeed in winning a seat in the legislature, the party must select a new leader who has won a seat; this can be on an interim basis if the leader is able to try again to win election. (One possibility is that another member who holds a "safe seat" agrees to resign and force a by-election.) As noted above, this is in contrast to presidential models, where the candidates for chief executive (president, governor, etc.) appear on all ballots for the entire jurisdiction. Conventionally, in a parliamentary model the chief executive (prime minister, premier, etc.) is the leader of the party that can command the "confidence" of the legislature; this is usually the party with the most seats. If that party holds a majority of the seats, that leader forms a *majority* government. If not, the leader forms a *minority* government, and is subject to being defeated should he/she lose the "confidence" of the legislature.

At the federal level in Canada, the legislature has two branches, an elected House of Commons and an appointed Senate. In theory, the existence of the Senate allows for including nonelected legislators within the Cabinet (e.g., if a government had too few elected members from a particular province); in practice, this tends to be relatively rare although not unheard of, particularly because such members would be handicapped by not being able to speak on behalf of their ministry in the House of Commons. At the federal level, there has been some pressure to move towards an elected Senate, to establish term limits, and/or to eliminate the Senate altogether. The provinces/territories do not have Senates; with only one branch of the legislature, all Cabinet members must have been elected within a constituency to be able to serve.

In contrast, most municipal governments in Canada tend to follow a more mixed model (with presidential elements). The mayor is elected by the entire municipality, and works with a council of elected representatives (often called *councillors*) who often represent geographical "wards" within that municipality (although in some jurisdictions, some representatives may also be elected "at large"). Depending on the municipality, these candidates may or may not be formally associated with a political party. There is also variation in how much power the mayor has; most Canadian jurisdictions use a "weak mayor" model where decisions must be made by the council, and the mayor's main power is the ability to persuade councillors to follow his/her agenda. In contrast, many US cities use a "strong mayor" model, where more power has been assigned to the mayor's office and to the civil service.

### 2.1.2 LEVELS OF GOVERNMENT

By definition, governments are geographically based. They accordingly exist at multiple levels (often called *orders*), of various sizes, with various powers and responsibilities associated with each level. In most countries, much power rests with the national government. Local activities usually are the responsibility of local governments. Between, there may (or may not) be regional governments, and/or other subnational entities (which may be called provinces, states, etc.).

Power can move to and from various levels, and involve different activities (e.g., planning, financing, managing, regulating, etc.). Again, multiple terms can be used to describe various models (Saltman et al., 2007). One common distinction is among deconcentration, delegation, and devolution. *Deconcentration* refers to the transfer of responsibility from central to peripheral offices of the same organization; it is sometimes referred to as *decentralization*. For example, a provincial Ministry of Health can shift some responsibilities to its branch offices. *Delegation* refers to the transfer of responsibility from a central agency to an organization independent of the central agency. For example, a Ministry of Health can transfer responsibilities to an autonomous public health agency. *Devolution* refers to the transfer of responsibility from central government agencies to lower-level, autonomous units of government through constitutional provisions (e.g., from the Ministry of Health to a local government authority). Note that *regionalization* may represent either decentralization or centralization, depending on where the powers had formerly been located.

The debate over centralization/decentralization relates to perceived advantages and disadvantages of the ability to tailor policies to local needs vs. the ability to ensure a uniform standard of services (or policies) in a larger jurisdiction. Issues of coordinating policies across jurisdictions may also arise.

### 2.1.3 FEDERAL VS. UNITARY MODELS

Another distinction relates to how to connect the various levels of government. Federalism divides authority among levels of government, and intentionally restricts the powers of the central government. There is a considerable literature examining various forms of federalism (Brooks, 2009; Cameron & Simeon, 2002; Lazar, 2010). For example, Lazar classified intergovernmental regimes using the following two sets of variables: the extent to which there is independence or interdependence between orders of government; and the extent to which a hierarchical or non-hierarchical relationship prevails. He used this to define four types of regimes, which he termed: *unilateral* (hierarchical, interdependent), *collaborative* (non-hierarchical, interdependent), *classical* (non-hierarchical, independent), and *beggar-thy-partner* (hierarchical, independent) (Lazar, 2006). In the classical (also termed disentangled) form of federalism, both levels of government carry out functions in the same policy area independently of one another. Key points differentiating various models include which responsibilities are decentralized, as well as the extent to which this division of power is constitutionally guaranteed. Political scientists have noted that federalism can be seen as a compromise between homogeneity and diversity, allowing individual jurisdictions to preserve elements of their own identity within the context of a larger nation. Indeed, *asymmetric federalism* allows each subnational unit to set up different agreements with the national government.

In Canada, federalism is a fundamental feature affecting many policies, and is particularly important in the area of health care (Banting & Corbett, 2002). The history can be traced back to the founding of Canada, and the way powers were constitutionally divided (see section 2.2.1, Federalism in Canada). Another possible model can be called a *confederal* relationship, referring to voluntary arrangements among various jurisdictions that can cross subnational borders. An example of such a quasi-national organization that is designed to operate at arm's length from both the federal and provincial/territorial governments is Canadian Blood Services (see Chapter 6, The Bite of Blood Safety), which acts as the national operator of the blood system; it follows national (federal) regulations, but is provincially funded, and has voluntary membership. (Quebec is not a formal member, but has its own blood agency that voluntarily cooperates with Canadian Blood Services.)

## 2.2 Institutions: The Case of Canada

### 2.2.1 FEDERALISM IN CANADA: THE *CONSTITUTION ACT, 1867*

The *Constitution Act, 1867* (formerly known as the *British North America Act*) is the legislative act that created Canada. It specifies the responsibilities of the national (federal) government in Ottawa, and of the provinces and territories (Department of Justice Canada, 1982).

Section 91 of the *Constitution Act* enumerates the powers given to the national government; it includes the residual power to legislate for the "peace, order, and good government of Canada" on matters not assigned to the provinces. One of the federal powers enumerated in this section was over "Quarantine and the Establishment and Maintenance of Marine Hospitals." Section 91 also gave the federal government the ability to raise money "by any Mode or System of Taxation."

Section 92 of the *Constitution Act* enumerates the exclusive powers of provincial legislatures. These include 92(7) "The Establishment, Maintenance, and Management of Hospitals, Asylums, Charities, and Eleemosynary Institutions in and for the Province, other than Marine Hospitals" and 92(16) "Generally all Matters of a merely local or private Nature in the Province." Subsequent court decisions have interpreted these clauses as placing most of health care under provincial jurisdiction. Other powers deemed to fall under provincial jurisdiction include education (which also encompasses professional training programs) and professional licensure; for that reason, health professionals are registered within a province/territory rather than at the national level. The provinces were also given jurisdiction over public lands and other natural resources in their area.

The constitution limited the provinces' power to raise money by restricting them to "Direct Taxation within the Province in order to the raising of a Revenue for Provincial Purposes." The provinces do have taxing power (clarified by a 1982 constitutional amendment) over natural resources. The resulting discrepancy in the ability of the different levels of government to raise revenue, along with differences in the wealth and population base of different provinces, led to what is often called "fiscal federalism," whereby the federal government has attempted to equalize the fiscal capacity across the country (see also section 7.1, Financing Health Care in Canada).

Section 95 of the *Constitution Act* gave "concurrent" powers to both levels of government for agriculture and immigration. It allows each province to "make Laws in relation to Agriculture in the Province, and to Immigration into the Province." However, it goes on to note that "it is hereby declared that the Parliament of Canada may from Time to Time make Laws in relation to Agriculture in all or any of the Provinces, and to Immigration into all or any of the Provinces; and any Law of the Legislature of a Province relative to Agriculture or to Immigration shall have effect in and for the Province as long and as far only as it is not repugnant to any Act of the Parliament of Canada." Thus, in the case of disagreement in these policy areas, the federal government would prevail. The federal government also retains the power to disallow any provincial statute, although it has not done so since 1943.

Constitutional responsibility for health protection/public health is accordingly somewhat ambiguous. Clauses that can be interpreted as making public health a primarily provincial concern include section 92(13) of the *Constitution Act*, which gives the provinces responsibility for "property and civil rights," and section 92(16), which gives them responsibility over matters of a "local or private nature" in the province. Subsequent legal interpretations have accordingly stated that the provinces have jurisdiction over public health, specifically over sanitation, and the prevention of communicable diseases. However, other clauses can be seen as giving some authority over health protection to the federal government. Section 91(27) of the *Constitution Act* gives the federal government power over criminal law, which would allow it to pass legislation to prevent the transmission of a "public evil" that is determined to be a danger to public health. Using this clause, the federal government has passed legislation to control transmission of health risks, particularly when they have the potential to cross provincial borders; examples include the *Food and Drugs Act* and the *Hazardous Products Act*. However, Supreme Court of Canada decisions have limited the scope of using the federal jurisdiction over criminal law to regulate in areas of health. One example was a 2011 confirmation that the federal government could not override the decision by a provincial government (in this case, British Columbia) to use its jurisdiction over health care to waive enforcement of drug laws and operate "harm reduction" facilities aimed at preventing overdose deaths among users of illegal drugs (Vancouver Coastal Health, 2012). Another was a 2011 decision striking down the ability of the federal government to regulate in vitro fertilization (see Chapter 14, Down the Tubes).

The federal government has further legislative power under the national concern section of the "peace, order and good government" power of the *Constitution Act*, which allows it to pass legislation to regulate matters of national health and welfare. To qualify under this section, intra- and extra-provincial implications of such issues must be linked, provinces must not be able to regulate effectively on their own, and failure of one province to regulate must be likely to affect the health of residents of other provinces. The federal government also retains authority over health protection through its powers over quarantine and over the regulation of trade and commerce of an interprovincial or international nature. As well, the federal government can involve itself nonlegislatively in public health by providing conditional funding for public health programs and/or by entering into legal contracts to develop public health initiatives.

The distribution of powers is a perennial issue in Canada, with provincial/territorial governments (particularly but not exclusively Quebec) being highly resistant to federal "intrusions" into those areas seen as being under provincial jurisdiction. One key implication for health care is that it is remarkably difficult for the federal government to play a national role, unless the provinces/territories agree to it. As noted above, one of the key vehicles has been fiscal federalism, whereby the federal government gives money to the provinces/territories for specified purposes, with or without strings attached (see section 7.1, Financing Health Care in Canada).

2.2.2 CHARTER OF RIGHTS AND FREEDOMS

In 1982, when the *BNA Act* was revised and renamed the *Constitution Act*, it was amended to add a Canadian *Charter of Rights and Freedoms* (Department of Justice Canada, 1982). These rights are not unconditional – the *Act* explicitly states that "The Canadian Charter of Rights and Freedoms guarantees the rights and freedoms set out in it subject only to such reasonable limits prescribed by law as can be demonstrably justified in a free and democratic society." The *Act* defines the following four "fundamental freedoms," which are said to apply to everyone: "(a) freedom of conscience and religion; (b) freedom of thought, belief, opinion and expression, including freedom of the press and other media of communication; (c) freedom of peaceful assembly; and (d) freedom of association."

The *Act* then lists a series of rights, which include: democratic rights (relating to the right to vote, and to how long legislatures could sit without having to call an election); mobility rights; legal rights; and equality rights. Mobility rights include the following provisions:

"Mobility of citizens
6. (1) Every citizen of Canada has the right to enter, remain in and leave Canada.

Rights to move and gain livelihood

    (2) Every citizen of Canada and every person who has the status of a permanent resident of Canada has the right (a) to move to and take up residence in any province; and (b) to pursue the gaining of a livelihood in any province. Limitation: (3) The rights specified in subsection (2) are subject to (a) any laws or practices of general application in force in a province other than those that discriminate among persons primarily on the basis of province of present or previous residence; and (b) any laws providing for reasonable residency requirements as a qualification for the receipt of publicly provided social services.

Affirmative action programs

    (4) Subsections (2) and (3) do not preclude any law, program or activity that has as its object the amelioration in a province of conditions of individuals in that province who are socially or economically disadvantaged if the rate of employment in that province is below the rate of employment in Canada."

The legal rights deal with "the right to life, liberty and security of the person" particularly as this applies to those involved with the justice system. Among the legal rights are the following:

"Life, liberty and security of person

    7. Everyone has the right to life, liberty and security of the person and the right not to be deprived thereof except in accordance with the principles of fundamental justice.

Treatment or punishment

    12. Everyone has the right not to be subjected to any cruel and unusual treatment or punishment."

Equality rights are defined in terms of "Equality before and under law and equal protection and benefit of law" and include the following:

"15. (1) Every individual is equal before and under the law and has the right to the equal protection and equal benefit of the law without discrimination and, in particular, without discrimination based on race, national or ethnic origin, colour, religion, sex, age or mental or physical disability.

Affirmative action programs

(2) Subsection (1) does not preclude any law, program or activity that has as its object the amelioration of conditions of disadvantaged individuals or groups including those that are disadvantaged because of race, national or ethnic origin, colour, religion, sex, age or mental or physical disability" (Department of Justice Canada, 1982).

### 2.2.3 THE ROLES OF LOCAL GOVERNMENT IN CANADA

Although provinces are further divided into geographical subunits (which may be called regions, municipalities, local governments, etc.), the Canadian constitution gave these subunits no independent authority other than what the provinces/territories chose to assign to them. These assignments can also be changed unilaterally by the province. According to Section 92(8) of the *Constitution Act*, 1867, "In each Province the Legislature may exclusively make Laws in relation to ... Municipal Institutions in the Province." There is considerable variation across Canada in how provinces relate to local governments (Young & Leuprecht, 2006). For more on the role of local government in Canada, see Sancton (2010).

### 2.2.4 REGIONAL AUTHORITIES IN CANADA

Beginning in the mid-1990s, most Canadian provinces have experimented with regional models for planning, managing, and/or funding health care. These regions would largely be classified as quasi-public (see section 6.1.1, Public and Private) and have varying responsibilities for the services in their catchment area. At the time of writing, all provinces using regional models have given them some responsibility for hospitals, while none had given them responsibility for physician services. (This may change; in 2012, Ontario announced its intentions to include certain primary health care services in its regional structures.) The handling of other services varies; for example, some but not all provinces/territories have placed community care, long-term care, and/or public health within the regional models. Regionalization thus has elements of both decentralization and centralization, because some of the activities for which the regional structures are responsible formerly lay with higher levels of government (e.g., provincial ministries), while others had formerly rested with individual communities and organizations (Kinnunen et al., 2007; Marchildon, 2010; Saltman et al., 2007). Alberta has moved towards more centralization; after eliminating most hospital boards and placing them within health regions, the province subsequently eliminated its regions in 2009, and moved much of the responsibility for planning and funding the province's hospitals and selected other services to a centralized provincial agency, Alberta Health Services, reporting directly to the provincial Minister of Health and Wellness.

Ontario's model was unusual within Canada, in that the regional bodies it set up did not directly deliver services. Ontario was also among the last to bring in regional models; its 14 Local Health Integration Networks (LHINs) were set up in 2006 as regional, not-for-profit corporations, and were explicitly prohibited from providing health services directly. Instead, local hospitals and other agencies have retained their own boards, although most of their provincial funding now flows through the LHINs. The LHINs assumed many functions from the Ministry of Health and Long Term Care (MOHLTC), and also took over the planning, management, and coordinating functions that had been the responsibility of the former District Health Councils. With the introduction of the LHINs, the Community Care Access Centres (CCACs), the agencies responsible for organizing and funding many community services, were realigned and merged to fit the new LHIN boundaries. At the time of writing, the local public health units had not yet been aligned with LHINs, although proposals to do so were made in 2012. LHINs were responsible for working with local health providers and community members to best determine the health service priorities of their geographic regions, including planning, integrating, and funding such local health services as: hospitals, CCACs, community support services, long-term care, mental health and addictions services, and community health centres (Ontario Ministry of Health and Long-Term Care, 2006). The MOHLTC retained a stewardship role and overall responsibility for such higher-level roles as establishing strategic direction and provincial priorities for the health system and developing legislation, regulations, standards, policies, and directives to support those strategic directions (Ontario Ministry of Health and Long-Term Care, 2013a). The LHINs have been seen by some as an added level of bureaucracy; indeed, one of Ontario's opposition parties, the Conservatives, under the leadership of Tim Hudak, had included a pledge to eliminate them in their October 2011 provincial election platform.

## 2.3  Historical Institutionalism, Path Dependency, and Policy Legacies

One set of political science theories points to the importance of previous policy decisions in constraining future activities. A variety of terms are used. *Historical institutionalism* stresses the importance of institutions (in the broader sense of including rules of the game) in influencing outcomes. The concept of *path dependency* emphasizes the extent to which prior policies may make it difficult (although not impossible) to reverse course. *Critical junctures* represent key decisions that help set future policies. The result is a series of *policy legacies*. Note that this set of theories does not help predict which paths will be taken; neither does it predict the occasions when decisions are revisited and modified and different paths taken. However, they can be helpful in clarifying barriers to policy change (Evans et al., 1985; Maioni, 1998; Pierson, 1993, 2000; Tuohy, 1999).

## 3. Ideas

Ideas affect how we think about politics, and what should happen. They structure how we see the world, and influence what we think is important. Indeed, the most important ideas are often "invisible" precisely because they are taken for granted. One clue that we are talking about ideas is that evidence is often irrelevant, because ideas about what policies or outcomes we would prefer cannot be proven to be right or wrong. When fundamental ideas differ, "evidence-based policymaking" is often an oxymoron; evidence can help clarify the facts, trade-offs, and the likely outcomes of particular policies, but it cannot dictate what people wish to achieve.

### 3.1 Ideologies, Paradigms, and Dominant Ideas

Some authors distinguish among categories of ideas based on how comprehensive they are (Brooks, 2009; Doern & Phidd, 1992; McLean & McMillan, 2003). At one extreme, an *ideology* is a set of interrelated beliefs that explains to its adherents how most things should work. Such ideologies as libertarianism or Marxism can provide tidy answers to most political questions, provided that one accepts the underlying premises of that ideology. *Paradigms* function similarly within particular policy arenas (e.g., the causes of ill health might be described differently by a biomedical model than by a social determinants of health framework). *Dominant ideas* are less all-encompassing, but highlight important (if often conflicting) goals. Specific objectives are even more specific than that. Note that ideas are also reflected in ethical frameworks (see section 3.6).

## 3.2  Role of the State

*Ideologies* can often be arrayed on a spectrum (conventionally described as stretching from "left" to "right"). Note that the terms used to describe particular ideologies may vary. For example, Europeans use the term "liberal" very differently than that term is used in North America; the European usage is closer to what North Americans call libertarianism. One key issue that distinguishes various ideologies relates to the balance between individual and societal *rights*, and the extent to which it is seen as appropriate for government to interfere with individuals. The term rights is used to refer to normative ideas about what people are entitled to, which can be based in legal, social, or ethical principles. Some rights are based on freedom from interference ("negative rights"), and others in terms of entitlement to basic necessities ("positive rights"). Scholars have suggested analyzing views about the appropriate role for governments on two dimensions: government's role in economic/business decisions (and the role for markets), and government's role in social/moral decisions (e.g., abortion, whether marijuana should be legalized, etc.). Examples can be found for most combinations of views on these two dimensions. Libertarians, for example, believe that government should play a minimal role on both types of issues. Social conservatives tend to want a minimal government role in economic decisions (allowing market forces to prevail), but are willing to have government enforce social/moral decisions (e.g., ensuring that abortion is not permitted). Similarly, some groups on the left may wish government to play a greater role in economic decisions (e.g., greater regulation and redistribution of income), but not in social issues (e.g., they may advocate legalizing such drugs as marijuana), whereas other groups also wish for activist government on both economic and social dimensions (e.g., they may want it to ban hate speech). Also note that most "positive rights" rest on legal/policy judgments and convey corresponding duties. For example, if I have a right to food or housing, then someone else must ensure that I get it, and must pay for it. Accordingly, positive rights are more difficult to enforce, and more susceptible to being modified when governments (and policies) change. In contrast, negative rights basically require that individuals should be left alone.

In general, most societies recognize that people may not always be able to take care of their own needs. In England, the poor law system, in place from the 16th until the mid-20th century, made a distinction between the "deserving poor" and the "undeserving poor." For example, the very old and the very young (as well as those with disabilities that would prevent them from working) will usually be dependent on others, usually family members, but if such family members are unwilling or unable to help, society may need to step in. This category of individuals is usually considered the "deserving" poor. In contrast, if people are able to work, society may feel that helping them encourages laziness; this group could be termed the "undeserving" poor. One influential school of work has identified three major models of the welfare state within capitalist societies, based on views about who is entitled to help, and under what circumstances (Esping-Andersen, 1990; Pierson & Castles, 2006). What is termed the *liberal welfare state* (where the term "liberal" is used in its European, libertarian sense) stigmatizes help. Aid is means-tested and relatively modest, social insurance plans tend to be relatively limited, and there is heavy reliance on market forces. The *corporatist welfare state* bases benefits in large part on perceived contributions to society, through such mechanisms as basing access to benefits on work/employment status. The *social-democratic welfare state* promotes equality and attempts to ensure that everyone has access to a high level of benefits; being unemployed in jurisdictions using this model is less likely to mean a dramatic drop in that person's ability to maintain a reasonable standard of living. Clearly, the costs of these various models differ considerably; a social democratic model requires a higher level of taxation, in exchange for a higher level of security for its citizens. A related body of work focuses on the total burden on state finances, and the extent to which "overload" can produce a "fiscal crisis" where demands for resources outweigh the ability to pay for them (O'Connor, 1973; Offe, 1984; Pierson & Castles, 2006). Again, different models will draw the line in different places.

## 3.3 Policy Goals

Some have noted that policy in most jurisdictions, including Canada, is often characterized by a number of "dominant ideas" (Doern & Phidd, 1992). They observe that policymaking often involves the need to balance multiple goals, all of which may be desirable, but which may not always be compatible. Deborah Stone has identified four dominant ideas, which she calls security, liberty, equity, and efficiency (Stone, 2002). As she notes, these objectives are not only potentially clashing but also prone to competing interpretations.

### 3.3.1 SECURITY

Stone (2002) defines security as the "satisfaction of minimum human needs" (p. 37). Much of the rationale for health policy arises from security as a policy goal. If someone is ill, that person wishes to know that he or she can receive help; if the illness strikes the main wage earner, that person may also want to know that his or her family will not starve. A similar rationale applies to systems of pensions, unemployment insurance, public housing, food aid, and other programs that attempt to construct a "floor" of basic benefits. As noted above (section 3.2, Role of the State), the nature of such programs, including who is entitled to what, clearly has ideological elements.

### 3.3.2 LIBERTY

Stone (2002) defines liberty as "do as you wish as long as you do not harm others" (p. 37). Liberty may thus clash with security, to the extent that an emphasis on liberty would imply that the state has no right to compel individuals to help others, or to regulate what the individuals do. Liberty would also argue for a low level of taxation. As noted above in section 3.1 (Ideologies, Paradigms, and Dominant Ideas), different ideologies may differ in the relative value placed on liberty as a policy goal.

### 3.3.3 EQUITY

Stone (2002) defines equity as "treating likes alike" (p. 37). This in turn leads to the question of how we define these terms. As she notes, "Ultimately, a policy argument must show a principled reason why it is proper to categorize cases as alike or different" (p. 53). This is far from simple. (See section 3.6 for a brief discussion of ethical frameworks.) Stone illustrates some different ways of interpreting equity through the example of dividing a chocolate cake. She begins by asking what an equitable way would be to divide a chocolate cake that has been brought to her policy class. The most obvious solution is to give an equal slice to everyone present. However, she notes that there are other ways to allocate resources. She notes that these approaches can be based on three basic criteria, which she terms recipients, items, and process.

The *recipients* criterion forces us to ask what the definition of membership should be – that is, to determine who should count as a member of the class of potential recipients. For example, because health care usually operates within a particular jurisdiction, determining a fair allocation of health care usually considers only the people who live there (if the plan is publicly financed), or those who are enrolled in a particular insurance plan (if it is privately financed). Even once the recipients have been defined, there are multiple ways of distributing the cake. For example, *rank-based distribution* contends that there are relevant internal divisions for distributing something, and is linked to concepts of horizontal and vertical equity (i.e., treat the same rank equally, and different ranks unequally). One example is workplace-based health insurance, which may give different benefits to full-time versus part-time workers. A similar concept is *distribution based on social cleavages* (i.e., age, gender, ethnic groups). For example, one may conclude that groups that have suffered historical disadvantages should receive distributive preference. Health coverage is commonly based on such criteria as age (e.g., seniors, children), place of employment, income, and/or disease group (e.g., special programs for those with particular illnesses, such as cancer).

The *items* criterion asks what is being distributed. In terms of the cake, should we consider the cake in isolation, or in the context of a larger meal? Should we consider one point in time, or a longer time frame? If somehow I had received a lesser share of a previous meal attended by the members of the class, does this mean that I should receive preference with respect to the cake? The items criterion also suggests that goods should be distributed based on value of the item to the individual. Diabetics, for example, would not be able to eat the cake. This concept is particularly relevant to health care, where need and ability to benefit are usually considered to be important aspects of resource allocation decisions.

The *process* criterion suggests that people are more willing to accept unequal results if the process is considered fair. This concept is particularly important in situations of shortage, when not everyone can be satisfied. For example, many people may need an organ transplant, but each organ can be used in only one recipient. This stress on process is a major component of the ethical theory *accountability for reasonableness* (see section 3.6.1). In her book, Stone discusses the implications of a number of possible processes that might be used to allocate scarce resources, including competition, lotteries, or elections; all have advantages and disadvantages.

### 3.3.4 EFFICIENCY

Stone (2002) defines efficiency as "getting the most out of a given input" or "achieving an objective at the lowest cost" (p. 61). At the societal level, efficiency is an ideal that can guide how society chooses to spend its money or allocate its resources in order to get the most value for these inputs. Note that this is a second-order policy goal, since efficiency is not relevant if one does not wish to gain a particular outcome in the first place. Economic analysis (see section 8.1) deals largely with efficiency.

## 3.4 Framing

The term *frames* is used to refer to mental structures that people use to provide categories and a structure for their thoughts. As Tversky and Kahneman (1981, 1986) noted, frames are extraordinarily powerful. *Framing* thus refers to the process of selectively using frames to control how a policy is perceived, and hence how it is evaluated. As one example, people will tend to support such policy goals as liberty and security, although they may differ in how to balance these goals if and when they clash. Framing theory highlights that the same set of facts can be manipulated (explicitly or implicitly) to serve different interests and to present different messages. One example would be whether to permit tobacco advertising on television. For many years, the tobacco industry portrayed such bans as an infringement on their right to communicate with their customers about a legal product; these arguments were framed to appeal to people's support of liberty in the form of free speech. Others framed restricting tobacco advertising as protecting children from adopting a potentially deadly habit, appealing to people's support of security as a policy goal. Similar battles about how to frame policy disputes can be found in many of the cases in this book.

Note that some theorists argue that framing is a rational decision, involving a conscious effort by stakeholders to frame an issue according to how they can best gain from influencing the situation's outcome. Others note that framing does have conscious elements, but may also be subjective and/or tacit; they stress that frames can tell us what goals stakeholders hold to be important and how stakeholders have made sense of a particular policy issue, in a way that expresses conscious as well as tacitly held beliefs. Frames may also appear in the form of policy stories (sometimes called causal stories), which can be important parts of policy discourse and debate (Stone, 1989).

Framing is also important because it can define which stakeholders participate. If the consequences of a certain policy problem are framed as affecting only a small range of individuals, then fewer stakeholders might be involved in discussing the options for moving forward. This also relates to the theory of scope of conflict discussed in section 4.3 (Schattschneider, 1975).

## 3.5 *Public Goods and Externalities*

The term *public good* (also referred to as collective goods), commonly used in the policy analysis and economics literature, is not the same as being "good for the public." Public goods (and their opposite, private goods) are defined in terms of two inherent characteristics, termed "rivalry in consumption" and "excludability in ownership in use."

*Rivalry* means that what one person consumes cannot be consumed by anyone else. *Excludability* means that some particular person has exclusive control over the good; it includes both physical and legal elements. For example, my sunglasses are private goods because when I wear them no one else can (rivalry in consumption) and, because I own them, I determine who gets to wear them at any particular time (excludability). Public goods are nonrivalrous and/or nonexcludable. If one person breathes clean air, that does not prevent others from doing so, so clean air meets the nonrivalrous criterion for being a public good. (In contrast, clean water may indeed be rivalrous; what one person drinks cannot be consumed by another.) Similarly, a nonexcludable good cannot be restricted to only those who wish to (or can) pay for it. For example, public roads are often nonexcludable, since after a road is built, people can go ahead and use it regardless of whether they have paid for it directly. However, a road can be made private by limiting its use to those who pay for it (e.g., a toll highway). National defence is an even clearer example of nonexcludability; one cannot say that only those willing to pay will be protected from foreign invasion.

Within public health, the phenomenon of *herd immunity* means that, once a high enough proportion of the population is protected from a communicable disease, the infectious agent becomes much less likely to be transmitted. In turn, this means that those coming in contact with the immune population are also protected from infection, regardless of whether they are personally immune. One ongoing policy problem is referred to as the *free rider* problem; purely rational individuals have an incentive to avoid paying for public goods, knowing that they will still be able to obtain the benefits as long as others agree to pay. For example, rational individuals would decline immunization, avoiding the personal costs and the potential risks of side effects, as long as enough of their neighbours were immunized to allow them to capture the benefits (in this case, through herd immunity).

This definition tells us that not everything that is good for the public would qualify as a public good. For example, having universal health care services financed by governments under a system of social insurance is sometimes referred to as a public good, but does not really meet the definition. It may be cost-effective to pool risks and resources, but most health care services to individuals are private goods. Although such traditional public health interventions as protecting the public from infectious diseases are indeed public goods, if I break my arm, treating me would not be deemed a public good; my care is both rival-rous and excludable. The category of "merit goods" or "club goods" is sometimes used to apply to goods and services, such as health care, that are not public goods, but are considered good for the public. One ratio-nale for defining merit goods arises where people are uncomfortable allowing others to suffer. However, as would be predicted from Stone's definitions of equity (see section 3.3.3), people may want to limit their help to recipients who satisfy certain conditions (e.g., citizenship).

A related concept is that of *externalities*, which can be either positive or negative. Externalities occur when private costs and benefits are not the same as social costs and benefits. Some of these externalities can be positive (e.g., herd immunity protects everyone in a community, regard-less of whether they were immunized). Some externalities can be nega-tive (e.g., pollution or global warming allows the polluters to transfer their costs to others). A key policy issue is that, without some mecha-nism to address externalities, there may be a tendency to underinvest in public goods with positive externalities, and to allow people to impose negative externalities on others. That is why even advocates of minimal government will usually accept government involvement in addressing public goods (e.g., national defence, protection against communicable diseases, prohibition against dumping polluting material into public waterways), both to deal with externalities and to prevent free riders. A number of policy instruments (see section 5.2) can be used to address externalities, including taxation and regulation (see section 5.2.1).

## 3.6  Ethical Frameworks

Deciding what is the "right" thing to do is not always obvious, and sometimes there are varying degrees of "right answers." The field of medical ethics often reflects more general philosophical doctrines, par-ticularly utilitarianism and deontology (Kuhse & Singer, 2009; Singer & Viens, 2008). *Utilitarian* or *consequentialist* theories posit that the deter-mination of whether an act is right or wrong (or even morally obliga-tory) is directly dependent on the resulting consequences produced by that action (or failure to act), whereas *deontological* theories argue that an action may be inherently moral or good, regardless of the consequences. These theories may link to discussions about such policy goals as liberty (see section 3.3.2), equity (see section 3.3.3), and efficiency (see section 3.3.4). *Normative ethics* attempts to ascertain which norms are considered to be moral and the reasons for their subsequent acceptance and strives to find agreement on the way things "should" be. However, there is no universally agreed-upon framework that can be used to determine the "correct" course of action or inaction (Daniels & Sabin, 2002). Bioethicists have outlined a number of guiding principles to assist in the decision-making process; these principles are designed to protect individuals' rights and freedoms, but may conflict and compete with one another. One widely used approach, commonly called *principlism*, was originally designed for use in biomedical research, but has been widely adopted in clinical and organizational ethics as well. It identifies the following four key principles: autonomy, beneficence, non-maleficence, and justice (Beauchamp & Childress, 2001). Principlism was codified in the 1979 Belmont Report, and these principles are often referred to as the Belmont Principles.

The principle of *autonomy* refers to respect for an autonomous individual's ability to deliberate and make decisions regarding personal goals and the freedom to pursue those goals. This principle encompasses other rights, including *respect for persons*, which affirms the notion that individuals should be treated as autonomous agents. A related view stresses that persons with diminished autonomy are entitled to protection. Indeed, the *harm principle* (associated with J.S. Mill) would stress that the only purpose for which power can be rightfully exercised over any member of a civilized community against his/her will is to prevent harm to others. Those accepting this principle would argue that a paternalist view that such actions would be for that person's own good, either physical or moral, is not sufficient. Another principle related to autonomy is *informed consent*, which argues that capable, informed individuals have the right to make decisions that affect them. In turn, this principle incorporates requirements for honesty and full information to ensure that such consent is truly informed. Another related principle is *confidentiality*, which requires that information be kept confidential from others, even including family members. (This is sometimes referred to in terms of *privacy*.)

The principle of *non-maleficence* stresses "first, do no harm."

The principle of *beneficence* stresses that providers should act in the best interests of their patients. This sometimes is used to suggest that benefits should be balanced against risks and costs (see also section 8.1, Economic Analysis). Note that this presents dilemmas when individuals make choices that may not be in their own best interests. Different ethical frameworks may make different recommendations about when such potentially suboptimal choices should or should not be respected.

The principle of *justice* stresses the fair distribution of benefits, costs, harms, and risks. For example, scholars often refer to *distributive justice* as representing a fair, equitable, and appropriate distribution (see also section 3.6.4). Note that fairness and justice can be viewed in both procedural and substantive terms (see also section 3.6.1, Accountability for Reasonableness).

Various combinations of these principles have been assembled into various ethical frameworks. Note that there are differences between frameworks addressing clinical decisions (which tend to concern themselves with implications for individual patients, often giving less attention to the implications for society as a whole), and those taking a more societal perspective. In the United Kingdom, the National Institute for Health and Clinical Excellence (NICE) explicitly states the "social value judgements" it uses as principles for the development of NICE guidance (National Institute for Health and Clinical Excellence, 2008). It begins with the four principles of bioethics noted above (respect for autonomy, non-malificence, beneficence, and distributive justice) but also notes the importance of procedural justice.

A growing body of work examines public health ethics. As one example, Gostin (2000) developed the following framework, which draws on the United Nations' Siracusa principles to justify public health interventions at a societal level:

1. Demonstrate risk (nature, duration, probability of harm, severity of harm);
2. Demonstrate intervention's effectiveness (effective risk reduction);
3. Assess economic costs (both direct and indirect);
4. Assess burden on individuals (invasiveness, frequency/scope of infringement, duration of infringement); and
5. Assess fairness of policy (benefits/services based on need, costs/burdens based on risks posed).

Another distinction, which is also used by legal scholars, is between *procedural justice* (which focuses on how decisions are made) and *substantive justice* (which focuses on the outcomes). We next briefly note two other widely used ethical frameworks: accountability for reasonableness and the precautionary principle.

### 3.6.1 ACCOUNTABILITY FOR REASONABLENESS

One influential (although controversial) approach argues that given disagreements about priority setting, one should focus on process rather than on outcomes. Daniels's accountability for reasonableness (A4R) framework argues that decisions are fair as long as the following four conditions are met, which he terms relevance, publicity, appeals/revision, and enforcement. *Relevance* is defined in terms of the rationales for decisions, which should "rest on evidence, reasons, and principles that all fair-minded parties … can agree are relevant to deciding how to meet the diverse needs of a covered population under necessary resource constraints" (Daniels & Sabin, 1998, p. 57). *Publicity* requires that the decisions, and the rationales for them, be publicly accessible. (Others refer to a similar requirement as transparency; that condition is satisfied if decisions are made in an open and accountable manner, with public participation.) There should be a mechanism for *appealing* decisions, and for revisiting them should additional evidence be forthcoming. Finally, there should be some mechanism for *enforcing* these decisions (Daniels, 2000; Daniels & Sabin, 1998; Martin et al., 2002). Gibson and Martin introduced an additional condition, the empowerment condition, which focuses on attempting to minimize power differences in the decision-making context and optimizing effective opportunities for participation (Gibson et al., 2005).

Resource allocation decisions have winners and losers. The A4R approach assumes that the losers will accept decisions as long as the process meets these fairness criteria. In contrast, scope of conflict theory (see section 4.3) would argue that losers might choose to revisit the decision, and may seek to select a venue and a set of rules to maximize their chance of winning.

### 3.6.2 THE PRECAUTIONARY PRINCIPLE

The precautionary principle argues that there is an obligation to protect populations against reasonably foreseeable threats, even under conditions of uncertainty (Kriebel & Tickner, 2001). This is a risk-averse concept, arguing that where the potential costs of inaction are high, it is the failure to implement preventive measures that requires justification. It has become influential in environmental science. There are several versions of the precautionary principle, which differ in how likely the risk must be to warrant taking action.

One key issue is the extent to which the precautionary principle should be applied to public health interventions. Some have noted that, if poorly applied, use of this concept risks doing more harm than good (Weir et al., 2010). The issue is not only the cost, which can be considerable, but also risks to future policy. Any preventive measure risks looking like the "boy who cried wolf"; to the extent that preventive measures prevent the adverse events from occurring, critics may well suggest that those interventions were not necessary. (The successful efforts to prevent computer systems from crashing for Y2K in 2000 are a classic example.) Others argue that all efforts should nonetheless be taken to avoid potential problems, however unlikely. After severe acute respiratory syndrome (SARS), Ontario explicitly incorporated the precautionary principle into the *Health Protection and Promotion Act*, albeit without being particularly clear about how, and under what circumstances, it would apply.

### 3.6.3  RESOURCE ALLOCATION / RATIONING

Resource allocation involves the distribution of goods and services to programs and people. Note that allocation decisions may occur at the *macro* level (e.g., resources given to health care vs. to other potential uses), the *meso* level (e.g., resources given to particular organizations and/or programs), and/or the *micro* level (e.g., allocations to specific individuals). In the context of health care, macro allocations of resources to various activities (health, education, roads, etc.) can be made by governments and/or by other decision makers (e.g., employers) at the national, provincial, and municipal level. Meso allocations are made at the level of institutions; for example, hospitals must decide how to allocate their resources across such programs as cancer treatment, cardiology, and dialysis. Micro allocations are made by providers and by payers at the level of the individual patient; this is sometimes referred to as "bedside rationing."

A number of approaches to resource allocation have been suggested. One way to categorize them is by the methods used. *Markets* ensure that those most willing to pay receive the resources. This may be seen as maximizing efficiency (see section 3.3.4) if one assumes that higher willingness to pay means that a higher value was assigned to that resource by the potential recipient (rather than it just reflecting differences in his/her disposable income). *Political* methods use societally determined guidelines, which preferably will be applied impartially (see section 3.6.1, Accountability for Reasonableness). *Lotteries* rely on chance. *Custom* continues business as usual.

The ethics of resource allocation are frequently considered in relation to the concept of *justice* and the physician's fiduciary duty towards the patient. Ongoing disputes concern the extent to which such considerations should be balanced against responsibility to others, including society as a whole. Some argue that human life is priceless; others focus on the fact that resources are limited, and on the *opportunity costs* (a term used by economists to refer to alternate uses which might be made of those resources). As Calabresi and Bobbit (1978) have noted, sometimes there is no clearly best alternative.

### 3.6.4 DISTRIBUTIVE JUSTICE

Underlying these disagreements are several related debates (Deber & Lam, 2009). One is ethical. In describing the failed attempt to reform health care under President Clinton, Stone (1993) has written about two visions of distributive justice. The *solidarity* principle assumes mutual responsibility, and seeks to distribute costs on the basis of ability to pay. *Actuarial fairness*, in contrast, rejects cross-subsidization; instead, it assumes that costs should be distributed based on expected utilization, where those with a higher likelihood of incurring costs should pay more, and those with a lower likelihood should pay less. For example, actuarial fairness would hold that those with a clean driving record should pay lower rates than those with a history of accidents; this means that risks should be pooled only among relatively homogeneous populations. Indeed, a libertarian viewpoint would argue that fairness not only precludes requiring individuals to subsidize others but also precludes mandating coverage at all (Stone, 2008). Canada, like most industrialized countries, has largely accepted a solidarity-based view for financing health care (Abelson et al., 2004; Mendelsohn, 2002; Soroka, 2007). In the United States, however, the debate continues, often vehemently. As Hacker (2008) has noted, greater emphasis on personal responsibility and an "ownership society" has eroded the safety net and led to what he terms the "great risk shift." Although data suggests that results, in terms of both costs and outcomes, are better in solidarity-based models of health insurance (see also section 5.9, Insurance, Elasticity, and Moral hazard), it is important to recognize that, to the extent this debate reflects underlying values about individual vs. mutual responsibility, such data is irrelevant (see section 3.2, Role of the State).

One influential approach in the ethics literature has been Aristotle's principle of *distributive justice*, which specifies that equals should be treated equally and those who are unequal should be treated unequally. (As noted in section 3.3.3, Equity, defining what is meant by "equal" can also be subject to dispute.) This approach would argue that unequal treatment is justified when resources are allocated based on morally relevant differences. Defining which differences so qualify, however, depends on values. Many would argue that characteristics pertaining to need or to the likely benefit from health services are morally relevant criteria for resource allocation, whereas such characteristics such as gender, sexual orientation, religion, level of education, or age alone are morally irrelevant. Others would disagree. Most ethicists argue that fair, open, and publicly defensible resource allocation procedures are also critical (see section 3.6.1, Accountability for Reasonableness). However, the lack of a comprehensive, widely accepted theory of justice gives rise to unresolved issues in rationing, including the following questions (Daniels, 1994):

The *fair chances vs. best outcomes* problem. To what degree should producing the best outcome be favoured over giving every patient an opportunity to compete for those limited resources?

The *priorities* problem. How much priority should we give to treating the sickest or most disabled patients?

The *aggregation* problem. When should we allow an aggregation of modest benefits to larger numbers of people to outweigh more significant benefits to fewer people?

The *democracy* problem. When must we rely on a fair democratic process as the only way to determine what constitutes a fair rationing outcome?

Another set of issues also relates to the ethical principles noted in section 3.6 (Ethical Frameworks), particularly beneficence. One question is who should make these decisions, and whether "patient empowerment" implies that patients should receive whatever treatment they desire, regardless of professional views about how likely it is to be effective. One suggestion is that patient participation can be divided into "problem solving" (which involves knowing the "right answer" about what the diagnosis is and what the likely effects of particular treatments would be) and "decision making" (which also involves patient preferences for particular outcomes), with most patients preferring to restrict their involvement to the decision-making elements (termed "shared decision making") (Deber et al., 1996).

A related question is whether this should depend on who is paying for the care, or whether the injunction for providers to do no harm
implies that such care should not be provided regardless of who is paying. Particularly given the power and knowledge imbalance that often
exists between physician and patient, to what extent is there a fiduciary duty on the physician's part to promote the patient's best interest?
The extent of this ethical duty, which is fundamental to the physician's
role in resource allocation, is a matter of controversy. Some argue that
physicians should do everything they believe might benefit a particular patient, without taking costs or other societal considerations into
account. A related principle is sometimes called the *Rule of Rescue*.
It refers to the injunction to rescue identifiable individuals in immediate peril, regardless of the cost. The tension between cost-effectiveness
and the Rule of Rescue can generate serious ethical and political difficulties for public policymakers faced with making resource allocation
decisions. The stress on identifiable individuals also tends to devalue
prevention; it is difficult to identify a specific person who did not catch
an infectious disease because he/she was immunized, or who was not
injured in an automobile accident because he/she was wearing a seat-
belt. Others may focus on opportunity costs and argue for the importance of balancing competing claims from other potential stakeholders,
including other potential patients who did not obtain the resources
used for the identified patient, as well as payers, and society as a whole
(McKneally et al., 1997). Others note the potential for a conflict of interest, particularly if payments are related to the decision about whether
to provide marginal therapies.

## 4. Interests

*Interests*, who are sometimes termed stakeholders, are key elements
of policymaking. They have a number of roles, including: articulating
political demands; seeking support for these demands among other
groups; attempting to transform these demands into authoritative
public policy by influencing the choice of political personnel, and the
processes of public policymaking and enforcement; and connecting
individuals to the political system via legitimate channels (as opposed
to having to riot in the streets). The political science theory of plural-
ism stresses that various groups are involved in attempting to influence
policy, and that power and influence thus vary depending on the issue
being examined.

Note that interests vary in how organized they are. At one extreme, *latent* interests may share similar concerns, but are not yet organized. *Solidarity groups* have moved to informal support of others with similar concerns, but do not yet have a formalized organizational structure. *Interest groups* (sometimes called *pressure groups*) have mobilized and organized, but vary in the resources they can bring to bear. Pross (1992) has defined interest groups as groups of people who have joined together to pursue common interests by attempting to influence decisions and/or influence the selection/election of decision makers. Pross has classified these groups on a number of dimensions, including their: objectives (broad vs. narrow; long-term vs. single interest); organization (the degree of continuity and cohesion); knowledge of government (minimal/naive vs. extensive); and membership (stable vs. fluid). At one end of the resulting continuum, *issue-oriented* groups are interested in particular objectives (e.g., stopping a construction project that might affect their neighbourhood). *Fledgling* groups are more organized, and *mature* groups more organized still. At the other end are what Pross called *institutionalized* groups, who have stable membership, strong organizational resources, and ongoing links to decision makers.

Another way of classifying interest groups is whether they are *economic* (producer) interest groups (e.g., business, service providers), or *social* (collective rights) associations (e.g., consumer groups, environmental groups, etc.) (Doern & Phidd, 1992). As noted in section 4.1, the economic interest groups, in general, are more likely to have *concentrated* interests; they will often use their resources to lobby, and to establish channels to government decision makers.

A related literature speaks of *advocacy coalitions*, defined as actors who share policy goals and/or basic beliefs, and try to manipulate rules, budgets, and people to achieve their goals (Sabatier & Jenkins-Smith, 1993).

There is also a considerable literature about political *participation* (Pateman, 1970). For example, Arnstein's Ladder of Participation discusses eight types of participation (Arnstein, 1969). At one end of this ladder is nonparticipation, with tokenism in the middle, and citizen power at the high end. Note that the literature may also differ in why participation is seen to be important. If it is seen as a means to making better decisions, one might focus on the actual decisions made. Under this view, participation is important to the extent that it affects the ultimate decision and ensures that the views of key stakeholders have been taken into account (see section 4.3, Scope of Conflict). If participation is also seen as an end, however, one might note that political participation can be a critical way of engaging individuals and making them feel like contributing members of society. If one accepts this view, participation is valuable in its own right, regardless of whether the ultimate decisions have changed.

There has been considerable focus in health care on using public engagement for decision making (Abelson & Eyles, 2004; Abelson et al., 2002; Rowe & Frewer, 2005). Chafe and colleagues (2008) have suggested the following series of questions that should be asked of all parties in evaluating a public participation exercise: (1) To what extent was the stated decision/issue clearly communicated to and understood by participants?; (2) To what extent was the desired level of public involvement achieved and what factors facilitated or hindered achievement of this objective?; (3) How did the final sample of participants compare to the intended sample and were the implications of any differences noted?; (4) Did the participants feel that they had sufficient background information to participate effectively in the exercise?; (5) What were the strengths and weaknesses of the methods used to analyze, summarize, and report the findings from the public participation exercise?; (6) What was the weight assigned to public input in the final decision-making process and was this consistent with the original intent of the exercise?; (7) To what extent did the outcomes meet the expectations of the organization and the participants?; (8) Were the methods used to engage the participants acceptable and effective for the intended purposes?; (9) Would all parties involved in the process agree to participate in a similar process in the future? Would they recommend participation in a similar process to a colleague, and/or to a family member?; and (10) What were the major lessons learned from the exercise?

### 4.1 Concentrated/Diffuse Interests

Another way to categorize interests is based on the intensity of their concern with a particular area. A *concentrated* interest has a strong stake in a particular issue; a *diffuse* interest is far less concerned about that issue. For example, producers of particular goods or services have a concentrated interest in how it will be priced or regulated; most of those who consume that good or service are unlikely to place as high a priority on that issue, because they consume many items and would not have the time to become involved in policies relating to them all. For that reason, "public forums" are less likely to attract the general public and tend to be dominated by the concentrated interests (Marmor & Morone, 1980). A related concept is the *astroturf* group, used to refer to groups which appear to be grass-roots organizations, but are in fact funded by concentrated (usually producer) interests (Lyon & Maxwell, 2004).

Despite the advantages that concentrated interests have in mobilizing for political activity, they do not always prevail over diffuse interests. Factors that facilitate the relative success of diffuse interests include having a large segment of the population paying attention to that policy issue (see section 5.1, Agenda Setting), and when the public does not trust the concentrated interests. Otherwise, policymaking often tends to be focused within policy communities.

## 4.2 Policy Communities

Political scientists use the term *policy community* to define "that part of a political system that has acquired a dominant voice in determining government decisions in a field of public policy ... by virtue of its functional responsibilities, its vested interests and its specialized knowledge" (Pross, 1992, p. 119). Policy communities can include government agencies, interest groups, media, and individuals that have an interest in a particular policy field. These policy communities can be loosely divided into the *sub-government*, which influences policy in that area, and the *attentive public*, who merely follows the debate (Coleman & Skogstad, 1990). Although they may disagree about policy details, members of a policy community do tend to share a "world view" and a vocabulary. For example, medicine, public health, and local government will usually form different, if potentially overlapping, policy communities. In general, concentrated interests are most likely to participate in the policy communities most closely related to their key concerns. Such participation, in turn, may be affected by what political scientists call the scope of conflict.

## 4.3 Scope of Conflict

*Scope of conflict* refers to a concept developed by Schattschneider, which stresses the importance of understanding who is involved in deciding about policies, which in turn is related to such elements as how policies are defined, who is at the table, and what the rules will be. For example, decisions about who should receive a particular clinical treatment may differ if they are made by individual clinicians, by public or private bureaucrats deciding on coverage policies, by regulators, or in a courtroom. In turn, the scope of conflict often helps determine the outcome (Schattschneider, 1975). If the consequences of a certain policy problem are framed as affecting only a small range of individuals, then fewer stakeholders might be involved. Schattschneider looked at why certain actors and groups do or do not participate in policy processes and suggested that policymakers tend to try to define policy conflicts in such a way that they can manage the scope of conflict and ensure resolution in their desired policy direction.

Schattschneider argues that, when analyzing the scope of conflict for a particular policy issue, it is important to determine why groups do or do not participate in the policy process. He pointed to three factors, which he termed visibility, intensity, and direction. *Visibility* refers to whether the group has information about the policy and knows whether it would be to its advantage to participate. Visibility accordingly favours groups that are sufficiently well organized and have the resources needed to ensure timely access to this information. *Intensity* refers to how attached the group is to the policy issue, and hence whether the group chooses to participate. *Direction* refers to the agenda of these groups and whether they see this as an important enough conflict for them to become involved with. In general, those with more resources are more likely to become involved, and to succeed in having the policies match their preferences. As Schattschneider (1975) observed, "The flaw in the pluralist heaven is that the heavenly chorus sings with a strong upper class accent" (pp. 34–35).

As noted in section 3.4 (Framing), policymakers will try to define conflicts in such a way as to manage the scope of conflict in order to ensure the adoption of their preferred policies. One key factor in determining whether a policy will be adopted is based on how the policy issues were defined. Schattschneider (1975) summarizes this as follows: "The definition of alternatives is the supreme instrument of power … He who determines what politics is about runs the country, because the definition of the alternatives is the choice of conflicts, and the choice of conflicts allocates power" (p. 66). When scope of conflict changes, different actors may be at the table, working under different rules; understanding who chooses to participate in trying to influence policy decisions is often critical to understanding policy formation (Kellow, 1988).

## 5. Some Additional Policy Concepts

### 5.1 Agenda Setting

Limits of time, money, and attention mean that not all potential problems can be dealt with. Political scientists use the term *agenda setting* to refer to the process of deciding what issues will be "on the table" at any given point in time (Baumgartner, 2001; Baumgartner & Jones, 1991; Fierlbeck, 2004; Kingdon, 2003; McCombs, 2002). There is a literature that focuses primarily on the role of the media (see section 5.8), but most scholars recognize that interests (see section 4), ideas (see section 3), and unexpected events may also play important roles in this process. In that connection, compelling stories can often attract media attention and place issues onto the agenda (Stone, 1989).

### 5.2 Policy/Governing Instruments

Government has an array of *instruments* it can use to achieve its goals. Doern and Phidd (1992) arrayed these in terms of the degree of coercion involved. At one extreme is what they term *exhortation*, whereby governments encourage stakeholders to act in a particular way. This may include information/education (e.g., encouraging healthy eating), and/or symbolic gestures (e.g., appointing the "first woman" to a particular role to show support for women). Next is the use of *expenditure*, where government provides funds for particular purposes. This may also include the use of *taxation* (tax policy), including giving tax breaks for certain activities. Next is *regulation*, where rules are established to encourage or penalize certain types of action (see also section 5.2.1). Finally, government can directly run an activity through *public ownership*. Another possibility, included in some frameworks, is to do nothing, and hope that the problem will solve itself without the need for government action.

Another formulation, which makes similar points in slightly different language, is Hood's NATO, which uses the terms nodality (information), authority, treasure, and organization (Hood, 1983). This approach can also be used to classify some instruments that government might use (Howlett et al., 2009). The *information*-based instruments include: information collection and release; advice and exhortation; advertising; and commissions and inquiries. The *authority*-based instruments include: command-and-control regulation; self-regulation; standard-setting and delegated regulation; and advisory committees and consultations. The *treasure*-based instruments include: grants and loans; user charges; taxes and tax expenditures; and interest group creation and funding. The *organization*-based instruments include: direct provision of goods and services and public enterprises; use of family, community, and voluntary organizations; and government reorganization.

### 5.2.1 REGULATION

The Organisation for Economic Co-operation and Development (OECD) (2002) has defined regulation as follows: "Regulation is broadly defined as imposition of rules by government, backed by the use of penalties that are intended specifically to modify the economic behaviour of individuals and firms in the private sector. Various regulatory instruments or targets exist."

Almost anything can be regulated. Regulations can be directed at individuals (e.g., specifying who can practice as a health professional), at activities (e.g., specifying allowed levels of emissions from industries), at prices, and so on. Justifications for regulation may include the need to protect the public, particularly when one is dealing with public goods (see section 3.5, Public Goods and Externalities), market failure (e.g., the presence of natural monopolies may justify regulating prices), and/or asymmetry of information (e.g., if one assumes that "consumers" are not sufficiently knowledgeable to judge the quality of those practicing a particular profession, one may use regulation to ensure that anyone practicing meets pre-specified standards; see also section 6.4, Professionalism).

One goal of regulation is to constrain behaviour that may be seen as not in the public interest. Regulation is thus highly contentious, and relates to views about the appropriate balance between individual action and state intervention (see section 3.2, Role of the State). Note that regulation is a high-coercion instrument, which has the additional feature of shifting the costs of compliance to those being regulated. Those with more libertarian views often criticize regulation for interfering with markets in such ways as imposing costs needed to comply with regulations on those being regulated, disallowing certain types of activities (e.g., minimum wage legislation may prevent employers from saving money through lowering their wage rates), and/or increasing costs through reducing competition by introducing barriers to entry for new providers (e.g., restricting the number of physicians licensed to practice).

## 5.3 Street-level Bureaucracy

As defined by Max Weber, *bureaucracies* were seen as a way of organizing activities (including those of the civil service) without the sorts of favouritism found in traditional societies. In an ideal bureaucracy, there would be clear lines of authority, clear rules and procedures, and neutral implementation. Someone seeking to renew a driver's license should not be treated differently because they were personal friends (or enemies) with the clerk in the licensing bureau. However, as pointed out by Lipsky (1980), this model of bureaucracy was not always feasible, and could sometimes be counterproductive. Lipsky coined the term *street-level bureaucrat* to refer to people who work on the front lines, directly interact with the public, and have considerable discretion in what they do and how they do it. Early examples described in the literature on street-level bureaucracy included police officers, parole officers, and social workers, but the concept was subsequently expanded to home care workers, nurses, salaried physicians, etc. The literature sometimes focuses on the possibilities that the street-level bureaucrat's decisions will violate policies of the organization, and sometimes on the need to ensure that these workers have the flexibility needed to address individual cases. Freidson (2001) suggested that professionalism (see section 6.4) could operate to ensure that the decisions made by street-level bureaucrats were not arbitrary, and were in the best interest of the public, particularly where it would be difficult or impossible to specify what decisions would be appropriate for particular cases.

## 5.4 Policy Implementation

Policies do not always achieve their intended results. The literature on *policy implementation* (usually associated with public administration) focuses on what is necessary to ensure that policy goals are achieved in practice (DiMaggio & Powell, 1983; March & Olsen, 1984; Matland, 1995; Sabatier, 1999; Sabatier & Mazmanian, 1980). Factors associated with policy failure could include having multiple and potentially conflicting goals, multiple actors (associated with the need for multiple decisions), and/or having key actors having different preferences, potentially held with different intensity (Pressman & Wildavsky, 1973). Setting up special purpose organizations may be helpful in facilitating policy implementation, but may also increase the amount of coordination needed and give additional potential blocking points at which policies can be delayed or altered.

A related literature discusses how individuals may react to policies they disagree with, including two key options: *exit* means that they withdraw from the organization, whereas *voice* means that they protest (Hirschman, 1970, 1980). This model stresses the importance of giving individuals a vehicle to change what an organization is doing peacefully, with one advantage being increased *loyalty*.

## 5.5 Globalization

*Globalization* refers to the increasing interdependence of the world. The global movement of goods, services, capital, and people presents both opportunities and risks (Smith, 2008). One obvious issue is governance; individual jurisdictions will be affected by the policies of other jurisdictions, but may have little ability to influence them (Courtney & Smith, 2010; Tindal & Tindal, 2008). One ongoing problem is the relative weakness of global governance, meaning that it is difficult to enforce policies to protect against externalities (see section 3.5, Public Goods and Externalities). For example, emissions from one country can travel across borders. Many cases in this book have globalization dimensions. People travel, and communicable disease can spread (see Chapter 2, Danger at the Gates, and Chapter 7, Looking for Trouble). Workers trained in one jurisdiction can seek to work in others (see Chapter 10, The Demanding Supply). Information can spread globally, making it difficult to regulate pharmaceutical advertising (see Chapter 16, Ask Your Doctor).

A number of international bodies, including the United Nations, the World Health Organization, the World Bank, and various trade bodies, have attempted to build an infrastructure for international governance; to date, this has proven relatively difficult. However, these bodies can be helpful both in collecting and providing information, and by providing opportunities for parties to meet and reach voluntary agreements.

## 5.6 Accountability

*Accountability* can be defined as having to be answerable to someone for meeting defined objectives (Emanuel & Emanuel, 1996; Fooks & Maslove, 2004; Marmor & Morone, 1980). It has financial, performance, and political/democratic dimensions (Brinkerhoff, 2004; Dobrow et al.,

2008) and can occur before (*ex ante*) or after (*ex post*) the fact. The actors involved may include various combinations of providers (public and private), patients, payers (including private insurers as well as the legislative and executive branches of government), the public, and regulators (governmental and/or professional); these actors can be connected in various ways (Shortt & Macdonald, 2002; Zimmerman, 2005). The tools for establishing and enforcing accountability are similarly varied, and require clarifying what is meant by accountability, including specifying for what, by whom, to whom, and how. Performance management and measurement are frequently suggested as important tools for improving systems of accountability. This can also be complex, and one size will rarely fit all. In a review, Deber and Schwartz (2011) have suggested that one key variable is the production characteristics of the goods and services being accounted for.

## 5.7 Production Characteristics

Goods and services can be seen as having *production characteristics* that will affect how performance can be measured and managed (Deber, 2004; Jakab et al., 2002; Preker & Harding, 2000, 2003; Preker et al., 2000; Rico & Puig-Junoy, 2002; Vining & Globerman, 1999). These include contestability, measurability, and complexity, which have been defined as follows (Preker & Harding, 2000).

*Contestable* goods are characterized by low barriers to entry and exit from the market, whereas non-contestable goods have high barriers such as sunk costs, monopoly market power, geographic advantages, and/or "asset specificity" (meaning that these resources cannot easily be used for other purposes). For example, the skills and resources needed for a hospital unit performing paediatric cardiac surgery cannot easily be deployed elsewhere, whereas laptop computers could be wiped of their contents and reused for other purposes.

*Measurability* relates to "the precision with which inputs, processes, outputs, and outcomes of a good or service can be measured" (Preker et al., 2000, p. 782). Monitoring performance is easiest when measurability is high. For example, it is relatively simple to specify the performance desired for conducting a laboratory test or collecting municipal garbage. In contrast, it would be more difficult to specify the activities to be expected of a general practitioner, and hence more difficult for an external body to monitor his/her performance and ensure quality.

*Complexity* refers not to how complex the particular goods and services are but to whether the goods and services stand alone or require coordination with other providers. For example, laboratory tests are highly measurable, but gain much of their value by being embedded within a system of care in which providers order tests appropriately, and are aided as required in interpreting and acting upon their results.

Additional insights arise from the theory of *transaction costs* and monitoring costs. This term refers to the costs of entering into an economic exchange; it includes the costs associated with obtaining the necessary information to find the desired goods and to compare prices, the costs of bargaining between potential buyers and sellers, and the costs associated with policing and enforcing contracts. Some of these issues have been addressed in economic theories relating to incomplete contracting, which is defined as contracts where all elements of the contract have not (and perhaps cannot) be defined in advance (Williamson, 1981, 1985, 1999).

## 5.8 Role of Media

When does something count as being newsworthy? News media usually see themselves as being in the business of telling stories. A number of factors have been identified which help define whether something is considered news (MediaCollege.com, 2011; Wikipedia, 2012). They include the following: (1) *timing* – news should be new; even important stories will not be considered "news" unless there are current developments; (2) *relevance* – this is defined both in terms of how many are affected (accidents with many casualties are deemed as more important than accidents which only kill a few), and how close to home the event is (events which happen locally, vs. those occurring in more distant locations, but also events happening to "people like us" rather than to those in different cultures); (3) *fame* – even minor events happening to celebrities may be seen as newsworthy; and (4) *human interest* – this is usually defined in terms of stories appealing to emotion.

## 5.9 Insurance, Elasticity, and Moral Hazard

Economics is based on the assumption that markets are the best way to allocate goods and services. In economics, price is the signal that ensures a balance between supply and demand. If demand exceeds supply, prices should rise until enough people are priced out of the market so that supply and demand are balanced. Market forces thus ensure that the scarce goods go to those who value them most, as demonstrated by their willingness to pay the higher price. In contrast, reducing price would be predicted to increase demand. Cost containment would accordingly discourage models that insulate people from the true costs of their purchasing decisions in favour of requiring consumers to pay for a greater share of the care they receive.

The concept *elasticity of demand* refers to the relationship between demand and price, commonly measured as the absolute value of the percentage change in quantity demanded divided by the percentage change in price. If the ratio is greater than one, demand is said to be price elastic. Conversely, if the ratio is less than one, demand is said to be inelastic. Clearly, if demand is inelastic, then market forces (in the form of prices) will not be effective ways of controlling costs.

Some theorists argue, on both ethical and empirical grounds, that utilization of health services differs from demand for consumer goods for a number of reasons. One key distinction is that it is (or at least should be) based on need rather than demand (Deber, 2003; Donaldson et al., 2005; Evans, 1984, 2004; Geyman, 2007; Herzlinger, 2004; Jost, 2007; Rice, 1998; Rosenthal & Daniels, 2006). These terms can be defined as follows: "In health economics, the term *demand* is the amount of a good or service consumers are willing and able to buy at varying prices, given constant income and other factors. Demand should be distinguished from *utilization* (the amount of services actually used) and *need* (which has a normative connotation and relates to the amount of goods or services which should be consumed based on professional value judgments)" (Academy Health, 2004).

*Information asymmetry* applies to situations where one party in a transaction has information not possessed by the other. Health care is characterized by considerable information asymmetry, in that most patients do not (and often cannot be realistically expected to) understand what is wrong with them, and what treatments might (or might not) help (Culyer, 1995; Evans, 1984; Getzen, 1997). Because need is defined by experts rather than by consumers, one might further argue that this undermines the underlying assumptions of a market. Those individuals receiving care are not always in the best position to decide what services they wish to purchase; information asymmetry reduces their ability to make truly informed decisions (Evans, 1996; Rice, 1997).

Another issue is the possibility that individuals may be faced with the possibility of very high costs beyond their ability to pay. *Insurance* is one way of dealing with the possibility of such high costs; individuals may choose to pool their risks, paying premiums to a third party (public or private) to generate sufficient funds to cover those affected in the event that these losses materialize. People may purchase fire insurance, hoping that they will never need to collect, but confident that should a disaster occur, the pooled resources from everyone in that insurance plan would generate enough money to pay their claim and allow them to start over. Several conclusions follow. First, insurance would not apply to a certainty; one could not expect to purchase fire insurance after one's house was already in flames. Second, *underwriting* is important; it would not seem fair to charge similar premiums to people with markedly different probabilities of loss. As one example, *actuarial fairness* would imply that those with poor driving records would pay higher rates, or even be unable to buy insurance at all. Third, one must decide how to deal with what is termed *moral hazard*, that is, to the prospect that insulating people from risk (a major purpose of insurance) may make them less concerned about the potential negative consequences of that risk than they otherwise might be. For example, those with flood insurance may be more willing to build in flood plains, in the confidence that insurance would cover their losses. Insurance plans often incorporate features to attempt to mitigate moral hazard. These may include co-payments (where claimants must still pay a portion of the losses they incur), deductibles (where claimants must pay for all loses up to a preset amount), and/or refusal to write policies at all to high-risk individuals.

There is considerable dispute as to the extent to which these underlying assumptions of market models apply to insurance for health care (Academy Health, 2004; Deber & Lam, 2009; Pauly, 1986). For example, if these market models do apply, it would imply that choice and competition should be encouraged, and that people should bear a significant portion of the costs of the care they use. In the "consumer-driven" model, wise consumers will shop around for the best buy, measured in terms of both quality and price. Financing should accordingly incorporate co-payments and deductibles to minimize moral hazard. Because severe illness can be very costly, with health care being a major cause of individual bankruptcy in the United States (Himmelstein et al., 2005), people may wish to purchase catastrophic coverage to cover claims above a predefined amount; such coverage may or may not incorporate additional co-payments, and/or caps on total coverage (Bloche, 2006; Herzlinger, 2004).

Closer analysis reveals that there are many problems with trying to apply this competitive market insurance model to health care. If one accepted this model, since one cannot insure against a certainty, one would not expect that people could buy coverage for care they knew they would need; accordingly, pregnant women should not be able to buy insurance to cover the certainty that they will need medical care to give birth. Actuarial fairness would also imply that those who have good genes, eat well, don't smoke, don't drink to excess, and exercise regularly should not have to subsidize those who do not. The least healthy should expect to pay the highest premiums, or even to be refused insurance should their anticipated costs be too high. In addition, to the extent that moral hazard exists, those with good health insurance, because they do not have to pay the full cost of any care they receive, would be predicted to have an incentive to overuse it; if that is true, cost control should therefore begin by ensuring that people have to bear a higher proportion of the consequences of their decisions. Advocates who support that position often quote the RAND health insurance study, which randomized families less than age 65 to different health insurance plans with different co-payments, and found that utilization for some services did indeed decrease among those with the higher co-payments. However, that study also found that health outcomes for those already poor and sick were worse (Newhouse, 2004; Newhouse & Insurance Experiment Group, 1993).

If competition is encouraged, one would expect that insurers would be influenced by the previous conclusions. Any insurer who charged the same to cover all individuals, regardless of their risk (often termed *community rating*) would not be competitive with plans which calibrated their premiums and could offer lower rates to lower-risk individuals. As these clients left, the more generous insurers would be left with higher-cost enrollees, and would have to increase their rates to cover this higher average cost. In what is often termed the adverse-selection *premium death spiral*, these insurers would be uncompetitive, and driven out of business (Fein, 2001). Without a level playing field, there is a substantial competitive advantage for plans that are able to select their clients.

In practice, this approach is indeed occurring. One example is the US group coverage market, which has often been employer-based and pools risks across the group of people working for those companies and receiving insurance coverage as one of their benefits. However, as the proportion of Americans with access to employer-based coverage decreased, more people were expected to buy insurance in the individual market. One study found that, between 2001 and 2007, nearly three-fourths of adults in the United States who tried to purchase coverage in the individual market never purchased a plan, either because the premiums were too high for them to afford, or because the insurers turned them down due to a pre-existing condition (Doty et al., 2009). Indeed, one major policy aim behind Obamacare was dealing with this population who would otherwise be uninsurable, although the extent to which the specific policies selected work was still undetermined at the time of writing. International studies have found that moves towards introducing more competition have found it difficult to accurately risk-adjust premiums, and the resulting incentives for insurers to avoid high-cost patients were leaving an increasing number of the most vulnerable people uninsured (Ellis & Vidal-Fernandez, 2007; Hsaio, 2007; Nicholson et al., 2003; van de Ven et al., 2003).

The concept of need has major implications for the ability to apply economic models. If one believes that people should receive needed care regardless of their ability to pay, they cannot be priced out of the market, and price signals cannot control costs. Instead, under those circumstances, there will be a floor price (whatever charity or government will pay) but no ceiling price; those who cannot afford care will drop down to the charity tier. Conversely, although market theory predicts that free care will, by definition, be abused, both evidence and logic suggest that this does not appear to apply to many health care services; few would want to receive services they do not need. One would expect a shoe store to advertise and market their products, and would not expect them to refuse to sell a potential customer a pair that they did not need. However, one would not expect a hospital to market half-price open heart surgery to anyone willing to pay for it, and few would argue that potential customers should be able to purchase open-heart surgery even if they were perfectly healthy (Deber, 2000; Donaldson et al., 2005; Evans, 2004). In an ideal system, receipt of care would be based on appropriateness (e.g., an expectation of benefit) rather than on consumer demand (Deber, 2008).

One indication that health care is indeed different from other markets is that few countries employ highly competitive models for health insurance. Even those countries that use social insurance financing approaches heavily regulate the insurers, often mandating the benefit package and who must be insured. As White (2007) has noted, these models achieve cost control by such mechanisms as "compulsory contributions and membership, contributions related to ability to pay, cost controls applied across the universe of providers, a very wide risk pool for beneficiaries ... and the resulting ability to be a price maker rather than a price taker" (p. 398).

As White (2007) further notes, "cost controls are good for payers and bad for providers (p. 409). Unsurprisingly, providers often resist such cost controls. In a competitive market, the goal is to be profitable, meaning that providers who are not competitive will, and should, be driven out of the market. Providers may react to competition by gaining market power, and indeed one trend in countries employing competing insurers (including the United States, but also social insurance models such as Germany) has been a consolidation among both providers and insurers (at the extreme, resulting in mergers to create local monopolies). Another strategy is to focus upon profitable clients and services and avoid serving those likely to generate a loss. Clients may not be profitable because they cannot afford to pay premiums, and one policy issue is the extent to which the poor should be subsidized to allow them to purchase insurance. Another reason for being unprofitable, however, results from the extent to which health expenditures are concentrated upon a small proportion of the population (see Chapter 18, Everybody Out of the Pool). To the extent that such concentration exists, it is far more difficult to achieve universal coverage and cost containment within a competitive market, because, as noted above, there are strong incentives for insurers to practice *risk selection* (often termed *cream skimming*) and avoid those most likely to be at the high end of the expenditure distribution. If costs are highly skewed, insurers will not have to avoid many clients to incur considerable savings (Deber & Lam, 2011a, 2011b).

## 5.10 Decision Making and Policy Change

Much of policy is related to decision making. A number of different models can be used. Economic analysis (see section 8.1) is based on rational decision-making theory, and assumes that a good decision will optimize (or maximize) outcomes. One variant, *bounded rationality*, takes into account the costs of doing the analysis required for maximizing outcomes, and recommends that it is sometimes more rational to select the first outcome that is "good enough," an approach that Simon named *satisficing* (Simon, 1978). Another approach, *incrementalism* (also called "muddling through"), noted that policymakers often continued on the same course until events forced them to change (Lindblom, 1959, 1979). A compromise position, *mixed scanning*, argued that the most rational approach was often to scan the environment and see which policy issues warranted further analysis (Etzioni, 1986).

A related set of theories examines how policies change over time, and how this is affected by prior policies (Currie, 2009; Hacker, 2004; Pierson, 1993). The *rational political model* combines rational decision making with scope of conflict theory (see section 4.3); it specifies policy options, policy goals, and potential stakeholders. A "fact matrix" gives the policy goals, and how likely each policy option is to achieve them; a "values matrix" gives the stakeholders and how important each policy goal is to each; and a "goal weights vector" indicates how important each potential stakeholder is, given the venue where that issue is being decided and the "rules of the game" there. One can then do the math to find the rational choice to maximize these weighted policy goals (Wiktorowicz & Deber, 1997).

## 6. Health Care Systems

### 6.1 Dimensions of Health Care Systems

There are a number of different elements to health care systems. The next sections define what is meant by public and private, distinguish between financing and delivery, and indicate possible combinations of these two dimensions. They next note the implication of different ways of paying providers. Note that precise details about how care is organized, delivered, and paid for may differ, not only across jurisdictions but also across types of services. Different models may exist in different jurisdictions, and may vary across such services as hospital care, physician services, pharmaceuticals, diagnostic imaging, long-term care, rehabilitation, dental care, vision care, home care, and so on.

#### 6.1.1 PUBLIC AND PRIVATE

The terms *public* and *private* apply to both how care is financed and how it is delivered (see section 6.1.2); the terms can each be divided into several categories (Deber, 2004; Evans, 1984). Public can refer to different levels of government, including national, state/provincial, regional, and local. Private can include: *corporate for-profit* business (which has a responsibility to maximize return to shareholders), *for-profit small business* (which also may include health care professional practices such as physician or physiotherapist offices, a category Evans calls "not-only-for-profit"), *not-for-profit* (NFP) organizations (both large and small organizations, including many hospitals and community agencies), and *individuals* and their families (who may pay for and provide many services). To this can be added *quasi-public* organizations, which are legally private, but heavily regulated, and span the boundary between public and private. The quasi-public category includes many of the Canadian regional health authorities referred to in section 2.2.4, many European sickness funds, and so forth.

Considerable research has been conducted on the relative efficiency and effectiveness of the private and public sectors in meeting health and social objectives. When performance standards and goals are easily specified and where programs are amenable to explicit arm's-length monitoring and control, private, for-profit delivery can be efficient, as would be predicted by the theory of markets (Bendick, 1989; Donahue, 1989), although other forms of delivery may also perform well. However, when goals are complex, the benefits of the private sector are less clear, particularly when other desired outcomes may be sacrificed to improve profitability.

*Privatization* refers to the movement from public to private. Weimer and Vining (1989) identify several meanings of the term, including: (1) the switch from direct public payment (which they call "agency subventions") to user fees; this financing switch may or may not incorporate subsidies and taxes to alter incentives; (2) the contracting-out of the provision of a good that was previously produced by a government bureau; (3) denationalization, or the selling of state-owned enterprises to the private sector; and/or (4) demonopolization, the process by which the government relaxes or eliminates restrictions that prevent private firms from competing with government bureaus or state-owned enterprises. Starr (1989) describes four types of privatization: (1) the termination of public programs and the disengagement of government from specific kinds of responsibilities (implicit privatization); an example would be Ontario's decision to no longer fund travel health clinics/ immunization clinics; (2) the transfer of public assets to private ownership; an example would be the sale of a government-owned railroad; (3) public financing of private service delivery instead of direct government service production; an example would be a privately run prison which was financed by a contract with the public justice system; and (4) the deregulation of entry by private firms into activities previously treated as public monopoly; an example might be private mail delivery.

A major trend towards privatization, or partial privatization, has developed over the last decade in a wide range of countries, including the United Kingdom, France, Canada, and New Zealand. One example is "public-private partnerships" (P3s, or PPPs), where private sector businesses participate with government in the delivery of infrastructure or services that had traditionally been provided by governments alone (see Chapter 5, Trouble on Tap).

### 6.1.2 FINANCING AND DELIVERY

As noted above, it is important to distinguish between how care is paid for ( *financing*) and how it is *delivered*. Various models exist, which reflect different roles for public and private. The OECD identifies four main types of funding for health services: public payment through *taxation / general revenues*; public / quasi-public payment through *social insurance*; *private insurance*, and direct *out-of-pocket* payments. As noted in section 5.9 (Insurance, Elasticity, and Moral Hazard), in the insurance models, premiums may be "risk-rated" (based on the expected costs of services required), or based on other factors, including age-sex group, income, and/or employment status. Internationally, there is considerable variation in the mix of funding approaches, which may also vary across type of service, and/or category of client (Allin et al., 2010; Colombo & Tapay, 2004; Deber & Lam, 2011a, 2011b; Docteur & Oxley, 2003). In turn, different funding models reflect different views about which costs should be born collectively, and which should be the responsibility of individuals and their families (see also section 3.2, Role of the State).

The providers delivering health care services may fall into a variety of these public-private categories. For example, a government-owned hospital would be classified as public delivery; this has been a common model in such countries as England, Australia, or Sweden. Most hospitals in such countries as Canada have fallen into the private, not-for-profit category. Physician offices in many jurisdictions are private, for-profit small businesses. Pharmaceutical companies are usually private, for-profit, investor-owned corporations. Note that many combinations are possible, particularly as countries experiment with alternative ways of delivering care.

### 6.1.3 MODELS OF HEALTH SYSTEMS

Health care systems thus may represent various combinations of public / private and financing / delivery, as shown in the 2 × 2 classification in Table 1.1.

Table 1.1. Classification of Health Care Systems

|  | Public financing | Private financing |
|---|---|---|
| Public delivery | National Health Service | User fees for public services |
| Private delivery | Public insurance (public contracting) | Private insurance |

Note that different models are used, not only in different jurisdictions but also for different categories of services and clients (Deber, 2004, 2009; Docteur & Oxley, 2003; Marchildon, 2013). The UK National Health Service (NHS) largely falls into the public financing–public delivery cell. In Canada, few services would fall into that category, with the exception of public health, and, in some provinces, government-run provincial psychiatric hospitals (almost all of which have been shifted to private NFP status). The private financing–public delivery cell is widely believed to be suboptimal for health care, and plays a minimal part in most developed countries, although it is still used in many developing countries which do not have the resources to publicly cover even medically necessary services. However, this category may be appropriate for other types of services. For example, in most countries, including Canada, much public transit would fall into the private financing–public delivery classification, since it is delivered by civil servants, but largely funded through the fare box. In Canada, the hospital and physician services falling under the *Canada Health Act* (see section 7.2) largely fall into the public financing–private delivery cell that the OECD calls *public contracting*, while such services as dental care and outpatient pharmaceuticals largely fall into the private financing–private delivery cell. Note that the United States has multiple models that fall into many of the cells of this table: the Veteran's Administration is public financing–public delivery; Medicare/Medicaid is public financing–private delivery; and most of those with private insurance fall into the private financing–private delivery category.

## 6.2 *Payment Mechanisms and Incentives*

A third dimension of health care systems can be called *allocation*; it deals with how resources flow from payers to providers, and the different incentives that go with different payment models. One categorization of approaches to paying providers uses two dimensions (Deber et al., 2008). The first is whether payment goes to individual providers or to provider organizations (e.g., hospitals, primary care organizations). The second dimension is the basis of payment, which can incorporate various combinations of: actual costs (e.g., drug plans may reimburse for the actual costs of pharmaceuticals plus a mark-up); time spent (e.g., wages); services provided (e.g., fee-for-service); population served (e.g., capitation); fixed/global budgets (which are often based on historical spending); and/or outcomes achieved. The basis for payment can make a difference, since different approaches have different incentive structures (Leger, 2008). For example, from a purely economic viewpoint, and recognizing that providers also seek to meet the needs of their patients, global budgets give an incentive to do as little as possible in order to ensure that the budget is not exceeded, fee-for-service (FFS) gives an incentive to deliver more services to increase revenues, and capitation gives an incentive to select the lowest-cost clients (and then to do as little as possible, subject only to ensuring that they are willing to remain in your practice). The appropriate model depends on both the *cost structures* involved and the desired patterns of servicing. For example, if *fixed costs* (e.g., rent, salaries) are a relatively high proportion of the total costs, then service-based funding models may be problematic, particularly given the potential for perverse incentives when the *marginal* costs added/saved from one more/fewer clients are smaller than the *average* costs incorporated into the funding formula. Problems thus may arise, both from inadequate funding in rural/remote areas where a facility must be staffed even if relatively few people use it, and from excessive payment to facilities that can attract additional clients. (School funding formulae based only on the number of students may present similar issues.) One approach that can be used is to tie payment models to the characteristics needed to ensure a high-quality, high-performing health system, with particular attention to whether there is *overuse, underuse,* or *misuse* of the particular services (Institute of Medicine, 2001). The choice of payment mechanisms is also related to views about government roles vs. the role of the market (see section 3.2, Role of the State), which in turn is related to views about what type of good health care is (see section 5.9, Insurance, Elasticity, and Moral Hazard).

Note that these fiscal incentives are often balanced by professionalism (see section 6.4); as professionals, providers are expected to ensure that appropriate care is given even if this would not maximize their profits.

However, most agree that it seems unwise to design incentives so that the best providers are punished financially for behaving professionally.

## 6.3   What Is Health?

As Chapter 3 (Making Canadians Healthier) notes, the definition of health has been somewhat contentious. One common definition from the World Health Organization (WHO) (1948) is that health is "a state of complete physical, mental and social well-being and not merely the absence of disease or infirmity." At the other extreme, some define health primarily in terms of delivering sickness care.

The Lalonde Report (Lalonde, 1974) argued that the health of populations was affected by four categories of factors (which it termed "fields"): *human biology, environment, lifestyle,* and *health care organization.* This report thus went beyond the traditional focus on providing clinical services (which it classified under health care organization) and on understanding the biological causes of disease (which it classified under human biology). The Lalonde Report used the term "environment" to refer to both physical and social environmental factors over which individuals would have little or no control, and the term "lifestyle" to refer to personal decisions that could contribute to illness or death. The report thus was among the first government documents to recognize the importance of a broader array of what soon came to be known as the *determinants of health* and to focus on how best to improve *population health.* The field of *health promotion* focuses on how best to help individuals improve their health, using mechanisms that often extend beyond the health care system.

Health care is not homogeneous; it can be subdivided into a number of sectors, which provide different sets of services. Because many of the cases in this volume deal with public health, we provide fuller detail on this subsector in section 6.3.1, and give some information about other subsectors as needed in the relevant cases.

### 6.3.1 PUBLIC HEALTH

As Shah (2003) has noted, "No common definition of public health is in use in Canada." Many, but not all, of the activities of *public health* deal with the health of populations. Much, but not all, of the focus is on disease prevention. Some, but not all, of the activities are carried out by organizations designated as "public health." These complexities mean that public health will always require communication and coordination among the many participants involved in potentially relevant activities. In addition, although public health in Canada is largely a provincial/territorial responsibility, much of public health does not deal with clinical services to individuals, and hence is not directly addressed by the terms of the *Canada Health Act* (see section 7.2).

One commonly used definition of public health is "public health is the combination of science, practical skills, and values directed to the maintenance and improvement of the health of all the people" (Last, 1988). This definition is close to that of *population health*, which the Public Health Agency of Canada (PHAC) (2012) defines as follows: "Population health is an approach to health that aims to improve the health of the entire population and to reduce health inequities among population groups. In order to reach these objectives, it looks at and acts upon the broad range of factors and conditions that have a strong influence on our health." Narrower definitions address *primary prevention* and encompass such core functions as population health assessment, surveillance, disease prevention, health protection, and health promotion (Health Disparities Task Group of the Federal/Provincial/Territorial Advisory Committee on Population Health and Health Security, 2004). A committee of Canada's Senate, led by Senators Kirby and LeBreton, reviewed public health infrastructure in Canada, with particular attention to the roles and responsibilities of various levels of government, and the adequacy of funding and resources. This group suggested not using the term public health (which they noted is often confused with publicly funded health care) and instead calling it "health protection and promotion," which they defined as encompassing the following activities: "disease surveillance, disease and injury prevention, health protection, health emergency preparedness and response, health promotion, and relevant research undertakings" (Standing Senate Committee on Social Affairs Science and Technology, 2003).

Yet public health goes beyond even these functions. It may also be heavily involved in provision of clinical services to target populations, usually for populations or services not covered by health insurance systems. In the United States, this means that public health is often responsible for the care of "indigent populations." In Canada, in addition to the health protection and promotion activities noted above, public health in many jurisdictions may also be involved in such activities as providing services to newborn children and their parents, sexual health education and family planning, preventive and clinical dental health services to vulnerable populations, and similar services.

One key aspect of public health in all jurisdictions relates to pre-venting and managing communicable diseases. Note that the control of infectious diseases clearly meets the definition of a public good (see section 3.5). Communicable diseases are caused by microorgan-isms, including bacteria, viruses, parasites, and fungi. They can result in infections of any organ of the human body, and may cause compli-cations arising from the infection and/or the host's immunological response to the infectious organism. Historically, infections have been the major cause of population mortality; however, in the 20th century a series of innovations, including the use of water sanitation (see Chap-ter 5, Trouble on Tap), better hygiene, vaccination, and antimicrobial drugs has resulted in a global reduction of infectious illness. Once such chronic diseases as cancer and cardiovascular illness had become the most frequent causes of death in most industrialized societies (see sec-tion 9.2, Comparative Health Data, and Chapter 3, Making Canadians Healthier), there was a premature belief that the era of infectious dis-eases was over. However, infectious disease has made a comeback over the last 50 years, with novel infections such as SARS (see Chapter 7, Looking for Trouble), West Nile virus (see Chapter 6, The Bite of Blood Safety), and human immunodeficiency virus (HIV), as well as resur-gence of "old" infections such as tuberculosis (see Chapter 2, Danger at the Gates).

Humans can acquire communicable diseases via four main routes of transmission (Hinman, 2003):

*Direct Transmission*: This category includes transmission from touch-ing (contact), sexual activity (sexually transmitted illnesses), and/or inhalation of large droplets over a short distance (less than 2 metres) from an affected person who is coughing or sneezing. Direct trans-mission occurs from person to person, and is the mode of transmis-sion in such diseases as viral gastroenteritis, HIV, and many viral and bacterial respiratory and skin infections. Influenza and SARS are primarily transmitted by direct mechanisms, but under some conditions might also be transmitted by the airborne route (see below).

*Indirect Transmission* (*Vehicle*): This category refers to diseases trans-mitted by contamination of inanimate objects such as food or water (e.g., salmonella, *E. coli*), or needles (e.g., HIV, hepatitis B). Other objects, such as children's toys that have not been washed, or cutting boards contaminated with food-borne organisms, can also transmit infection in this way. Note that some of these diseases (including HIV and hepatitis B) can also be transmitted directly by sexual intercourse.

*Indirect Transmission* (*Vector*): This category refers to diseases transmitted by living animals such as mosquitoes (malaria, West Nile virus), ticks (Lyme disease), or fleas (plague). Usually, these "vector" animals pick up the virus from the host (a bird, mammal, or human), and transfer it to another person or animal.

*Airborne*: Diseases such as measles, chicken pox, and tuberculosis are caused by organisms that can be suspended in the air and carried long distances; these may often result in outbreaks whose origins are difficult to trace, due in part to the large numbers of affected people. As noted above, some respiratory viruses normally transmitted by the direct route may sometimes become aerosolized and become capable of travelling longer distances.

Outbreaks of communicable diseases may be described as *epidemics* when there are more cases of that disease than normal, or as *pandemics* if there are worldwide epidemics of that disease (World Health Organization, 2009).

### 6.3.2 SICKNESS CARE SUBSECTORS

Various sickness care subsectors are addressed in many of the cases.

The terms "primary care" and "primary health care" are commonly used to designate the initial point of entry into a health care system, often including the role of the primary care provider as gatekeeper and coordinator of care. The term *primary care* (PC) tends to be focused on the provision of services to diagnose, treat, and manage health conditions, usually (although not exclusively) performed by physicians. As used in the World Health Organization's Alma Ata Declaration (World Health Organization, 1978), the term *primary health care* (PHC) is defined more broadly as the "first level of contact of individuals, the family and community with the national health system," and as including not only primary care clinical services but also health promotion, disease prevention, and rehabilitation. As such, there may be some overlap with certain aspects of public health (see section 6.3.1). PHC is often delivered by a multidisciplinary team. Note that PC and PHC have attracted considerable attention internationally from health reformers, with such scholars as Starfield (2009) presenting evidence that they are essential for a high-performing health care system. In Canada, physician services are fully covered under the terms of the *Canada Health Act* (see section 7.2), whereas non-hospital services provided by other team members may or may not be. The assortment of PC delivery models is addressed in Chapter 11 (Primary Health Care in Ontario).

*Hospitals* provide more specialized care. Depending on how specialized it is, such care may be described as secondary, tertiary, or quaternary. Hospitals in Canada are largely not-for-profit, private organizations. They are heavily funded from public sources. In many provinces, they have been subsumed into regional health authorities (see section 2.2.4). Note that medically necessary hospital services in Canada must be fully insured to comply with the conditions of the *Canada Health Act* (see section 7.2). Chapters 8 (Filling in the Gaps) and 13 (What to Do with the Queue) are among the cases that focus on aspects of hospital care.

*Long-term care* (LTC) refers to a set of health, personal care, and social services. Unlike acute care, which is required for a relatively short time, LTC services are often (but not always) required on a sustained basis. LTC may be delivered within a specialized facility (e.g., nursing homes, homes for the aged) and/or in the community (e.g., in-home services, community support services, supportive housing). Most community-based LTC services are provided by family members, friends, and volunteers, but there is also a strong role for paid workers. LTC is sometimes divided into three functions: *acute care substitution* allows people to be discharged from acute hospitals; *long-term care substitution* serves those who might otherwise be in long-term care institutions, and *prevention/maintenance* keeps people healthy enough to remain out of institutions (Dumont-Lemasson et al., 1999). LTC is the focus of Chapters 19 (Long Term Care Reform in Ontario) and 20 (Depending on How You Cut It).

*Rehabilitation* refers to treatments designed to facilitate recovery, including physical therapy, occupational therapy, and speech language therapy. It can be delivered in inpatient, LTC, or outpatient settings (including the home). Note that rehabilitation outside hospitals is not required to be covered by the *Canada Health Act*, although provinces/territories may choose to do so. Rehabilitation is dealt with (in passing) in Chapter 17 (Rehabilitating Auto Insurance).

*Pharmaceuticals* are an important element in preventing, treating, and managing disease, and account for a considerable proportion of health expenditures. Pharmaceutical issues are addressed in Chapters 12 (At Any Price), 15 (Prescription for Conflict), and 16 (Ask Your Doctor).

## 6.4 Professionalism

Much of health care is delivered by professionals. Although there is some dispute as to precisely what defines a *profession*, most agree that they have the following characteristics: (1) they possess *specialized knowledge*, attained through established training programs, and attested to through certification procedures; (2) they provide *services* to members of the public; (3) there is a *risk* to the public if the services are not done properly; and (4) the clients who receive these services are often not in a position to judge quality, or even whether the services are necessary; accordingly, there is an *agency* relationship with the clients receiving the service (i.e., *caveat emptor* is not an appropriate way to manage the relationship).

Because only those with that specialized knowledge can assess competence, professions tend to be *self-regulating* (Freidson, 1986, 2001). Long-standing examples of professions are medicine, law, and engineering. More recently, other occupations have been recognized as professions (see section 7.3 for the health professions regulated in Ontario at the time of writing). There can be considerable variation in which professions are regulated where. Different jurisdictions may take different approaches to regulating professions, and the approach may also vary by profession. One element that may be incorporated is *protection of title*; where this exists, one cannot claim to be a member of that profession unless one is registered with the local regulatory college. Another possible element is the regulation of *controlled acts*, defined as acts where there is a perceived danger if these are performed by unqualified individuals. One example of a controlled act would be performing surgery. Note that these approaches are not mutually exclusive. In most cases, professional *colleges* are given the responsibility for regulating their profession. Practicing as a professional in any jurisdiction will accordingly require recognition/certification of that person's credentials, which is usually tied to professional licensure/registration.

There are a number of trade-offs inherent in professional self-regulation. In most cases, the regulatory college is supported through dues charged to those registered with it. This can be expensive (particularly for small professions). There may also be perceptions of conflict of interest between the interests of the profession and those of the public. Restricting who can practice a profession may be seen as a mechanism for "keeping the competition out." This can be entirely appropriate (in terms of ensuring that the public is protected from unqualified providers), but may also help protect the income of providers. Professionalism also incorporates elements of autonomy (to the extent that professional judgment is required), and hence works on the assumption that these providers will practice ethically. The regulatory colleges accordingly act as a "backstop" to enforce standards of competence, including handling complaints and, in the worst case, removing that person's license to practice that profession.

## 7. Health Care in Canada

As noted in section 2.2.1 (Federalism in Canada), Canada does not and cannot have a national health care system, because constitutional responsibility for health care largely rests at the provincial/territorial level (Marchildon, 2013). About 70% of health expenditures are paid from public sources – including almost all hospital and physician costs (Canadian Institute for Health Information, 2013c). As noted in section 6.1 (Dimensions of Health Care Systems), even within these publicly funded sectors, Canada uses what the OECD calls a public-contract model (Docteur & Oxley, 2003), meaning that even publicly financed services are almost entirely delivered by private providers. This introduces the potential for substantial variation among providers in where and how they practice, even within a single jurisdiction.

Another set of issues is evident in the area of public health (see section 6.3.1). To the extent that public health involves public goods and externalities (see section 3.5), a strong case can be made for ensuring that policies are coordinated at the national or even global level (see section 5.5, Globalization). Although public health, like health care, is a largely provincial responsibility, the different provinces have chosen to handle it in different ways. Many have devolved responsibility for some public health activities to local/regional units (see also section 2.2.4), while others have retained control at the provincial level. In Ontario, public health was traditionally the responsibility of a series of local boards of health (also called public health units). However, the province could, and did, set requirements for what services needed to be delivered. It also paid a portion of the costs, although, unlike other provinces, it has required municipal governments to share the costs of these public health units (Deber et al., 2006).

As noted in section 7.2 (*Canada Health Act*), to receive full federal transfers, provincial/territorial health insurance plans must comply with the terms of the federal *Canada Health Act* (CHA). The *CHA* is a floor, not a ceiling; provinces are able to fund beyond these requirements should they wish to do so. Accordingly, there is considerable variability across jurisdictions in the extent of publicly financed coverage for out-of-hospital care delivered by non-physician providers (including outpatient pharmaceuticals, rehabilitation, long-term care, etc.). There is also considerable variability in how services are managed and delivered, albeit with many commonalities amid these variations. As noted below, for historical reasons, the *CHA* requirements focus on services to individuals (specifically, hospitals and doctors) rather than on public health or other determinants of health.

However, differences in fiscal capacity across the country have led the federal government to provide financial assistance to the provincial/territorial governments to allow them to set up roughly equivalent coverage in many (but not all) areas, particularly those services falling under the requirements of the *CHA* (see section 7.2).

## 7.1 Financing Health Care in Canada: Fiscal Federalism

An issue in most federal systems is how to deal with differences in the economic capacity of different regions, including deciding when, and how, to ensure that all residents of a particular nation have access to roughly equal levels of key services regardless of the ability of that region to pay for them. Different jurisdictions vary in which services are seen as requiring national standards, but health care and education usually qualify. In Canada, both of these programs fall under provincial jurisdiction. One common mechanism, called *fiscal federalism*, involves various forms of transferring resources from the national government to subnational jurisdictions to help equalize their fiscal capacity to provide roughly comparable services (Oates, 1999). The formulas vary. One key distinction is whether the funds are in the form of *cash* grants, or in the form of *tax room* (also called *tax points*). Tax room refers to an agreement whereby the senior level of government decreases its tax rate, leaving room for the subnational units to increase their tax rates (should they choose to do so) without increasing the total tax burden on the individual taxpayer. Note that tax points cannot be taken back, and (unlike cash payments) do not give the senior level of government any power to enforce how those resources are used. The value of tax points is also related to the economic health of a particular jurisdiction; if residents do not have much taxable income, then tax points cannot yield much revenue. In contrast, cash grants can be tied to conditions, and withheld should those conditions be violated. Note that the level of transfers can be based on various combinations of how much is actually being spent on particular programs, the population of that jurisdiction (which may or may not be adjusted for such factors as age distribution, perceived needs, etc.), and/or differences in fiscal capacity across jurisdictions. In Canada, as in many federal states, these arrangements have long been contentious (Lazar, 2010).

Approaches to financing health care in Canada have evolved over time, and used a variety of mechanisms (Marchildon, 2013; Taylor, 1978). Health coverage in Canada evolved gradually, with different provinces setting up various programs. Starting in 1948, the federal government provided cash payments to provincial/territorial governments for selected programs (e.g., hospital construction) through the National Health Grants program. In 1957, the federal government passed the *Hospital Insurance and Diagnostic Services Act* (*HIDS*) with all-party approval; this provided federal funds to the provinces/ territories to cover about half the costs of their hospital insurance programs as long as they complied with national conditions. (The formula was more complex than a simple cost-shared model, since it was based on both national and provincial spending.) In 1966, the federal *Medical Care Act* provided similar cost sharing for provincial insurance plans for physician services. By cost sharing only hospital and physician services, health care delivery in most provinces became focused on those forms of delivery, since community-based care provided by non-physicians would not attract federal matching funds. Note that, unlike the National Health Service in the United Kingdom (which delivered services using public hospitals), the model Canada employed involved public payment for private delivery, in what the OECD has called a public contracting model (see section 6.1.3, Models of Health Systems).

To obtain matching federal funds, all provinces eventually set up complying insurance plans, first for hospital care (under *HIDS*), and then for physician services (under the *Medical Care Act*). When *HIDS* began on July 1, 1958, only five provinces (Newfoundland, Manitoba, Saskatchewan, Alberta, and British Columbia) had set up hospital insurance programs, but all provinces were participating by January 1961. Similarly, all provinces had implemented full insurance coverage for medically necessary hospital and physician services by 1971; this coverage is commonly referred to as Medicare. The funding model was modified in 1977 with passage of the *Federal-Provincial Fiscal Arrangements and Established Programs Financing Act* (known as *EPF*); this legislation grouped the federal transfers for *HIDS*, the *Medical Care Act*, plus a third cost-shared program that had helped the provinces to fund post-secondary education (which was also under provincial jurisdiction) into a new transfer using a new payment model. Rather than cost-share spending, *EPF* computed an entitlement for each province based on its population (rather than on its actual spending for those programs), and, as noted above, changed the formula to transfer some of the money in the form of *tax points* (whereby the federal government lowered its tax rates and allowed the provincial/territorial governments to occupy the vacated tax room). Only the residual difference between the provincial entitlement and the amount deemed to have been yielded from the tax points was given in the form of cash. These transfers went directly into provincial budgets, freeing the provinces to deliver these services in the manner they saw as best. Although the *per capita* entitlement was supposed to increase each year at the rate of inflation, in subsequent years economic difficulties led the federal government to unilaterally alter the formula, eventually removing all inflation adjustment. One consequence was the erosion of the cash contribution, since the tax points remained unchanged. To preserve federal cash transfers (and federal ability to influence provincial policy), in 1996 *EPF* was combined with the 1966 *Canada Assistance Plan*, another federal transfer to the provinces, which had helped pay the costs for certain non-universal social programs; the new transfer was renamed the *Canada Health and Social Transfer*. In 2004 this was split into two transfers, renamed the *Canada Health Transfer* and the *Canada Social Transfer*.

That 1977 shift in how federal transfers were paid (from cost sharing to per capita entitlements) has resulted in a separation between the legislation setting out how much money provincial/territorial governments would receive, and the legislation specifying what, if any, conditions would need to be met to receive the money (Fard, 2009). It is notable that, although funding for health, post-secondary education, and social welfare programs was incorporated into these transfer programs, federal conditions exist only for health insurance, in the form of the 1984 *Canada Health Act* (*CHA*). The *CHA* was largely based on the earlier cost-sharing legislation for *HIDS* and the *Medical Care Act*; it set up explicit terms and conditions with which the provinces/territories would have to comply in order to receive full federal transfers. One attempt to update these programs occurred through meetings of the federal/provincial/territorial governments, resulting in the 2004 First Ministers' Accord on Health Care Renewal (commonly called the

*Health Accord*). This set out the amount of the transfer, and suggested some general future priorities, albeit with few mechanisms for enforcement. Note that this agreement is due to expire in 2014, and the extent to which the current model will be retained remains to be seen. At the time of writing, the federal government had unilaterally announced what the transfers would be for the next agreement, and indicated that it would not set any new conditions on these funds. Another proposal, floated by some government advisors, was to convert all of the federal transfer to tax points. Should this occur, the *CHA* would become unenforceable, and, since tax points cannot be taken back, the policy shift could not be reversed by subsequent governments.

## 7.2  Canada Health Act

The *Canada Health Act* (*CHA*) sets up the terms and conditions that must be met by provincial/territorial insurance plans to qualify for a full cash contribution from the federal government (Flood & Choudhry, 2004; Flood et al., 2005; Madore, 2005). It includes the following five conditions:

1. *Public Administration*: This requirement says nothing about how care should be delivered. It requires that the provincial/territorial insurance plan must be administered and operated on a non-profit basis by a public authority, designated by the province. The public authority can, with conditions, designate an agency to receive payments to the provincial health care insurance plan, and/or to carry out on its behalf responsibilities in connection with receipt or payment of accounts for insured health services.
2. *Comprehensiveness*: This condition requires the provincial/territorial plan to insure all "insured health services" (defined below) that are provided to "insured persons" by hospitals and doctors, and where the law of the province so permits, similar or additional services of other health care practitioners.
3. *Universality*: This condition states that the plan must cover all insured health services for all insured persons in that province/territory under uniform terms and conditions.
4. *Portability*: Because plans are set up on a provincial basis, this requirement specifies what would happen when someone insured in one province needs care while outside that jurisdiction. The condition specifies that the waiting period before a new resident

in that province/territory is eligible for insured health services cannot exceed three months (see also Chapter 2, Danger at the Gates). It further requires certain coverage when insured residents are temporarily out of province. For care provided in another province/territory within Canada, payment will be at the rate that is approved by the plan of the province in which the services are provided, although provinces are able to negotiate alternate arrangements should they wish to do so. For care provided outside of Canada, however, provinces must pay only the amount that they would have paid for a similar service provided within their province. Individuals travelling to jurisdictions where care is likely to be costlier (e.g., the United States) will therefore need to have additional private travel health insurance. The portability condition also specifies what will happen when residents move from one province to another. If provinces chose to impose a minimum waiting period (which can be up to three months), the costs of any "medically necessary" care they receive will still be the responsibility of the "sending" province for that time period; this enables people to visit other parts of the country for a short time period without imposing costs on the location they are visiting, but may cause problems for new immigrants, since they do not have a "sending" province (see Chapter 2, Danger at the Gates). After the waiting period, the person is deemed to have moved, and the "receiving" province will then assume responsibility for the costs of insured care. To minimize problems of people moving across provincial boundaries to gain access to services that may not be covered in the "sending" province, provincial insurance plans have the right to require that prior permission be obtained before paying for "elective insured services" out of province. Emergency services, however, must be covered.

5. *Accessibility*: This condition requires that the provincial plan provide insured health services to insured persons on uniform terms and conditions. These insured services must be "reasonably" accessible to all insured persons; direct or indirect impediments (including user charges) to insured persons for insured services are explicitly prohibited. This condition also requires that the provincial plans must provide *reasonable compensation* to practitioners for all insured health services they provide to insured persons; this will usually be determined through negotiations between the province and the provincial organization representing the medical

practitioners. Disputes are to be settled through conciliation or binding arbitration. Similarly, the provincial plan must provide reasonable payment to hospitals to cover the cost of insured health services provided to insured persons.

The *CHA* specifies that "If a provincial health care plan does not meet the above stated criteria it will be subject to reduced or complete withholding of cash contributions or any amounts payable to them by Canada." As defined, complying with these criteria thus includes pro-hibitions on extra billing or user fees for insured services; however, fees for services not meeting the definition of insured services (including accommodation and meals for those people in chronic care facilities) are permitted. There is also a requirement to provide the federal health minister with the information set out in the regulations on a yearly basis, and for the provincial/territorial health plans to give recognition for the contributions and payments made by Canada under the *CHA* in any public documents, advertising, and promotional material relating to insured health services and extended health care services in the province.

The question of defining what is meant by medical necessity is a perennial issue (Charles et al., 1997). As noted above, the *CHA* deals with it by speaking of *insured services*, which the *Act* has defined as follows:

Insured health services: includes hospital services, physician services and surgical dental services provided to insured persons, but does not include any health services that a person is entitled to and eligible for under any other Act of Parliament or under any Act of the legislature of a province that relates to workers' or workmen's compensation.

The CHA defines these three categories of insured services as follows:

*Hospital services*: includes any of the following services provided to in-patients or out-patients at a hospital, if the services are medically necessary for the purpose of maintaining health, preventing disease or diagnosing or treating an injury, illness or disability namely:

Accommodation and meals at the standard or public ward level and preferred accommodation if medically required;
Nursing service;

Laboratory, radiological and other diagnostic procedures, together with the necessary interpretations;

Drugs, biologicals and related preparations when administered in the hospital;

Use of operating room, case room and anaesthetic facilities, including necessary equipment and supplies;

Medical and surgical equipment and supplies;

Use of radiotherapy facilities;

Use of physiotherapy facilities, and;

Services provided by persons who receive remuneration therefore from the hospital but do not include services that are excluded by the regulations.

*Physician services*: means any medically required services rendered by medical practitioners.

*Surgical dental services*: means any medically or dentally required surgical-dental procedures performed by a dentist in a hospital, where a hospital is required for the proper performance of the procedures. (Government of Canada, 1984)

In practice, almost no dental services meet this criteria; dental care is almost entirely privately financed in Canada (see also section 9.1, Canadian Data).

The CHA distinguishes between insured services and "extended health care services" (e.g., intermediate care in nursing homes, adult residential care service, home care service, and ambulatory health care services). Extended health care services are not subject to the CHA terms and conditions; people can be charged for using them (Madore, 2005).

Note that these terms and conditions have several implications for Canadian health policy. First, as described above, the portability provisions have been interpreted as allowing provinces to wait up to three months before extending coverage to new arrivals; provinces varied in the extent to which they were taking advantage of this provision and requiring immigrants to wait for health care access (see Chapter 2, Danger at the Gates). Second, the definition of insured services means that, once non-physician care shifts from hospitals, these services are no longer required to be insured, even though they may still be viewed as medically necessary. This has been particularly problematic for outpatient pharmaceuticals (since drugs for inpatients are included within the CHA definition), outpatient rehabilitation, primary care by non-physician providers, and home care. Provinces are free to extend such coverage, but do not have to. The definition of comprehensiveness includes the provision "and where the law of the province so permits, similar or additional services of other health care practitioners." Although this provision allows provinces to designate other providers as falling under this provision, this has rarely been done; however, some provinces have so designated midwifery (see Chapter 9, Midwifery: Special Delivery). If so designated, such providers will be publicly paid for these insured services, but will not be able to extra bill beyond the fee schedule. Third, enforcement of the *CHA* conditions depends on the existence of a cash contribution (since tax points cannot be withheld), and on the willingness of the federal government to enforce the *Act*. Neither can be taken for granted, particularly given the unwillingness of some provinces to cede control to the federal government over areas they deem to be under provincial jurisdiction.

## 7.3  Regulating Health Professionals

In Canada, most health professionals are regulated by governing bodies, often called professional *colleges*, which are responsible for registration, protection of public, complaints, and maintenance of competency. The precise professions that are registered vary somewhat by province. For example, Ontario's *Regulated Health Professionals Act, 1981* (*RHPA*), sets a framework that regulates the scope of practice of the following colleges governing health professions in Ontario: College of Audiologists and Speech-Language Pathologists of Ontario; College of Chiropodists of Ontario; College of Chiropractors of Ontario; College of Dental Hygienists of Ontario; Royal College of Dental Surgeons of Ontario; College of Dental Technologists of Ontario; College of Denturists of Ontario; College of Dietitians of Ontario; College of Massage Therapists of Ontario; College of Medical Laboratory Technologists of Ontario; College of Medical Radiation Technologists; College of Midwives of Ontario; College of Nurses of Ontario; College of Occupational Therapists of Ontario; College of Opticians of Ontario; College of Optometrists of Ontario; Ontario College of Pharmacists; College of Physicians and Surgeons of Ontario; College of Physiotherapists of Ontario; College of Psychologists of Ontario; and College of Respiratory Therapists of Ontario. In addition, the *RHPA* legislates the Transitional Council of the College of Traditional Chinese Medicine Practitioners and Acupuncturists of Ontario. Another Act, the *Drugless*

*Practitioners Act*, regulates the board of directors of Drugless Therapy – Naturopathy (Ontario Ministry of Health and Long-Term Care, 2013b). In general, certain professions (e.g., medicine, nursing) are registered in all provinces. The provincial/territorial colleges regulating each profession usually work together in national associations, and have sought to standardize requirements and ease the ability of professionals registered in one province to be registered should they move to another Canadian jurisdiction.

## 8. Some Useful Tools

### 8.1 Economic Analysis: Cost-effectiveness

*Economic analysis* is a series of methods for comparing the *costs* and *consequences* of different policy alternatives. Although there are many complexities, they share a basic approach. First, they involve comparing alternatives. One cannot speak of something as being *cost-effective*; it is always more or less cost-effective than the available alternatives to which it is being compared. Second, they require the ability to compute the costs and consequences. An economic analysis involves calculating the difference in costs between the alternatives being compared (net costs) and dividing these by the difference in their outcomes (net effectiveness). One can thus compute the incremental price of obtaining a unit of benefit (e.g., dollars per year of life gained). This is rarely simple. One set of questions is whose costs and consequences count; analyses can be done from various perspectives (commonly, patients, providers, payers, and/or society). Another set of issues relates to how these costs and consequences will be determined. The resulting family of economic analysis approaches includes cost-minimization, cost-benefit, cost-effectiveness, and cost-utility analysis.

If consequences are identical for both alternatives, it is not necessary to compute these consequences at all. This allows use of *cost-minimization*, the simplest form of economic analysis, where one needs only to compute the costs and then select the lowest-cost alternative. One example might be decisions about what brand of an otherwise identical product to purchase.

If consequences differ, but can all be expressed in monetary terms, then one can perform *cost-benefit* analysis, where one prices out the costs and consequences and then looks at the monetary return on the money invested.

If consequences cannot be expressed in monetary terms, but can be translated into a single common metric, one can do a *cost-effectiveness* analysis (CEA). For example, one can compute the number of life years gained, or the number of cases detected by a screening program, and then compute the cost for each unit of benefit.

*Cost-utility* analysis is closely related to CEA; it expresses consequences in terms of a common metric (in this case, life years gained), but then adjusts these for the *quality*. Commonly, quality is measured on a scale from 0 (worst) to 1 (best). For example, one might decide that living one year in perfect health would be rated as 1, death would be rated as 0, whereas living but being unable to get out of bed would have a rating somewhere in the middle. The resulting score (on the 0 to 1 scale) is called the *utility* of that health state. One could then multiply the number of years in each health state by the quality of each, to compute the number of quality-adjusted life years (QALYs) obtained.

How to compute these quality ratings is highly controversial. The most methodologically accepted method, the *standard gamble*, asks respondents to compare a *sure thing* (usually, living for a fixed period of time in a particular health state) against a gamble with two possible outcomes, specified as cure (valued at 1), or instant death (valued at 0). One then systematically varies the probability of the two possible outcomes of the gamble until the respondent is *indifferent* between the gamble and the health state being evaluated. For example, if someone says that he or she would be equally willing to risk a 20% chance of death or to live in a particular health state, you can then say that the value attached to that health state would be 0.8. Another approach, the *time trade-off* (TTO), eliminates the risk element, and asks respondents how many years in perfect health they would deem equivalent to a fixed period of time in that health state. For example, if they would see 15 years in perfect health as equivalent to 20 years with the given health state, the utility attached to that state would be 15/20, or 0.75. A third approach asks respondents to directly value the health state (e.g., on a scale from 0 to 100), which can then be translated into a utility score. A fourth approach asks for *willingness to pay* (WTP) for a particular outcome, measured in monetary terms. There is also some variability in whose responses are used to compute utilities; these may come from the general public, or from people who actually live with the particular condition being assessed. (In general, those with more experience with the health condition tend to assign higher values to that health state than do the general population.) Note that there is considerable dispute as to whether assigning a lower value to life with a disability devalues the lives of persons who must live with that condition. On the other hand, without such quality adjustments, no value is placed on interventions that may not improve life expectancy but can greatly enhance quality of life.

Another issue relates to how to treat costs and consequences that occur at a future time. The conventional approach is to *discount* these future consequences. The choice of discount rate clearly can have an impact, particularly for outcomes occurring many years in the future. This is particularly consequential when dealing with disease prevention.

A number of classic texts address how to perform economic analysis (Drummond et al., 2005; Gold et al., 1996; Kattan, 2009).

## 8.2  Screening

A number of the cases deal with efforts to detect conditions before they are symptomatic. They accordingly require some knowledge about where *screening* is or is not useful.

Screening was defined by the 1951 US National Conference on Chronic Disease as the presumptive identification of unrecognized disease or defect by the application of tests, examinations, or other procedures which can be applied rapidly to sort out apparently well persons who probably have a disease from those who probably do not. A screening test is not intended to be diagnostic. Persons with positive or suspicious findings must be referred to their physicians for diagnosis and necessary treatment (Wilson & Jungner, 1968).

### 8.2.1  CRITERIA FOR SCREENING

The criteria for determining when screening programs are considered useful have been well developed by epidemiologists. One widely used model, developed by Wilson and Jungner for the World Health Organization, argues that screening programs are justified only when all of the following apply (Andermann et al., 2008; Wilson & Jungner, 1968).

1. The condition sought is an important health problem.
2. There is an accepted treatment for patients with recognized disease.
3. Facilities for diagnosis and treatment are available.
4. There is a recognizable latent or early symptomatic stage.
5. There is a suitable test or examination.
6. The test is acceptable to the population.

7. The natural history of the condition, including development from latent to declared disease, is adequately understood.
8. There is an agreed policy on whom to treat as patients.
9. The cost of case finding (including diagnosis and treatment of patients diagnosed) is economically balanced in relation to possible expenditure on medical care as a whole.
10. Case finding is a continuing process and not a "once and for all" project.

Note that these criteria justify screening entirely in terms of benefit to the individual affected. However, in cases of communicable disease, there may also be a rationale for identifying cases even if they cannot be treated, in order to protect others from disease transmission. (This was a heated debate in the early years of HIV/AIDS, in terms of whether benefit to others who might be at risk would justify screening, even if the individuals affected could not yet be treated.)

8.2.2 ASSESSING SCREENING TESTS (TEST/TRUTH)
Table 1.2 illustrates a simple way to look at the outcomes of a screening test by comparing the *truth* (where + means that disease is present, and − means that it is absent) with the results of a *test* (which can be positive or negative). The resulting 2 × 2 table yields four possibilities. Reading down the columns, those with the disease (Truth: +) can be identified by the test (true positive), or missed (false negative); those without disease (Truth: −) can still test positive (false positive) or be correctly identified as not having that condition (true negative).

Ideally, one would wish to minimize both the number of false positives and of false negatives. A test that said that everyone was positive would be guaranteed to have no false negatives, but would also generate a considerable amount of unnecessary follow-up testing and treatment for false positives, and might do far more harm than good. Assessing *test performance* is thus a crucial aspect of making decisions about when to use screening or diagnostic tests.

There are two complementary ways of looking at test performance. One focuses on the columns, and looks at sensitivity and specificity. These terms are defined as follows.

*Sensitivity* is the ability to correctly pick up positive cases, and is computed by dividing the number of true positives by the total with disease (Truth: +). *Specificity* is the ability to correctly rule out disease, and is computed as the number of true negatives divided by the total without

Table 1.2. Test vs. Truth

|             | Truth: +            | Truth: −                | Total                   |
| ----------- | ------------------- | ----------------------- | ----------------------- |
| Test: +     | True positive       | False positive          | Total testing positive  |
| Test: −     | False negative      | True negative           | Total testing negative  |
| Total       | Total with disease  | Total without disease   | Total                   |

disease (Truth: −). Ideally, a screening test would have 100% sensitivity and 100% specificity. In practice, no tests are that accurate. There is accordingly a trade-off in determining the *cut-off* value where a test result is deemed to be positive (e.g., what level of blood pressure will be defined as high?). One can reduce false negatives by indicating that more people have disease; this will also increase the rate of false positives. The converse also applies. Determining the appropriate cut-off thus depends on balancing the consequences of failing to detect a case against the consequences of incorrectly identifying one.

The second element to judging test performance focuses on the rows and looks at positive and negative *predictive value*. These terms are defined as follows: Positive predictive value is the probability that a person truly has the disease given that he or she tests positive, and is computed as true positives divided by the total testing positive. Negative predictive value is the probability that a person truly does not have the disease given that he or she tests negative, and is computed as true negatives divided by the total testing negative. It is important to recognize that the predictive value of a screening test depends on not only sensitivity/specificity but also the *prevalence* of that condition in the population.

### 8.2.3 THE ROLE OF PREVALENCE

*Prevalence* refers to the proportion of people in a given population who have a given condition, meaning that they fall into the column (Truth: +). In laboratory settings, most people tested are likely to come from high-prevalence populations, which is why they were sent to have the test in the first place. Once tests move into community settings, prevalence is usually far lower. This can make a significant difference in test performance. The following three examples begin with a test with 95% sensitivity and 95% specificity (higher than most) and construct test vs. truth tables for a population of 10,000 people, varying the

Table 1.3. Example 1: If Prevalence Is 50%

|         | Truth: + | Truth: − | Total  |
|---------|----------|----------|--------|
| Test: + | 4,750    | 250      | 5,000  |
| Test: − | 250      | 4,750    | 5,000  |
| Total   | 5,000    | 5,000    | 10,000 |

Table 1.4. Example 2: If Prevalence Is 5%

|         | Truth: + | Truth: − | Total  |
|---------|----------|----------|--------|
| Test: + | 475      | 475      | 950    |
| Test: − | 25       | 9,025    | 9,050  |
| Total   | 500      | 9,500    | 10,000 |

Table 1.5. Example 3: If Prevalence Is 0.2%

|         | Truth: + | Truth: − | Total  |
|---------|----------|----------|--------|
| Test: + | 19       | 499      | 518    |
| Test: − | 1        | 9,481    | 9,482  |
| Total   | 20       | 9,980    | 10,000 |

prevalence. In example 1 (Table 1.3), prevalence is 50%, which means that 5,000 have the condition. In example 2 (Table 1.4), prevalence is 5%, which would yield 500 cases. In example 3 (Table 1.5), prevalence is .2%, which would yield 20 cases. We leave as an exercise for the observer what would happen if prevalence were even lower than that, noting that this is frequently the case. For example, the Ontario Newborn Screening Program estimated the prevalence among babies born in Ontario of several conditions they do screen for; congenital hypothyroidism was 1 in 3,000 to 4,000; phenylketonuria (PKU) was 1 in 12,000; and tyrosinemia (Type 1) was 1 in 100,000 (see Chapter 23, Screen Tests).

In Example 1, the predictive value of a positive test is thus 4,750 / 5,000 = 95%, while the predictive value of a negative test is 4,750 / 5,000 = 95%.

In Example 2, the predictive value of a positive test is now 475 / 950 = 50%, while the predictive value of a negative test is 9,025 / 9,050 = 99.7%.

In Example 3, the predictive value of a positive test in this low-prevalence population is 19 / 518 = 3.7%, while the predictive value of a negative test is 9,481 / 9,980 = 99.99%.

Low prevalence means inefficient screening. As illustrated by Example 3, if prevalence is low, even a good test with high sensitivity and high specificity would generate mainly false positives. Whether a test is worth doing thus depends on the consequences, not only to the true positives (which is what is usually emphasized) but also to the false positives (which is usually neglected).

## 8.3  Heuristics and Biases in Decision Making

An extensive literature has clarified that people tend to use various cognitive shortcuts (*heuristics*) in making decisions (Kahneman et al., 1982). While often helpful, such heuristics can also cause people to make systematic errors. Some of the key heuristics particularly germane to how people perceive risks include the following.

*Availability*: People judge an event to be likely if it is easy to recall (or imagine) instances of it. This can be misleading, particularly given the extent to which people base these perceptions on media reports (see section 5.8, Role of Media). For example, one classic study asked people to estimate how many deaths per year occurred from various causes, and compared this to the actual number as reported in public health statistics (Slovic et al., 1980). This study confirmed that people tend to overestimate rare, publicized events (e.g., airplane accidents), and to underestimate common ones (e.g., diabetes). Indeed, the availability heuristic creates the dilemma that even discussing a low probability hazard may increase its judged probability. However, it is worth noting that the same study found that being struck by lightning qualified as one of the most underestimated causes of death, being far more common than its popular use to denote an extremely rare event would suggest.

*Anchoring and adjustment*: Studies have confirmed that people tend to adjust estimates based on an initial starting estimate. If this first estimate is inaccurate, the resulting estimates are also likely to be inaccurate.

*Overconfidence:* People tend to think they know more than they do, and to be overly confident in their estimates. In effect, we all tend to think that we are above average.

*Desire for certainty*: People tend to be uneasy with uncertainty. This can be particularly problematic when dealing with scientific estimates, since scientists are reluctant to claim certainty.

### 8.3.1 PROSPECT THEORY

Kahneman and Tversky (1979) also confirmed that people tend to react differently to gains than to losses. People tend to be far more risk-averse when speaking of losses than of gains. People will buy lottery tickets (showing risk seeking for gains) but also buy insurance against unlikely events (showing risk aversion for losses).

In turn, this implies that framing can alter how a gamble is perceived (see section 3.4, Framing). One classic experiment indeed found that people evaluated the attractiveness of surgery, relative to radiation therapy, differently depending on, among other variables, whether the problem was framed in terms of the probability of living or in terms of the probability of dying (McNeil et al., 1982). This has affected how many hospitals word their consent form (usually, they will include both ways of framing the probabilities). Another common example can be seen in flyers for pizza shops, which may advertise "free delivery" and then add "10% discount for pickup." Although this offer indicates that delivery is not in fact free, it recognizes that people often react differently to not receiving a discount than to having to pay directly.

### 8.3.2 RISK PERCEPTION

Many decisions involve *risk*. Policy issues involve deciding what risks are acceptable, and who should decide. Even the definition of risk has many meanings (and can thus generate considerable confusion). A simple definition of risk refers to *uncertainty* in what might happen, as opposed to dealing with a certain outcome. However, some scholars distinguish between situations where the probabilities of various possible outcomes are known and measurable (which are described using the term *risk*), and those where the probabilities are unknown (which are described using the term *uncertainty*). An additional distinction is the source of these known probabilities, which can be based on prior probabilities, or on subjective estimates (which will often increase the uncertainty of the estimates). Estimating such probabilities is an inherent element of most economic analysis (e.g., how likely are particular outcomes); see also section 8.1 (Economic Analysis) and Chapter 12 (At Any Price).

A number of studies analyzing how people perceive risk were conducted in an effort to clarify why people found nuclear power plants much riskier than coal-generated power, even though far more people had died from the latter (Fischhoff et al., 1981; Schwing & Albers, 1980; Slovic, 1987; Slovic et al., 1981). They found that the perception of risk was systematically related to a number of factors, particularly to how well the risk was understood, the extent to which it evoked a feeling of dread, and how many people were exposed to that risk. Their studies confirmed that people tended to see risk as higher (and as less acceptable) if it was classified as follows: *involuntary* (e.g., second-hand smoke) vs. voluntary (e.g., sky diving); *dread* (e.g., airplane crashes) as opposed to common (e.g., traffic accidents); and/or *catastrophic* (e.g., SARS epidemic) as opposed to common (e.g., diabetes). Other important factors included whether the condition was certainly fatal (e.g., HIV/AIDS in the early years); whether people knew that they were exposed; whether the risk was immediate or delayed; whether the risk was seen as controllable; whether it was known to science; and whether the number of fatalities per event was large or small. Media attention could increase perceived risk. Risks with identifiable victims (particularly children) were seen as more severe than those with statistical victims.

## 8.4  Health Human Resources

A variety of trained professionals are required to deliver health care services. Some, but not all, are health professionals (see section 6.4, Professionalism). As noted in section 9.1 (Canadian Data), the Canadian Institute for Health Information (CIHI) tracks data for many health occupations (24 at the time of writing), reporting "their counts, practice settings, regulatory environment, and trends in supply, demographics, and education" through the Canada's Health Care Providers series, collected through the Health Personnel Database (HPDB). They devote particular attention to physicians, nurses, and (since 2005) such professionals as occupational therapists, pharmacists, physiotherapists, medical radiation technologists, and medical laboratory technologists. Data is available on the CIHI website (Canadian Institute for Health Information, 2008, 2013a, 2013d).

### 8.4.1  PROJECTING SUPPLY AND DEMAND

A review of planning approaches clarified that there is no single accepted approach to planning health human resources (HHR) (Deber et al., 2010). Planning requires that indicators be projected to ascertain future supply and demand. Such projections are notably difficult, particularly since other things rarely remain equal. In general, the time horizons used by most predictive models are usually relatively short (often 10 years), although both supply and demand operate over a far longer time period. The main forecasting approaches include: supply projection; demand-based; needs-based; and benchmarking against health systems with similar populations and health profiles (Roberfroid et al., 2009).

One common way of projecting future supply is to use a *stock and flow* model. One begins with a stock of providers, usually measured as full-time equivalents (FTEs), which in turn requires determining how much work would constitute full-time. New providers are added to the existing stock through new graduates emerging from training programs, immigration, and increased labour force participation (e.g., return to work, increasing numbers of hours worked). They are subtracted through death, retirement, emigration, and decreased labour force participation (Maynard, 2006). Other things being equal, one can thus project the future workforce, and simulate the likely impact of different policy levers.

Assessment of *needs* for health human resources can be undertaken at varying levels of complexity. All have advantages and limitations. *Utilization-based* requirement planning, based on an established provider-to-population ratio, is a frequently employed methodology. In this approach, the current population of a society is related to the total pool of practicing providers through a caregiver-to-population ratio. Changes in population and provider attrition rates are then estimated so that future requirements can be calculated. More complex models include adjustments for changes in the ratio of male/female providers, deviations in work patterns, and shifts in patient demographics, such as aging or prevalence of disease. Because utilization-based models discount improvements in productivity, ignore alternative provider sources, and are divorced from measures of outcome efficacy, they may miscalculate HHR requirements.

*Needs-based* planning methodologies also factor in normative assessments of the care that should be consumed by a population into provider-to-population ratios. Population needs can be estimated by expert opinion, Delphi assessment, and/or epidemiologic surveys. While simple, because needs are defined by providers rather than consumers, needs-based assessments may overestimate consumer demand for services. These estimates may also be affected by changes in such factors as disease rates and in how diseases are managed (including technological developments).

*Demand-based* approaches to manpower planning determine the number of providers required to meet the demand for services generated by a given population of individuals. Demand for medical services, in this approach, is viewed as a multivariate function relating the quantities of services a population desires to the cost of those goods and services, the available financial resources, the psychological wants of the population, and the availability of providers. Demand, in such models, depends on such factors as the underlying health status of a population, the population's perception of the efficacy of medical care, and the cost of obtaining that care. In such models, demand for medical services is typically less than need, since potential patients may decide not to seek out treatments that may involve out-of-pocket costs, travel and waiting time, lost wages, and emotional suffering for individuals, even in environments with comprehensive medical insurance. Note that this approach is often plagued by data availability issues. Discrepancies between need and demand (including needs for which individuals do not seek care, needs which cannot be satisfied for technological reasons, and demands for services not based on need) may also be difficult to address.

*Benchmarking* compares HHR supply in a particular jurisdiction with other jurisdictions, where the benchmarks can be established in various ways (e.g., efficiency, outcomes, etc.).

The supply of HHR in a given region is thus a function of educational output, attrition (death, retirement, and emigration), and inflow (immigration). Growth in population, changes in provider-to-population ratios, and relative earning power of providers may all influence the number of individuals who enter clinical education programs and the number of trained professionals who immigrate to, or emigrate from, a region. Because of the manner in which powers are distributed within the Canadian federation, provinces are generally able to control only the educational component of HHR supply. As noted in section 2.2.1, although immigration is officially a "concurrent power," it is largely controlled by the federal government (see also Chapter 10, The Demanding Supply).

## 9. Some Data

### 9.1 Canadian Data

The Canadian Institute for Health Information (CIHI) publishes information about such topics as health expenditures, the public-private mix, and the supply of health providers. The reader is referred to the

CIHI website for up to date information. A wide variety of useful reports and data files are also available for download (Canadian Institute for Health Information, 2013b).

One key database tracks health expenditures. For 2011, for example, CIHI noted that total spending on health care in Canada was forecasted to be $200.5 billion, or approximately $5,800 per capita. About 70% of this spending came from public sources, and 30% from private sources. CIHI divides health spending into the following "uses of funds": hospitals, other institutions, physicians, other professionals, drugs, capital, public health, administration, and other health spending (see also Chapter 18, Everyone Out of the Pool). Note that not all health expenditures represent clinical services; for example, the "other" category also captures health research. By "use of funds" the most recent data at the time of writing was for 2009; the largest share was for hospitals, but this was about 29% (and down considerably from what it had been several decades ago); outpatient pharmaceuticals came second (16%) and physicians third (14%). Public spending varied considerably by subsector, accounting for about 99% of physician services, 90% of hospital services, 71.5% of the costs of other institutions (which includes some LTC facilities), but 39% of outpatient drugs (inpatient drugs are included in hospital budgets) and 8.2% of other FFS professionals (recognizing that many of non-physician professionals delivering services within hospitals do not charge FFS, but are paid from the hospital budget). Health spending accounted for about 40% of provincial budgets, although this varies somewhat by province (and by what other services are contained in provincial, as opposed to local, budgets). In contrast to the 1998–2008 period, when average annual growth in health spending was 7.4%, the growth rate had decreased, and was estimated at 4.0% for 2011. This growth was still somewhat higher than inflation and population growth, but lower than the growth in the overall economy. As a result, health care was forecast to drop from its peak of 11.9% (in 2009 and 2010) to 11.6% of Canada's gross domestic product (GDP) (Canadian Institute for Health Information, 2013c).

## 9.2 Comparative Health Data

OECD Health Data provides standardized data for its member countries over time. Information is available from its website (Organisation for Economic Co-operation and Development, 2012).

At the time of writing, the most recent data had been released in October 2012. The website also includes, in downloadable form, frequently requested data, a selection of key indicators from OECD Health Data organized by main themes, as well as briefing notes for the 34 OECD member countries (including Canada), and a full list of indicators in the database. It includes the following variables:

*Health expenditure.* Because different countries use different currencies, the OECD standardizes expenditure data in a number of ways. One is to convert to purchasing power parities (PPP), expressed in US dollars. Another is to compute proportions (e.g., of gross domestic product, of total expenditures). The *expenditure* variables provided in the database include the following:

- Total expenditure on health, percentage of gross domestic product
- Total health expenditure per capita, US$ PPP
- Total health expenditure, average annual growth rate per capita
- Public health expenditure, average annual growth rate per capita
- Public expenditure on health, percentage of total expenditure on health
- Public health expenditure per capita, US$ PPP
- Out-of-pocket expenditure on health, percentage of total expenditure on health
- Out-of-pocket expenditure on health, US$ PPP
- Pharmaceutical expenditure, percentage of total expenditure on health
- Pharmaceutical expenditure per capita, US$ PPP

*Health care resources* variables include the following:

- Physicians, density per 1,000 population
- Nurses, density per 1,000 population
- Medical graduates, density per 100,000 population
- Nursing graduates, density per 100,000 population
- Hospital beds, density per 1,000 population
- Acute care beds, density per 1,000 population
- Psychiatric care beds, per 1,000 population
- MRI units, per million population
- CT scanners, per million population

Health care *activities* variables include the following:

- Doctor consultations per capita
- MRI exams, per 1,000 population
- CT scanner exams, per 1,000 population
- Hospital discharge rates, all causes, per 100,000 population

- Average length of stay, all causes, days
- Average length of stay for acute myocardial infarction (AMI), days
- Average length of stay for a normal delivery, days
- Caesarean sections, per 1,000 live births
- Pharmaceutical consumption, antibiotics, defined daily dose

Health status (*mortality*) variables include the following:

- Life expectancy at birth, females, males, and total population
- Life expectancy at 65 years old, females and males
- Infant mortality rate, deaths per 1,000 live births
- Potential years of life lost (PYLL), all causes, females and males
- Causes of mortality, suicides, deaths per 100,000 population

*Risk factors* variables include the following:

- Tobacco consumption, percentage of females, males, and adult population who are daily smokers
- Alcohol consumption, litres per population aged 15+
- Obesity, percentage of females, males, and adult population with a BMI > 30 kg/m$^2$, based on self-reports
- Obesity, percentage of females, males, and adult population with a BMI > 30 kg/m$^2$, based on measures of height and weight

Although not all data is available for all countries and for all years, the spreadsheets in the 2012 release gave data from 1960 to 2011 (where available) for the following countries: Australia, Austria, Belgium, Canada, Chile, Czech Republic, Denmark, Estonia, Finland, France, Germany, Greece, Hungary, Iceland, Ireland, Israel, Italy, Japan, Korea, Luxembourg, Mexico, the Netherlands, New Zealand, Norway, Poland, Portugal, Slovak Republic, Slovenia, Spain, Sweden, Switzerland, Turkey, the United Kingdom, and the United States.

This data can be helpful in placing particular countries in international perspective. For example, examination of the public and private shares of health expenditures reveals that Canada's public share (at about 70% of health expenditures), far from representing "socialized medicine," was relatively low internationally.

REFERENCES CITED AND FURTHER READING

Abelson, J., & Eyles, J. (2004). Public participation and citizen governance in the Canadian health system. In P.-G. Forest, G.P. Marchildon, & T. McIntosh

(Eds.), *Changing health care in Canada: Romanow papers* (Vol. 2, pp. 279–311). Toronto, ON: University of Toronto Press.

Abelson, J., Forest, P.-G., Eyles, J., Smith, P., Martin, E., & Gauvin, F. (2002). Obtaining public input for health systems decision making: Past experiences and future prospects. *Canadian Public Administration, 45*(1), 70–97. http://dx.doi.org/10.1111/j.1754-7121.2002.tb01074.x

Abelson, J., Mendelsohn, M., Lavis, J.N., Morgan, S.G., Forest, P.-G., & Swinton, M. (2004). Canadians confront health care reform. *Health Affairs, 23*(3), 186–93. http://dx.doi.org/10.1377/hlthaff.23.3.186

Academy Health. (2004). *Glossary of terms commonly used in health care.* Academy Health, Advancing Research, Policy and Practice. http://www.academy health.org/files/publications/glossary.pdf

Allin, S., Stabile, M., & Tuohy, C.H. (2010). *Financing models for non-Canada Health Act services in Canada: Lessons from local and international experiences with social insurance.* Canadian Health Services Research Foundation (CHSRF) Series of Reports on Financing Models: Paper 2, Ottawa, ON. http://www.cfhi-fcass.ca/sf-docs/default-source/commissioned-research-reports/CHSRF_4FinancingModels_En-final2.pdf?sfvrsn=0

Andermann, A., Blancquaert, I., Beauchamp, S., & Dery, V. (2008). Revisiting Wilson and Jungner in the genomic age: A review of screening criteria over the past 40 years. *Bulletin of the World Health Organization, 86*(4), 317–19. http://dx.doi.org/10.2471/BLT.07.050112

Arnstein, S.R. (1969). Ladder of citizen participation. *Journal of the American Institute of Planners, 35*(4), 216–24. http://dx.doi.org/10.1080/019443669089 77225

Bachrach, P., & Baratz, M.S. (1962). Two faces of power. *American Political Science Review, 56*(4), 947–52. http://dx.doi.org/10.2307/1952796

Bachrach, P., & Baratz, M.S. (1963). Decisions and non-decisions: An analytical framework. *American Political Science Review, 57*(3), 632–42. http://dx.doi .org/10.2307/1952568

Banting, K.G., & Corbett, S. (2002). *Health policy and federalism: A comparative perspective on multi-level governance.* Montreal: McGill-Queen's University Press.

Baumgartner, F.R. (2001). Agendas: Political. In N.J. Smelser & P.B. Baltes (Eds.), *International encyclopedia of the social & behavioral sciences* (pp. 288–91). Oxford, UK: Elsevier. http://dx.doi.org/10.1016/B0-08-043076-7/01092-5

Baumgartner, F.R., & Jones, B.D. (1991). Agenda dynamics and policy subsystems. *Journal of Politics, 53*(4), 1044–74. http://dx.doi.org/10.2307/2131866

Beauchamp, T.L., & Childress, J.F. (2001). *Principles of biomedical ethics* (5th ed.). New York: Oxford University Press.

Bendick, M., Jr. (1989). Privatizing the delivery of social welfare services: An ideal to be taken seriously. In S.B. Kamerman & A.J. Kahn (Eds.), *Privatization and the welfare state* (pp. 97–120). Princeton, NJ: Princeton University Press.

Bloche, M.G. (2006). Consumer-directed health care. *New England Journal of Medicine, 355*(17), 1756–9. http://dx.doi.org/10.1056/NEJMp068127

Brinkerhoff, D. (2004). Accountability and health systems: Toward conceptual clarity and policy relevance. *Health Policy and Planning, 19*(6), 371–9. http://dx.doi.org/10.1093/heapol/czh052

Brooks, S. (2009). *Canadian democracy: An introduction* (7th ed.). Toronto: Oxford University Press.

Brooks, S., & Miljan, L. (2003). *Public policy in Canada: An introduction* (6th ed.). Don Mills, ON: Oxford University Press.

Calabresi, G., & Bobbit, P. (1978). *Tragic choices: The conflicts society confronts in the allocation of tragically scarce resources.* New York: W.W. Norton.

Cameron, D., & Simeon, R. (2002). Intergovernmental relations in Canada: The emergence of collaborative federalism. *Publius: The Journal of Federalism, 32*(2), 49–71. http://dx.doi.org/10.1093/oxfordjournals.pubjof.a004947

Canadian Institute for Health Information. (2008). *The Health Personnel Database technical report.* Ottawa, ON. http://tools.hhr-rhs.ca/index.php?option=com_mtree&task=att_download&link_id=5964&cf_id=68&lang=en

Canadian Institute for Health Information. (2013a). *Canada's health care providers, 1997 to 2011: A reference guide.* Canadian Institute for Health Information (CIHI). https://secure.cihi.ca/estore/productFamily.htm?pf=PFC2161&lang=en&media=0

Canadian Institute for Health Information. (2013b). *Home page.* http://www.cihi.ca/CIHI-ext-portal/internet/EN/Home/home/cihi000001

Canadian Institute for Health Information. (2013c). *National health expenditure trends, 1975–2011.* https://secure.cihi.ca/estore/productFamily.htm?locale=en&pf=PFC2400&lang=en

Canadian Institute for Health Information. (2013d). *Regulated nurses: Canadian trends, 2007 to 2011.* https://secure.cihi.ca/estore/productFamily.htm?locale=en&pf=PFC2016&lang=en

Chafe, R., Neville, D., Rathwell, T., & Deber, R. (2008). A framework for involving the public in health care coverage and resource allocation decisions. *Healthcare Management Forum, 21*(4), 6–13. http://dx.doi.org/10.1016/S0840-4704(10)60050-6

Charles, C.A., Lomas, J., Giacomini, M., Bhatia, V., & Vincent, V.A. (1997). Medical necessity in Canadian health policy: Four meanings and … a funeral? *Milbank Quarterly, 75*(3), 365–94. http://dx.doi.org/10.1111/1468-0009.00060

Coleman, W.D., & Skogstad, G. (1990). *Policy communities and public policy in Canada: A structural approach.* Mississauga, ON: Copp Clark Pitman.

Colombo, F., & Tapay, N. (2004). *Private health insurance in OECD countries: The benefits and costs for individuals and health systems.* OECD Health Working Papers, No. 15, Paris, France: OECD. http://dx.doi.org/10.1787/5272110 67757

Courtney, J.C., & Smith, D.E. (Eds.). (2010). *The Oxford handbook of Canadian politics.* Oxford: Oxford University Press. http://dx.doi.org/10.1093/oxfor dhb/9780195335354.001.0001

Culyer, A. (1995). Need: The idea won't do – but we still need it. *Social Science & Medicine, 40*(6), 727–30. http://dx.doi.org/10.1016/0277-9536(94)00307-F

Currie, W.L. (2009). From professional dominance to market mechanisms: Deinstitutionalization in the organizational field of health care. *Information Systems Outsourcing, 4,* 563–89. http://dx.doi.org/10.1007/978-3-540-88851-2_25

Daniels, N. (1994). Four unsolved rationing problems: A challenge. *Hastings Center Report, 24*(4), 27–29. http://dx.doi.org/10.2307/3562841

Daniels, N. (2000). Accountability for reasonableness. *British Medical Journal, 321*(7272), 1300–1. http://dx.doi.org/10.1136/bmj.321.7272.1300

Daniels, N., & Sabin, J. (1998). The ethics of accountability in managed care reform. *Health Affairs, 17*(5), 50–64. http://dx.doi.org/10.1377/hlthaff .17.5.50

Daniels, N., & Sabin, J.E. (2002). *Setting limits fairly: Can we learn to share medical resources?* Oxford: Oxford University Press. http://dx.doi.org/10.1093/acprof:oso/9780195149364.001.0001

Deber, R. (2000). Getting what we pay for: Myths and realities about financing Canada's health care system. *Health Law in Canada, 21*(2), 9–56.

Deber, R. (2003). Health care reform: Lessons from Canada. *American Journal of Public Health, 93*(1), 20–4. http://dx.doi.org/10.2105/AJPH.93.1.20

Deber, R. (2004). Delivering health care services: Public, not-for-profit, or private? In G.P. Marchildon, T. McIntosh, & P.-G. Forest (Eds.), *The fiscal sustainability of health care in Canada: Romanow papers* (Vol. 1, pp. 233–96). Toronto: University of Toronto Press.

Deber, R. (2008). Access without appropriateness: Chicken Little in charge? *Health Policy (Amsterdam), 4*(1), 12–18.

Deber, R. (2009). Canada. In J. Rapoport, P. Jacobs, & E. Jonsson (Eds.), *Cost containment and efficiency in national health systems: A global comparison* (pp. 15–39). Weinheim, Germany: Wiley-VCH Verlag GmbH.

Deber, R., Baumann, A., Gamble, B., & Laporte, A. (2010, May 2–5). *Supply and demand of health workers in an economic downturn.* Paper presented at the 12th Annual International Medical Workforce Collaboration, New York City.

http://rcpsc.medical.org/publicpolicy/imwc/2010-IMWC12/IMWC10
deber.pdf

Deber, R., Hollander, M.J., & Jacobs, P. (2008). Models of funding and reimbursement in health care: A conceptual framework. *Canadian Public Administration, 51*(3), 381–405. http://dx.doi.org/10.1111/j.1754-7121.2008.00030.x

Deber, R., Kraetschmer, N., & Irvine, J. (1996). What role do patients wish to
play in treatment decision making? *Archives of Internal Medicine, 156*(13),
1414–20. http://dx.doi.org/10.1001/archinte.1996.00440120070006

Deber, R., & Lam, K.C.K. (2009). *Handling the high spenders: Implications of the
distribution of health expenditures for financing health care, 2009 Annual Meeting &
Exhibition*. American Political Science Association. http://papers.ssrn.com/
sol3/papers.cfm?abstract_id=1450788

Deber, R., & Lam, K.C.K. (2011a). *Experience with medical savings accounts in
selected jurisdictions* (Paper 4). CHSRF Series of Reports on Financing Models.
http://www.cfhi-fcass.ca/SearchResultsNews/11-07-21/ae5a6480-4a76-
4066-a7cc-d71f4f98c5ed.aspx

Deber, R., & Lam, K.C.K. (2011b). *Medical savings accounts in financing healthcare*
(Paper 3). CHSRF Reports on Financing Models. http://www.cfhi-fcass.ca/
sf-docs/default-source/commissioned-research-reports/RAISA3-Medical
SAcc_EN.pdf?sfvrsn=0

Deber, R., Millan, K., Shapiro, H., & McDougall, C.W. (2006). A cautionary tale
of downloading public health in Ontario: What does it say about the need
for national standards for more than doctors and hospitals? *Health Policy
(Amsterdam), 2*(2), 56–71.

Deber, R., & Schwartz, R. (2011). *Change towards outcome based performance
management: An expedited synthesis final report*. CIHR Expedited Knowledge
Synthesis Program. http://www.approachestoaccountability.ca/reports/
ESfinal.pdf

Department of Justice Canada. (1982). *A consolidation of the Constitution Acts,
1867 to 1982*. Consolidated as of January 1, 2013. http://laws-lois.justice
.gc.ca/PDF/CONST_E.pdf#page=69

DiMaggio, P.J., & Powell, W.W. (1983). The iron cage revisited: Institutional
isomorphism and collective rationality in organizational fields. *American
Sociological Review, 48*(2), 147–60. http://dx.doi.org/10.2307/2095101

Dobrow, M.J., Sullivan, T., & Sawka, C. (2008). Shifting clinical accountability
and the pursuit of quality: Aligning clinical and administrative approaches.
*Healthcare Management Forum, 21*(3), 6–12. http://dx.doi.org/10.1016/
S0840-4704(10)60269-4

Docteur, E., & Oxley, H. (2003). *Health-care systems: Lessons from the reform experience* (OECD Health Working Paper No. 9). http://www.oecd.org/health/
health-systems/22364122.pdf

Doern, G.B., & Phidd, R.W. (1992). *Canadian public policy: Ideas, structure, process* (2nd ed.). Toronto: Nelson Canada.

Donahue, J.D. (1989). *The privatization decision: Public ends, private means.* New York: Basic Books.

Donaldson, C., Gerard, K., Jan, S., Mitton, C., & Wiseman, V. (2005). *Economics of health care financing: The visible hand* (2nd ed.). Basingstoke, UK: Palgrave/ Macmillan.

Doty, M.M., Collins, S.R., Nicholson, J.L., & Rustgi, S.D. (2009, July). *Failure to protect: Why the individual insurance market is not a viable option for most U.S. families* (Issue Brief No. 1300). The Commonwealth Fund. http://www.common wealthfund.org/~/media/Files/Publications/Issue%20Brief/2009/Jul/ Failure%20to%20Protect/1300_Doty_failure_to_protect_individual_ins_ market_ib_v2.pdf

Drummond, M.F., Sculpher, M.J., Torrance, G.W., O'Brien, B.J., & Stoddart, G.L. (2005). *Methods for the economic evaluation of health care programmes* (3rd ed.). Toronto: Oxford University Press.

Dumont-Lemasson, M., Donovan, C., & Wylie, M. (1999). *Provincial and territorial home care programs: A synthesis for Canada.* Minister of Public Works and Government Services Canada: Health Canada. http://www.hc-sc.gc.ca/ hcs-sss/pubs/home-domicile/1999-pt-synthes/index-eng.php

Ellis, R.P., & Vidal-Fernandez, M. (2007). Activity-based payments and reforms of the English hospital payment system. *Health Economics, Policy, and Law, 2*(4), 435–44. http://dx.doi.org/10.1017/S1744133107004276

Emanuel, E.J., & Emanuel, L.L. (1996). What is accountability in health care? *Annals of Internal Medicine, 124*(2), 229–39. http://dx.doi.org/10.7326/0003-4819-124-2-199601150-00007

Esping-Andersen, G. (1990). *The three worlds of welfare capitalism.* Princeton, NJ: Princeton University Press.

Etzioni, A. (1986). Mixed scanning revisited. *Public Administration Review, 46*(1), 8–14. http://dx.doi.org/10.2307/975437

Evans, P.B., Rueschemeyer, D., & Skocpol, T. (Eds.). (1985). *Bringing the state back in.* New York: Cambridge University Press. http://dx.doi.org/10.1017/ CBO9780511628283

Evans, R.G. (1984). *Strained mercy: The economics of Canadian health care.* Toronto: Butterworths.

Evans, R.G. (1996). Going for the gold: The redistributive agenda behind market-based health care reform. *Journal of Health Politics, Policy and Law, 22*(2), 427–65.

Evans, R.G. (2004). Financing health care: Options, consequences, and objectives for financing health care in Canada. In G.P. Marchildon, T. McIntosh, &

P.-G. Forest (Eds.), *The fiscal sustainability of health care in Canada: Romanow Papers* (Vol. 1, pp. 139–96). Toronto: University of Toronto Press.

Fard, S.M. (2009). *The Canada Health Transfer.* Government of Canada, Parliamentary Information and Research Service. http://www.parl.gc.ca/Content/LOP/researchpublications/prb0852-e.pdf

Fein, R. (2001). *Medical care, medical costs: The search for a health insurance policy.* Cambridge, MA: Harvard University Press.

Fierlbeck, K. (2004). Paying to play? Government financing and agenda setting for health care. In G.P. Marchildon, T. McIntosh, & P.-G. Forest (Eds.), *The fiscal sustainability of health care in Canada: Romanow papers* (Vol. 1, pp. 340–65). Toronto: University of Toronto Press.

Fischhoff, B., Lichtenstein, S., Slovic, P., Derby, S.L., & Keeney, R.L. (1981). *Acceptable risk.* Cambridge, MA: Cambridge University Press.

Flood, C.M., & Choudhry, S. (2004). Strengthening the foundations: Modernizing the Canada Health Act. In T. McIntosh, P.-G. Forest, & G.P. Marchildon (Eds.), *The governance of health care in Canada: Romanow papers* (Vol. 3, pp. 346–87). Toronto: University of Toronto Press.

Flood, C.M., Roach, K., & Sossin, L. (2005). *Access to care, access to justice: The legal debate over private health insurance in Canada.* Toronto: University of Toronto Press.

Fooks, C., & Maslove, L. (2004). *Rhetoric, fallacy or dream? Examining the accountability of Canadian health care to citizens* (Health Care Accountability Paper No. 1). Canadian Policy Research Networks. http://www.cprn.org/documents/27403_en.pdf

Freidson, E. (1986). *Professional powers: A study of the institutionalization of formal knowledge.* Chicago: University of Chicago Press.

Freidson, E. (2001). *Professionalism, the third logic.* Chicago: University of Chicago Press.

Getzen, T.E. (1997). *Health economics: Fundamentals and flow of funds* (2nd ed.). New York: John Wiley and Sons.

Geyman, J.P. (2007). Moral hazard and consumer-driven health care: A fundamentally flawed concept. *International Journal of Health Services, 37*(2), 333–51. http://dx.doi.org/10.2190/J354-150M-NG76-7340

Gibson, J., Martin, D., & Singer, P. (2005). Evidence, economics and ethics: Resource allocation in health service organizations. *Healthcare Quarterly, 8*(2), 50–9. http://dx.doi.org/10.12927/hcq..17099

Gold, M.R., Siegel, J.E., Russell, L.B., & Weinstein, M.C. (1996). *Cost-effectiveness in health and medicine.* New York: Oxford University Press.

Gostin, L.O. (2000). *Public health law: Power, duty, restraint.* Berkeley: University of California Press.

Government of Canada (1984). *Canada Health Act, Bill C-3*. Statutes of Canada, 1984 (R.S.C. 1985, c. 6; R.S.C. 1989, c. C-6). http://laws-lois.justice.gc.ca/PDF/C-6.pdf

Hacker, J.S. (2004). Privatizing risk without privatizing the welfare state: The hidden politics of social retrenchment in the United States. *American Political Science Review, 98*(2), 243–60. http://dx.doi.org/10.1017/S0003055404001121

Hacker, J.S. (2008). *The great risk shift*. New York: Oxford University Press.

Health Disparities Task Group of the Federal/Provincial/Territorial Advisory Committee on Population Health and Health Security. (2004). *Reducing health disparities – Roles of the health sector: Discussion paper*. http://www.phac-aspc.gc.ca/ph-sp/disparities/ddp-eng.php

Herzlinger, R.E. (2004). *Consumer-driven health care: Implications for providers, payers, and policymakers*. San Francisco: Jossey-Bass.

Himmelstein, D. U., Warren, E., Thorne, D., & Wollhandler, S. (2005). Market watch: Illness and injury as contributors to bankruptcy. *Health Affairs*. doi: 10.1377/hlthaff.w5.63

Hinman, A. (2003). *Infectious disease control* (2nd ed.). New York: Delmar Learning.

Hirschman, A.O. (1970). *Exit, voice and loyalty: Responses to decline in firms, organizations, and states*. Cambridge, MA: Harvard University Press.

Hirschman, A.O. (1980). Exit, voice and loyalty: Further reflections and a survey of recent contributions. *Milbank Memorial Fund Quarterly: Health and Society, 58*(3), 430–53. http://dx.doi.org/10.2307/3349733

Hood, C.C. (1983). *The tools of government*. Chatham, NJ: Chatham House.

Howlett, M., Ramesh, M., & Perl, A. (2009). *Studying public policy: Policy cycles & policy subsystems* (3rd ed.). Don Mills, ON: Oxford University Press.

Hsaio, W.C. (2007). Why is a systematic view of health financing necessary? *Health Affairs, 26*(4), 950–61. http://dx.doi.org/10.1377/hlthaff.26.4.950

Institute of Medicine. (2001). *Crossing the quality chasm: A new health system for the 21st century*. Washington, DC: National Academic Press.

Jakab, M., Preker, A., Harding, A., & Hawkins, L. (2002). *The introduction of market forces in the public hospital sector: From new public sector management to organizational reform*. World Bank's Human Development Network, Health, Nutrition, and Population. http://siteresources.worldbank.org/HEALTHNUTRITIONANDPOPULATION/Resources/281627-1095698140167/Jakab-TheIntroductionof-whole.pdf

Jenkins, W.I. (1978). *Policy analysis: A political and organizational perspective*. London: M. Robertson.

Johnson, P.M. (2005). *A glossary of political economy terms*. Auburn University. http://www.auburn.edu/~johnspm/gloss/index

Jost, T.S. (2007). *Health care at risk: A critique of the consumer-driven movement.* Durham, NC: Duke University Press.

Kahneman, D., Slovic, P., & Tversky, A. (Eds.). (1982). *Judgment under uncertainty: Heuristics and biases.* Cambridge, MA: Cambridge University Press. http://dx.doi.org/10.1017/CBO9780511809477

Kahneman, D., & Tversky, A. (1979). Prospect theory: An analysis of decision under risk. *Econometrica, 47*(2), 263–91. http://dx.doi.org/10.2307/1914185

Kattan, M.W. (2009). *Encyclopedia of medical decision making* (Vols. 1–2). London: SAGE.

Kellow, A.J. (1988). Promoting elegance in policy theory: Simplifying Lowi's arenas of power. *Policy Studies Journal: The Journal of the Policy Studies Organization, 16*(4), 713–24. http://dx.doi.org/10.1111/j.1541-0072.1988.tb00680.x

Kingdon, J.W. (2003). *Agendas, alternatives, and public policies* (2nd ed.). New York: Longman.

Kinnunen, J., Danishevski, K., Deber, R.B., & Tulchinsky, T.H. (2007). Effects of decentralization on clinical dimensions of health systems. In R.B. Saltman, V. Bankauskaite, & K. Vrangbaek (Eds.), *Decentralization in health care* (pp. 167–88). Berkshire, UK: Open University Press.

Kriebel, D., & Tickner, J. (2001). The precautionary principle and public health: Reenergizing public health through precaution. *American Journal of Public Health, 91*(9), 1351–5. http://dx.doi.org/10.2105/AJPH.91.9.1351

Kuhse, H., & Singer, P. (Eds.). (2009). *A companion to bioethics* (2nd ed.). Mississauga, ON: John Wiley and Sons. http://dx.doi.org/10.1002/9781444307818

Lalonde, M. (1974). *A new perspective on the health of Canadians: A working document.* Minister of Supply and Services Canada. http://www.phac-aspc.gc.ca/ph-sp/pdf/perspect-eng.pdf

Lasswell, H.D. (1958). *Politics: Who gets what, when, how.* New York: Meridian Books, World Publishing.

Last, J.M. (1988). *A dictionary of epidemiology* (2nd ed.). New York: Oxford University Press.

Lazar, H. (2006). The intergovernmental dimensions of the Social Union: A sectoral analysis. *Canadian Public Administration, 49*(1), 23–45. http://dx.doi.org/10.1111/j.1754-7121.2006.tb02016.x

Lazar, H. (2010). Intergovernmental fiscal relations: Workhorse of the federation. In J.C. Courtney & D.E. Smith (Eds.), *The Oxford handbook of Canadian politics* (pp. 111–30). Oxford: Oxford University Press. http://dx.doi.org/10.1093/oxfordhb/9780195335354.003.0007

Leger, P.T. (2008). Physician payment mechanisms. In M. Lu & E. Jonsson (Eds.), *Financing health care: New ideas for a changing society* (pp. 149–76). Weinheim, Germany: Wiley-VCH Verlag GmbH, KGaA.

Lindblom, C.E. (1959). The science of "muddling through." *Public Administration Review, 19*(2), 79–88. http://dx.doi.org/10.2307/973677

Lindblom, C.E. (1979). Still muddling, not yet through. *Public Administration Review, 39*(6), 517–26. http://dx.doi.org/10.2307/976178

Lipsky, M. (1980). *Street-level bureaucracy: Dilemmas of the individual in public services*. New York: Russell-Sage Foundation.

Lyon, T.P., & Maxwell, J.W. (2004). Astroturf: Interest group lobbying and corporate strategy. *Journal of Economics & Management Strategy, 13*(4), 561–97. http://dx.doi.org/10.1111/j.1430-9134.2004.00023.x

MacLean, G.A., & Wood, D.R. (2010). Studying politics. In G.A. MacLean & D.R. Wood (Eds.), *Politics: An introduction* (pp. 23–45). Don Mills, ON: Oxford University Press.

Madore, O. (2005). *The Canada Health Act: Overview and options* (Current Issue Review 94–4E). Library of Parliament. http://www.parl.gc.ca/Content/LOP/ResearchPublications/944-e.htm

Maioni, A. (1998). *Parting at the crossroads: The emergence of health insurance in the United States and Canada*. Princeton, NJ: Princeton University Press.

March, J.G., & Olsen, J.P. (1984). The new institutionalism: Organizational factors in political life. *American Political Science Review, 78*(3), 734–49. http://dx.doi.org/10.2307/1961840

Marchildon, G.P. (2010). Health care. In J.C. Courtney & D.E. Smith (Eds.), *The Oxford handbook of Canadian politics* (pp. 111–30). Oxford: Oxford University Press. http://dx.doi.org/10.1093/oxfordhb/9780195335354.003.0024

Marchildon, G.P. (2013). *Health systems in transition: Canada* (2nd ed.). Toronto: University of Toronto Press.

Marmor, T.R., & Morone, J.A. (1980). Representing consumer interests: Imbalanced markets, health planning and the HSAs. *Milbank Memorial Fund Quarterly: Health and Society, 58*(1), 125–65. http://dx.doi.org/10.2307/3349709

Martin, D.K., Giacomini, M., & Singer, P. (2002). Fairness, accountability for reasonableness, and the views of priority setting decision-makers. *Health Policy (Amsterdam), 61*(3), 279–90. http://dx.doi.org/10.1016/S0168-8510(01)00237-8

Matland, R.E. (1995). Synthesizing the implementation literature: The ambiguity-conflict model of policy implementation. *Journal of Public Administration: Research and Theory, 5*(2), 145–74.

Maynard, A. (2006). Medical workforce planning: Some forecasting challenges. *Australian Economic Review, 39*(3), 323–9. http://dx.doi.org/10.1111/j.1467-8462.2006.00422.x

McCombs, M. (2002). Agenda setting. In N.J. Smelser & P.B. Baltes (Eds.), *International encyclopedia of the social & behavioral sciences* (pp. 285–8). New York: Elsevier.

McKneally, M.F., Dickens, B.M., Meslin, E.M., & Singer, P.A. (1997). Bioethics for clinicians: 13. Resource allocation. *Canadian Medical Association Journal*, 157(2), 163–7.

McLean, I., & McMillan, A. (2003). *Concise dictionary of politics* (2nd ed.). Oxford: Oxford University Press.

McNeil, B.J., Pauker, S.G., Sox, H.C., Jr., & Tversky, A. (1982). On the elicitation of preferences for alternative therapies. *New England Journal of Medicine*, 306(21), 1259–62. http://dx.doi.org/10.1056/NEJM198205273062103

MediaCollege.com. (2011). *What makes a story newsworthy?* Wavelength Media. http://www.mediacollege.com/journalism/news/newsworthy.html

Mendelsohn, M. (2002). *Canadians' thoughts on their health care system: Preserving the Canadian model through innovation.* Queen's University. http://www.queensu.ca/cora/_files/MendelsohnEnglish.pdf

National Institute for Health and Clinical Excellence. (2008). *Social value judgements: Principles for the development of NICE guidance* (2nd ed.). http://www.nice.org.uk/media/C18/30/SVJ2PUBLICATION2008.pdf

Newhouse, J.P. (2004). Consumer-directed health plans and the RAND health insurance experiment. *Health Affairs*, 23(6), 107–13. http://dx.doi.org/10.1377/hlthaff.23.6.107

Newhouse, J.P., & Insurance Experiment Group. (1993). *Free for all? Lessons from the RAND health insurance experiment.* Cambridge, MA: Harvard University Press.

Nicholson, S., Bundorf, M.K., Stein, R.M., & Polsky, D. (2003). *The magnitude and nature of risk selection in employer-sponsored health plans* (National Bureau of Economic Research Working Paper 9937). http://www.nber.org/papers/w9937

Oates, W.E. (1999). An essay on fiscal federalism. *Journal of Economic Literature*, 37(3), 1120–49. http://dx.doi.org/10.1257/jel.37.3.1120

O'Connor, J. (1973). *The fiscal crisis of the state.* New York: St. Martin's Press.

Offe, C. (1984). *Contradictions of the welfare state.* Cambridge, MA: MIT Press.

Ontario Ministry of Health and Long-Term Care. (2006, March 15). *Local health integration networks (LHINs): Building a true system* (Bulletin 21). Ontario Ministry of Health and Long-Term Care. http://www.ontla.on.ca/library/repository/ser/247449/2006/2006no21.pdf

Ontario Ministry of Health and Long-Term Care. (2013a). *About the ministry.* Ontario Ministry of Health and Long-Term Care. http://www.health.gov.on.ca/en/common/ministry/default.aspx

Ontario Ministry of Health and Long-Term Care. (2013b). *Health care professions: Regulation.* http://www.health.gov.on.ca/en/pro/programs/hhrsd/about/regulated_professions.aspx

Organisation for Economic Co-operation and Development. (2002). *Glossary of statistical terms*. http://stats.oecd.org/glossary/detail.asp?ID=3295

Organisation for Economic Co-operation and Development. (2012). *OECD health data 2012*. http://www.cihi.ca/CIHI-ext-portal/internet/EN/Home/home/cihi000001

Pateman, C. (1970). *Participation and democratic theory*. Cambridge, MA: Cambridge University Press.

Pauly, M.V. (1986). Taxation, health insurance, and market failure in the medical economy. *Journal of Economic Literature, 24*(2), 629–75.

Pierson, C., & Castles, F.G. (2006). *The welfare state reader* (2nd ed.). Malden, MA: Polity Press.

Pierson, P. (1993). When effect becomes cause: Policy feedback and political change. *World Politics, 45*(4), 595–628. http://dx.doi.org/10.2307/2950710

Pierson, P. (2000). Increasing returns, path dependence, and the study of politics. *American Political Science Review, 94*(2), 251–67. http://dx.doi.org/10.2307/2586011

Preker, A.S., & Harding, A. (2000). *The economics of public and private roles in health care: Insights from institutional economics and organizational theory* (Health, Nutrition and Population Discussion Paper). Human Development Network, International Bank for Reconstruction and Development / World Bank. http://siteresources.worldbank.org/HEALTHNUTRITIONAND POPULATION/Resources/281627-1095698140167/Preker-TheEconomicsOf Public-whole.pdf

Preker, A.S., & Harding, A. (Eds.). (2003). *Innovations in health service delivery: The corporatization of public hospitals*. Washington, DC: World Bank. http://dx.doi.org/10.1596/0-8213-4494-3

Preker, A.S., Harding, A., & Travis, P. (2000). "Make or buy" decisions in the production of health care goods and services: New insights from institutional economics and organizational theory. *Bulletin of the World Health Organization, 78*(6), 779–89.

Pressman, J.L., & Wildavsky, A. (1973). *Implementation: How great expectations in Washington are dashed in Oakland* (3rd ed.). Berkeley: University of California Press.

Pross, A.P. (1992). *Group politics and public policy* (2nd ed.). Toronto: Oxford University Press.

Public Health Agency of Canada. (2012). *What is the population health approach?* http://www.phac-aspc.gc.ca/ph-sp/approach-approche/index-eng.php

Rice, T. (1997). Can markets give us the health system we want? *Journal of Health Politics, Policy and Law, 22*(2), 383–426.

Rice, T. (1998). *The economics of health reconsidered* (2nd ed.). Chicago: Health Administration Press.

Rico, A., & Puig-Junoy, J. (2002). What can we learn from the regulation of public utilities? In R.B. Saltman, R. Busse, & E. Mossialos (Eds.), *Regulating entrepreneurial behaviour in European health care systems* (pp. 73–90). Buckingham, UK: Open University Press.

Roberfroid, D., Leonard, C., & Stordeur, S. (2009). Physician supply forecast: Better than peering in a crystal ball? *Human Resources for Health, 7*(10), 1–13.

Rosenthal, M., & Daniels, N. (2006). Beyond competition: The normative implications of consumer-driven health plans. *Journal of Health Politics, Policy and Law, 31*(3), 671–85. http://dx.doi.org/10.1215/03616878-2005-013

Rowe, G., & Frewer, L.J. (2005). A typology of public engagement mechanisms. *Science, Technology & Human Values, 30*(2), 251–90. http://dx.doi.org/10.1177/0162243904271724

Sabatier, P. (1999). *Theories of the policy process.* Boulder, CO: Westview Press.

Sabatier, P., & Mazmanian, D. (1980). The implementation of public policy: A framework of analysis. *Policy Studies Journal: The Journal of the Policy Studies Organization, 8*(4), 538–60. http://dx.doi.org/10.1111/j.1541-0072.1980.tb01266.x

Sabatier, P.A., & Jenkins-Smith, H.C. (1993). *Policy change and learning: An advocacy coalition approach.* Boulder, CO: Westview Press.

Saltman, R.B., Bankauskaite, V., & Vrangbaek, K. (2007). *Decentralization in health care.* Berkshire, UK: Open University Press.

Sancton, A. (2010). Local government. In J.C. Courtney & D.E. Smith (Eds.), *The Oxford handbook of Canadian politics* (pp. 111–30). Oxford: Oxford University Press. http://dx.doi.org/10.1093/oxfordhb/9780195335354.003.0008

Schattschneider, E.E. (1975). *The semisovereign people: A realist's view of democracy in America* (3rd ed.). New York: Holt, Rinehart and Winston.

Schwing, R.C., & Albers, W.A., Jr. (1980). *Societal risk assessment: How safe is safe enough?* (Part 2). New York: Plenum Press.

Shah, C.P. (2003). *Public health and preventive medicine in Canada* (5th ed.). Toronto: Elsevier Canada.

Shortt, S.E.D., & Macdonald, J.K. (2002). Toward an accountability framework for Canadian healthcare. *Healthcare Management Forum, 15*(2), 24–32. http://dx.doi.org/10.1016/S0840-4704(10)60577-7

Simon, H. (1978). Rationality as process and as product of thought. *American Economic Review, 68*(2), 1–33.

Singer, P.A., & Viens, A.M. (Eds.). (2008). *The Cambridge textbook of bioethics.* Cambridge, UK: Cambridge University Press. http://dx.doi.org/10.1017/CBO9780511545566

Slovic, P. (1987). Perception of risk. *Science, 236*(4799), 280–5. http://dx.doi
.org/10.1126/science.3563507

Slovic, P., Fischhoff, B., & Lichtenstein, S. (1980). Facts and fears: Understanding
perceived risk. In R.C. Schwing & W.A. Albers, Jr., (Eds.), *Societal risk assessment: How safe is safe enough?* (Part 2, pp. 181–216). New York: Plenum Press.

Slovic, P., Fischhoff, B., Lichtenstein, S., & Roe, F.J.C. (1981). Perceived risk:
Psychological factors and social implications (and discussion). *Proceedings
of the Royal Society of London, Series A, Mathematical and Physical Sciences,
376*(1764, The Assessment and Perception of Risk), 17–34.

Smith, R. (2008). Globalization: the key challenge facing health economics in
the 21st century. *Health Economics, 17*(1), 1–3. http://dx.doi.org/10.1002/
hec.1335

Soroka, S.N. (2007, February). *Canadian perceptions of the health care system.*
Health Council of Canada. http://healthcouncilcanada.ca/rpt_det.php?
id=126

Standing Senate Committee on Social Affairs Science and Technology. (2003,
November). *Reforming health protection and promotion in Canada: Time to act,
Ottawa, ON.* Parliament of Canada. http://www.parl.gc.ca/Content/SEN/
Committee/372/soci/rep/repfinnov03-e.htm

Starfield, B. (2009). Toward international primary care reform. *Canadian Medical
Association Journal, 180*(11), 1091–2. http://dx.doi.org/10.1503/cmaj.090542

Starr, P. (1989). The meaning of privatization. In S.B. Kamerman & A.J. Kahn
(Eds.), *Privatization and the welfare state* (pp. 15–48). Princeton, NJ: Princeton
University Press.

Stone, D. (2008). *The Samaritan's dilemma: Should government help your neighbor?*
New York: Nation Books.

Stone, D.A. (1989). Causal stories and the formation of policy agendas. *Political
Science Quarterly, 104*(2), 281–300. http://dx.doi.org/10.2307/2151585

Stone, D.A. (1993). The struggle for the soul of health insurance. *Journal of
Health Politics, Policy and Law, 18*(2), 287–317. http://dx.doi.org/10.1215/
03616878-18-2-287

Stone, D.A. (2002). *Policy paradox: The art of political decision making* (3rd ed.).
New York: W.W. Norton.

Taylor, M.G. (1978). *Health insurance and Canadian public policy: The seven decisions that created the Canadian health insurance system* (2nd ed.). Montreal:
McGill-Queen's University Press.

Tindal, C.R., & Tindal, S.N. (2008). *Local government in Canada: An introduction*
(7th ed.). Scarborough, ON: Nelson College Indigenous.

Tuohy, C.H. (1999). *Accidental logics: The dynamics of change in the health care arena
in the United States, Britain, and Canada.* New York: Oxford University Press.

Tversky, A., & Kahneman, D. (1981). The framing of decisions and the psychology of choice. *Science, 211*(4481), 453–8. http://dx.doi.org/10.1126/science.7455683

Tversky, A., & Kahneman, D. (1986). Rational choice and the framing of decisions. *Journal of Business, 59*(4, Pt. 2), S251–78. http://dx.doi.org/10.1086/296365

Vancouver Coastal Health. (2012). *Legal status.* http://supervisedinjection.vch.ca/legal_status/

van de Ven, W.P.M.M., Beck, K., Buchner, F., Chernichovsky, D., Gerdiol, L., Holly, A., et al. (2003). Risk adjustment and risk selection on the sickness fund insurance market in five European countries. *Health Policy (Amsterdam), 65*(1), 75–98. http://dx.doi.org/10.1016/S0168-8510(02)00118-5

Vining, A.R., & Globerman, S. (1999). Contracting-out health care services: A conceptual framework. *Health Policy (Amsterdam), 46*(2), 77–96. http://dx.doi.org/10.1016/S0168-8510(98)00056-6

Weimer, D.L., & Vining, A.R. (1989). *Policy analysis: Concepts and practice.* Englewood Cliffs, NJ: Prentice Hall.

Weir, E., Schabas, R., Wilson, K., & Mackie, C. (2010). A Canadian framework for applying the precautionary principle to public health issues. *Canadian Journal of Public Health, 101*(5), 396–8.

White, J. (2007). Markets and medical care: The United States 1993–2005. *Milbank Quarterly, 85*(3), 395–448. http://dx.doi.org/10.1111/j.1468-0009.2007.00494.x

Wikipedia. (2012). *News values.* http://en.wikipedia.org/wiki/News_values

Wiktorowicz, M., & Deber, R. (1997). Regulating biotechnology: A rational-political model of policy development. *Health Policy (Amsterdam), 40*(2), 115–38. http://dx.doi.org/10.1016/S0168-8510(96)00889-5

Wildavsky, A. (1979). *Speaking truth to power: The art and craft of policy analysis* (2nd ed.). Boston, MA: Little, Brown.

Williamson, O.E. (1981). The economics of organization: The transaction cost approach. *American Journal of Sociology, 87*(3), 548–77. http://dx.doi.org/10.1086/227496

Williamson, O.E. (1985). *The economic institutions of capitalism.* New York: Free Press.

Williamson, O.E. (1999). Public and private bureaucracies: A transaction cost economics perspective. *Journal of Law Economics and Organization, 15*(1), 306–42. http://dx.doi.org/10.1093/jleo/15.1.306

Wilson, J.M.G., & Jungner, G. (1968). *Principles and practice of screening for disease* (Public Health Paper No. 34). World Health Organization. http://whqlibdoc.who.int/php/WHO_PHP_34.pdf

World Health Organization. (1948). *Preamble to the Constitution of the World Health Organization as adopted by the International Health Conference.* http://www.who.int/about/definition/en/print.html

World Health Organization. (1978). *Declaration of Alma-Ata.* WHO Regional Office for Europe. http://www.euro.who.int/en/who-we-are/policy-documents/declaration-of-alma-ata,-1978

World Health Organization. (2009). *Pandemic influenza preparedness and response.* http://www.who.int/influenza/resources/documents/pandemic_guidance_04_2009/en/

Young, R., & Leuprecht, C. (2006). *Canada: The state of the federation 2004: Municipal-federal-provincial relations in Canada.* Montreal: McGill-Queen's University Press.

Zimmerman, S.V. (2005). *Mapping legislative accountabilities* (Health Care Accountability Paper No. 5). Canadian Policy Research Networks. http://www.cprn.org/documents/35118_en.pdf

# 2 Danger at the Gates?

## Screening for Tuberculosis in Immigrants and Refugees

*MICHAEL GARDAM, MARISA CREATORE, AND*
*RAISA B. DEBER*

In the spring and summer of 1999, more than 200 people of Tibetan descent crossed the New York-Ontario border into Canada and asked for refugee status. Five of the Tibetans were found to have active pulmonary tuberculosis (TB), a contagious disease, with the infecting bacteria resistant to all of the front-line medications initially used to treat TB. Media coverage on radio, national newspapers, and television ensued, much portraying the Tibetan situation as an example of how the Canadian immigration system was flawed, and was potentially putting Canadians at risk of contracting a deadly disease. This case addresses several policy issues, including: screening for communicable diseases, immigration policy, risk perception, and federal-provincial relations.

### Appendices

Appendix A: A Medical Overview of TB
Appendix B: Canadian Immigration Policy
Appendix C: Screening for TB
Appendix D: References Cited and Further Reading

### The Case

In the spring and summer of 1999, more than 200 people of Tibetan descent crossed the New York-Ontario border into Canada claiming refugee status. They were placed in a crowded refugee shelter in downtown Toronto until their claims could be assessed. As part of the application process, most of the claimants underwent a physical examination and a chest radiograph searching for evidence of active pulmonary tuberculosis (TB). Within weeks of arrival, five claimants were found to be suffering from active, contagious TB and were started on antituberculosis therapy. Subsequent investigations revealed that the infecting bacteria were resistant to all of the front-line medications used to treat TB. This story was picked up by the media, including radio reports, and a front-page story in a major national newspaper, the Toronto *Globe and Mail*. Immigration had already been a hot media topic over the summer of 1999; Kosovar refugees had been airlifted to Canada, and several boatloads of illegal Chinese migrant workers had landed in British Columbia and had asked for refugee status. The Tibetan situation was thus portrayed as yet another example of how the Canadian immigration system was flawed, and in this instance, was potentially putting Canadians at risk of contracting a deadly disease. Suddenly, public health, the Ontario health care system, and the federal government were under attack for allowing this perceived threat to Canadians to occur. The Canadian Broadcasting Corporation ran stories about how Toronto was now the TB capital of Canada. Immigration border guards threatened to walk off the job. A senior member of their union was quoted as saying, "Without proper controls either in the States before they come to Canada, or at the Canadian border, there may well be people released into the Canadian public who pose a health threat to people they meet on the street, people who get on the subways, the streetcar, bus, shopping plazas, whatever" (see Chapter 1, section 8.3.2, Risk Perception). Comparisons were made to the high costs that New York City had incurred from TB in its population.

## TB

TB is a common and deadly infectious disease. Once known as consumption, it was a major cause of death among the urban poor in North America and Europe. With the discovery of the tubercle bacillus *Mycobacterium tuberculosis* in 1882, improved public health measures, and development of the BCG vaccine in 1921 and potent antituberculosis drugs in the latter half of the 20th century, many experts believed that TB would be eradicated by the year 2000. That has not happened, and the rise of drug-resistant strains suggests it will be difficult if not impossible to do so. Developed countries have indeed seen an impressive drop in TB cases over the past 50 years, but the disease has continued to run rampant through the majority of the world's population.

Currently, TB causes more adult deaths than any other infectious disease worldwide other than HIV/AIDS. In 1993 the World Health

Organization (WHO) declared TB a global emergency. The WHO has estimated that one-third of the world's population is infected with TB and that over 8 million new active cases are diagnosed each year. However, as a result of strong public health programs, improvements in living conditions, and effective treatments, TB incidence (i.e., new cases), prevalence (i.e., total number of cases), and death rates appear to be stable or in decline. The vast majority of active cases occur in the developing world. Additional information about TB is provided in Appendix A.

Canada boasts one of the lowest rates of TB in the world. The incidence of Canadian cases peaked at the end of World War II in 1945, at 120 cases per 100,000 and then rapidly declined in subsequent years; the incidence rate was estimated as 4.7 cases per 100,000 in 2007 and has continued to fall (Public Health Agency of Canada 2012). TB among nonimmigrant Canadians disproportionately affects already vulnerable populations, including: Aboriginal populations, particularly those living on reserve; homeless persons; intravenous drug users; and those with underlying medical conditions (notably HIV/AIDS).

As TB rates within Canada have fallen, an increasing proportion of Canadian cases originate from travellers and immigrants arriving from countries with a relatively high incidence of the disease. This is particularly noticeable in cities. In Toronto, the majority of new immigrants to Toronto now come from countries with high rates of TB. Accordingly, although the overall number of TB cases reported annually among foreign-born populations in Canada has not increased substantially in the last 40 years, the relative proportion of TB cases that occur among foreign-born persons in Canada has. Over 90% of the new TB cases diagnosed each year now occur in the foreign-born, with the majority of these cases among recent immigrants (living in Canada for < 10 years prior to being diagnosed). At the time of the case, the city of Toronto was home to about 25% of the annual Canadian TB cases, with the incidence of TB in the city approaching 21 per 100,000 population. Almost all of the drug-resistant TB cases in Canada have been diagnosed in Toronto.

## Canadian TB Screening Policy for Refugees and Immigrants

Immigration policy in most countries attempts to balance a number of goals, both humanitarian and economic. An ongoing policy debate concerns how many immigrants to admit, and the basis on which to admit them. People may be admitted because they bring needed skills, to facilitate family reunification, and/or because they are refugees in need of protection. The process of immigration screening involves the decision of who should be allowed/denied entry to Canada and what conditional requirements should be met before allowing entry (Appendix B provides additional information about Canada's immigration policy at the time of the case).

Among the government's policy goals was to minimize the exposure of Canadians to imported infectious diseases. At the time of the case, there were two processes in place in order to achieve this: screening for active disease at the time of entry; and post-landing surveillance (now referred to as medical surveillance) for those at high risk for developing reactivation disease. Both processes involve logistic and legal/ethical challenges. In the case of TB, it was recognized that time-of-entry screening would generally detect applicants with active TB at the time of application, but would not detect those with inactive disease. (Appendix C gives some information about the available screening tests and which were being used.) Accordingly, the time-of-entry approach cannot prevent the arrival of those at high risk of developing active disease within a few years of landing in Canada, or even in the period between the immigration medical examination and arrival in Canada. Medical surveillance, however, involves both imposing demands on individuals after they had been given landed immigrant status and ensuring that individuals adhere to these demands. To the extent that such demands differ from those expected of Canadian citizens, legal and ethical problems may arise.

**Jurisdictional Issues**

*Federal (Citizenship and Immigration Canada)*

At the time of the case, the federal government intended to accept between 200,000 and 225,000 immigrants to Canada per year, including approximately 25,000 refugees. The federal government noted that it sought to balance the economic needs of Canada, humanitarian concerns, a respect for diversity, and a need to minimize perceived (and real) abuses of the system by criminals, human traffickers, migrant workers, and potential terrorists. The medical screening process was a low priority.

Members of the Toronto working group for multidrug-resistant tuberculosis approached the federal government seeking funds for the management of TB in new immigrants and refugees. The federal Minister of Health responded that, with the exception of the Interim Federal Health Program (IFHP), which paid for limited care for qualifying refugees, the provision of funding for health care was a provincial responsibility. However, although provincial insurance plans are required to fully cover all medically necessary physician and hospital services to all legal residents of Canada, the portability provisions of the *Canada Health Act* allow the provinces to impose a three-month waiting period before this coverage takes effect (see Chapter 1, section 7.2, *Canada Health Act*). Ontario was one of the provinces taking advantage of this provision.

## Provincial (Ontario Ministry of Health and Long-Term Care)

At the time of the case, the province of Ontario received between 50% and 60% of all immigrants to Canada. The provincial Ministry of Health shared Toronto Public Health's frustration with the immigration TB screening process, and agreed that there was inadequate social support for new immigrants and refugees. The province argued that, since Toronto's TB problem was largely a result of immigration, the necessary financial resources for the treatment, care, and social support of patients with TB should be provided by the federal government.

## Local (Toronto Public Health Department)

As noted in Chapter 1, section 2.2.1 (Federalism in Canada), public health in Canada is largely seen as being under provincial/territorial jurisdiction. However, at the time of the case, the approach taken by Ontario (and most other provinces) was to delegate much of this authority to a series of local public health departments, each governed by a local Board of Health (many of whose members are local elected politicians). The City of Toronto was the sixth largest government in Canada, larger than many provinces. Toronto Public Health, its municipal public health department, was the largest health unit in the country. The city was reluctant to pay for what they believed should be federal or provincial responsibilities.

### Stakeholder Views

## TB Specialists

TB specialists voiced several concerns regarding the existing state of TB diagnosis and management. They noted that most TB cases in Toronto were diagnosed when people sought treatment for symptoms rather than being detected as a result of screening. Delays in diagnosis and inappropriate treatment are well-known risks for increased transmission in the community, and for development of drug resistance. As the incidence of TB had waned in Canada over the past few decades, education surrounding the diagnosis and management of TB was mostly dropped from medical school curricula. Thus, there was a perception that many recent graduates were ill-prepared to manage cases appropriately, and that even older physicians might be lacking the knowledge necessary to treat drug-resistant cases. This was a particular concern in the Greater Toronto area, where the majority of drug-resistant cases were concentrated.

Concern was also voiced over the public health unit's practice of referring TB cases and their contacts to family physicians rather than directly to specialists; TB specialists believed that the resulting quality of care was both uneven and potentially dangerous. They also voiced concerns over the lack of resources available to most clinicians to adequately manage the often complicated social, psychological, and pharmacological issues that can arise with TB patients. The specialists called for the development of a centralized network of dedicated multidisciplinary TB clinics, to which front-line physicians or public health could refer any TB cases as well as their contacts (since these contacts would also be at risk of catching TB).

*The Media*

Immigrant and refugee issues figured prominently in the Canadian media at the time of the case. The images of Kosovar refugees being airlifted to Canada, boatloads of illegal migrants off the coast of British Columbia, and the laying of criminal charges against refugee claimants evoked powerful albeit different emotions in Canadians. In opinion polls, Canadians had consistently ranked immigration as one of the top issues facing Canada. However, the media do more than reflect the interests of their readers; they often shape public opinion and in turn help to shift political agendas (see Chapter 1, section 3.4, Framing). Immigration policy is often contentious. One newspaper story included the suggestion that "Ottawa's immigration and refugee incompetence is killing Canadians" and made references to "typhoid Marys," and refugees, immigrants, and visa students arriving with "grave and communicable diseases."

*Immigrants and Refugees*

TB in Canada is by and large a disease of marginalized populations who typically do not have an organized voice. Would-be immigrants and refugee claimants were the group most directly affected by immigration medical screening, yet there was no organized pressure group focused on their interests. This was in sharp contrast to some other infectious diseases, such as HIV/AIDS, around which many highly influential pressure groups had formed. Many refugees have experienced significant human rights abuses and traumatic events prior to arrival and may fear contact with the health system or any official government body. They may fear that diagnosis of TB will result in the refusal of their refugee claim and thus may avoid seeking care when ill. Once diagnosed with TB, immigrants and refugees may be hesitant to speak out as they often face discrimination from within their own cultural group and may fear deportation. For the same reasons, those deemed at-risk for developing TB may avoid medical surveillance, especially if they fear the consequences of a positive diagnosis.

Canada is also a multicultural nation. By the 2006 census, almost 20% of the population of Canada was foreign-born. About one-third of Canada's population lived in the three metropolitan areas of Toronto, Montreal, and Vancouver, and these cities were home to over two-thirds of the recent immigrants. The World Health Organization has called Toronto the most multicultural city in the world, with more than 50% of the city's population being foreign-born. Immigrant groups – and indeed most Canadians – were understandably hostile to policy moves seen to be discriminatory.

**The Task Force**

As noted, in response to the Tibetan crisis, the Toronto Public Health department created a Toronto working group on multidrug-resistant tuberculosis in June 1999. The group included provincial public health and Ministry of Health officials, clinicians with expertise in TB, and a designated medical practitioner. (There was no member representing Citizenship and Immigration Canada, which is part of the federal government.) This group identified several issues that it considered important to controlling TB in the city. They recommended that the highest priority should be to improve the TB screening program for new arrivals. Other issues identified included the lack of system-wide coordination, a lack of hospital facilities to deal with infectious cases, limited clinical guidelines, a lack of surgical facilities, limited number of clinicians with expertise in treating drug-resistant TB, delays in the immigration/refugee screening process, and inadequate housing and shelters for new immigrants and refugees. The committee also pointed out that Ontario's policy of not providing health insurance coverage for the first three months after being granted Landed Immigrant status (see Chapter 1, section 7.2, *Canada Health Act*) might stop some individuals with active TB from seeking and/or receiving medical care during this waiting period. After meeting with the Toronto Board of Health on the TB issue, the mayor of Toronto stated that if the federal government was going to continue to accept immigrants and refugees at current levels, it must be willing to provide additional funds to the City of Toronto to help with their housing and settlement. The federal government disagreed, reiterating its understanding that these issues were under provincial jurisdiction.

DECISION POINT

You are the Medical Officer of Health for the city of Toronto. You note that there is a substantial TB problem in your city. What should you do? What should you urge others to do?

SUGGESTED QUESTIONS FOR DISCUSSION

1. What are the possible policy alternatives for TB screening? Discuss their strengths and weaknesses.
2. How much of a public health risk does TB pose? How does it compare with other communicable diseases (e.g., influenza, or HIV/AIDS)?
3. Discuss when screening is justified and how it should be implemented. Is screening for latent TB disease among recent immigrants justified? Among other Canadians judged to be at higher risk? Among all Canadians?
4. What are the goals of immigration policy? How should these be balanced?
5. Discuss the roles and responsibilities of the various levels of government in controlling TB. Who is responsible for the health of recent immigrants? Is TB a local or a national problem?

6. Discuss the ethical issues involved in balancing control of infectious diseases with civil rights.
7. Discuss the role of the media.

## APPENDIX A: A MEDICAL OVERVIEW OF TB

### Infection and Progression to Active Disease

TB is a systemic infectious disease caused by the bacteria *Mycobacterium tuberculosis*, often referred to as tubercle bacilli. TB is transmitted by the airborne route (see Chapter 1, section 6.3.1, Public Health); when an infected person coughs, *M. tuberculosis* bacilli are dispersed in the air on microscopic droplets, which may then be inhaled by others. Although it is theoretically possible to develop TB after inhaling one infectious organism, in reality, most infections occur after prolonged exposure to highly infectious cases, with household contacts of an infectious case of TB at highest risk.

Once deposited in the lungs, tubercle bacilli multiply and then disseminate throughout the body in an often asymptomatic process termed *primary infection*. Approximately 2–8 weeks after inhaling the organisms, the cellular immune system usually halts the infectious process and the only evidence of infection may be a positive tuberculin skin test or, rarely, scarring on a chest radiograph; only 5% of infected patients will have an abnormal chest radiograph (see Appendix C for more details about these tests). This state of asymptomatic infection is termed *latent infection*. Most infected people will remain in this state for their whole life and never become sick. However, in roughly 10% of otherwise healthy cases, *reactivation* may occur, meaning that latent infection may progress to contagious, symptomatic pulmonary infection (*active disease*). Most of this risk occurs within the first two years of becoming infected. This risk is greatly increased in individuals with certain underlying medical conditions (e.g., HIV/AIDS, chronic renal failure). Similarly, children less than five years of age frequently do not mount an adequate immune response to the primary infection and may develop a disseminated, often fatal form of active TB.

TB can reactivate in any part of the body, but most commonly reactivates in the upper segments of the lungs. Reactivation pulmonary TB is typically more contagious than primary infection because of the large number of organisms present in a patient's sputum and the propensity of reactivation TB to cause pulmonary cavities (tubercles) that become filled with infectious organisms.

Individuals suffering from active TB often have symptoms for months before they are diagnosed. The reasons for this delay have included the unavailability of sensitive and specific diagnostic tests, the vagueness and slow onset of the symptoms, and physician inexperience in diagnosing TB. It is estimated that in this infectious period prior to diagnosis, the average case of TB will infect 15 other individuals. In Ontario, the provincial *Health Protection and Promotion Act* required that all cases of TB must be reported to the local public health department. (Chapter 7, Looking for Trouble, deals with issues around surveillance for infectious diseases.)

The treatment of active TB can be challenging for both patients and their health care providers. At the time of the case, the standard regimen involved the use of four drugs (isoniazid, rifampin, pyrazinamide, and ethambutol) for two months (intensive phase of treatment) until the results of sensitivity testing were known, followed by isoniazid and rifampin for an additional four months (the continuation phase) if the *M. tuberculosis* strain was fully sensitive to those drugs. When the medications are prescribed and taken appropriately, the cure rate for drug-sensitive TB is greater than 97%. Unfortunately, poor adherence to treatment not only is the most common cause of treatment failure but also can contribute to the development of drug-resistant TB. Each of these medications can have significant serious side effects, which in turn often discourages compliance with all six months of therapy. For example, the risk of serious clinical hepatitis due to isoniazid is about 0.2%–0.5% in those under the age of 35, and increases with age over 35. Fortunately, about 90% of those who develop clinical hepatitis will see the symptoms slowly resolve. However, the remaining 10% develop fulminant hepatitis, which has a high fatality rate and may require liver transplantation.

**Preventive Treatment for Infected Individuals**

Drug therapy is also recommended for individuals with latent TB infection who are at high risk for progression to active disease. If individuals with inactive TB are treated with isoniazid therapy for 6 to 12 months, the risk of reactivation decreases (estimates are that the risk drops by 75%–93%). Accordingly, at the time of writing, both the American Thoracic Society and Health Canada recommended that such individuals be treated for nine months. As is the case with treatment of active TB, however, the success of the drug regimen in preventing TB disease depends on adherence. In practice, most individuals in this category do not take the drug, usually because they were never offered it. It is understandably difficult to convince people who feel healthy to take a potentially toxic drug for preventive purposes. The best compliance rates seen in randomized controlled trials approach 80%; it is assumed that compliance in real-life settings is considerably less than this.

### Who Is at Risk?

The World Health Organization has released an extensive series of reports on TB, including a brief fact sheet (World Health Organization, 2012). In general, TB is a major cause of death worldwide; the WHO estimated that in 2009, there were 9.4 million new cases, of which a high proportion occurred in Asia and sub-Saharan Africa. Deaths were estimated at 1.7 million people. Although certain countries have a much higher burden of disease, risk is associated with being immunocompromised (with HIV infection being a major factor), as well as with poverty and poor, crowded living conditions.

Health Canada and the Public Health Agency of Canada have noted that, although the risk of developing TB is very low for most Canadians, there were still about 1,600 new cases reported annually in Canada. TB is classified as moderately contagious; casual contact is not particularly risky, but those having frequent exposure are at risk of infection. They noted that those with HIV/AIDS are particularly at risk, as are residents of some Aboriginal communities with high rates of disease, the poor (particularly the urban homeless), and residents of long-term care and correctional facilities, as well as the staff who work there. Other risk factors include certain cancers, diabetes, and cigarette smoking (Health Canada & Public Health Agency of Canada, 2012).

### Emergence of Multidrug-resistant TB

*Multidrug-resistant TB* (MDR-TB) is defined as resistance to at least isoniazid and rifampin, the two primary antituberculosis drugs. Patients infected with multidrug-resistant strains usually require therapy for more than two years and often require the surgical excision of infected tissue in order to bring about a cure. The overall cure rate after prolonged therapy is also reduced, although it is still approximately 70%.

There are few therapeutic options available for highly resistant strains, and clinicians often have to use highly toxic, relatively poorly effective medications. Most patients with MDR-TB in Toronto are hospitalized for several months during the start of their treatment, sometimes against their will, as a public health precaution and to ensure that they are compliant with therapy. It has been estimated that each case of MDR-TB costs the Canadian health care system approximately $250,000.

People can become infected with drug-resistant TB through one of two general mechanisms; they can acquire a drug-resistant strain from someone else (*primary resistance*), or they can initially have a drug-sensitive strain which, through the selective pressure of ineffective or inappropriate therapy, develops resistance (*acquired*, or *secondary resistance*).

The incidence of drug-resistant and multidrug-resistant strains has been increasing in many parts of the world, including Canada. In Canada, almost all multidrug-resistant cases have been found among foreign-born patients in the greater Toronto area. Based on a 1999 multidrug-resistance rate of 3%, the WHO identified Toronto as a hotspot for MDR-TB.

A more recent development has been the emergence *of extensively drug-resistant TB* (XDR-TB). Unlike MDR-TB, XDR was essentially untreatable at the time of writing, and is seen by the WHO as a major potential threat.


APPENDIX B: CANADIAN IMMIGRATION POLICY

Canada is a country of immigrants, but immigration policy has varied considerably over time. At the time of writing, Canada's immigration policy was governed by the 2002 *Immigration and Refugee Protection Act* (*IRPA*), which replaced the previous *Immigration Act* of 1976. The Canadian government noted that the legislation was "designed to ensure that the movement of people into Canada contributes to the country's social and economic interests, and meets its humanitarian commitments while protecting the health, safety and security of Canadians." It set forth several admissible categories of immigrants, which can be categorized into three main elements: *economic class* (which in turn includes a number of categories of skilled workers, professionals, and investors); *family class* (includes the spouse, common-law partner, dependent children, and parents of Canadians); and *refugees and persons in need of protection class.*

In addition, people can be admitted as *temporary workers*, without a clear path to citizenship. This category has grown significantly since the time of the case. At the time of writing, Canada had moved from a single set of entry admission criteria to a system with multiple entry points, each with different rules, including provision for provinces to nominate immigrants, and employers to recruit foreign workers. They have also expanded the number of temporary foreign workers admitted to Canada, and made it more difficult to qualify under the family class or as refugees.

Within the economic class, a point system gave points for a set of criteria, such as education, experience, and facility in official languages. Note that these rules are subject to change, as are the caps on how many can be admitted, by category of immigrant and/or country of origin.

Any foreign resident wishing to live, work, or study in Canada had to apply for entry via Citizenship and Immigration Canada (CIC). For the most part, those applying as immigrants or sponsored refugees must do so from their country of origin or of current residence (i.e., the application could not be made on Canadian soil). Section 19 of the *Immigration Act* also listed various classes of persons who were inadmissible; this encompassed not only those with criminal records, with involvement with espionage and terrorism, or likely to be a "Public Charge" (defined as likely to be unable or unwilling to support themselves and persons depending on them for care), but also those not meeting the medical requirements specified in the legislation and accompanying regulations. People were medically inadmissible if they were seen as posing a danger to public health, to public safety, or were likely to make "excessive" demands on health or social services.

Once the application had been submitted, all applicants and their dependents were required to undergo and pass a medical examination (which included both a physical examination and certain laboratory testing) to screen applicants for both chronic and communicable diseases. The exam had to be conducted by a designated medical practitioner (DMP), usually in their country of current residence (i.e., before the applicants could enter Canada), although applicants could select their DMP. The results of the examination would then be forwarded to a medical officer (part of the Canadian immigration process), who would determine whether the applicants were admissible. The results of the examination were valid for 12 months. Under some circumstances, individuals would be refused entry into Canada if they suffered from a medical condition that would be considered as placing an undue burden on the Canadian health care system (e.g., schizophrenia, chronic renal failure requiring dialysis, etc.) or if they had a communicable disease which would pose a threat to the well-being of Canadians (which would include active TB). However, under the revised *Immigration and Refugee Protection Act*, in effect at the time of the case, Family Class sponsored spouses, their dependent children, convention refugees and persons in need of protection, and their dependents would not necessarily be refused entry even if they had such a health condition that would be deemed to place "excessive demand" on health or social services. That decision would be made by the visa officer, although those decisions were subject to appeal.

There were some differences in how various categories of new entrants to Canada would be processed. In particular, individuals who claimed refugee status upon landing on Canadian soil (refugee claimants) belonged to a different category than sponsored refugees, since refugees usually would not have undergone medical examinations before arriving in Canada. A refugee claimant was still required to have an examination by a DMP, but this would happen in Canada. The regulations specified that this should occur within 60 days of arriving in Canada, but this was not always enforced. The exact process has varied somewhat; for example, in some periods, the medical examination was carried out only after a formal hearing took place to establish the validity of the refugee claim, a process that may take several weeks or even months. An additional difference between immigrants and refugees is that the medical screening process and chest radiograph for refugee claimants not only were performed in Canada but also were paid for by the federal government, with refugees found to have active TB then referred for treatment. (In 2012, the federal government made significant cuts to the Federal Interim Health Program, although it still offered coverage for urgent conditions that offered a risk to public health or safety. This policy change has evoked considerable concern among the physicians and other providers who treat refugee claimants.)

Note also that the process for seeking refugee status has changed somewhat since the time of the case, and that these new procedures would probably have prevented these claimants in this case from seeking refugee status. A document on the CIC website (Citizenship & Immigration Canada, 2008) noted, "Under an agreement with the United States, refugee claimants must seek asylum (protection) in the first safe country where they arrive. For example, if you entered Canada at a land border from the United States, you will not be able to claim refugee protection in Canada. Sometimes there are exceptions (such as those who already have family in Canada)."

APPENDIX C: SCREENING FOR TB

**Available Tests**

As noted in Chapter 1, section 8.2 (Screening), there is a difference between screening and testing. The term *screening* is applied to situations where tests are used on people without symptoms; *testing* is used to attempt to diagnose those who already show symptoms that might be compatible with particular diagnoses. The diagnosis of TB is often difficult because the clinical manifestations are typically vague and nonspecific and because there is no reliable, accurate diagnostic test. The diagnosis is thus based on a synthesis of available clinical and laboratory data. The ways to test for TB at the time of the case are indicated below.

Although the manifestations of TB are highly variable, certain key historical clues have been identified as helpful in suggesting a diagnosis of TB. These include: coming from an endemic area, being a close contact of someone known to have TB, having taken TB medications in the past, and weight loss. Such *clinical suspicion* would then have to be followed by one or more of the specific tests described below.

The *tuberculin skin test*, also referred to as the Mantoux screening test, the Tuberculin Sensitivity Test, the Pirquet test, or the PPD (purified protein derivative), has been used for over a century to diagnose TB infection. The test involves injecting a small amount of purified protein derivative obtained from *M. tuberculosis* under the skin in the forearm. Patients previously infected with TB will develop an area of swelling (induration) at the infection site, whereas those with no history of infection will either develop an insignificant degree of swelling or exhibit no reaction at all.

There are several problems with this test. The test itself can be difficult to perform correctly. Interpretation requires that the patient come back to the testing facility 48 to 72 hours after the injection to have his/her test read by an experienced health care worker. The tuberculin skin test also does not distinguish between active disease and asymptomatic infection. The test is approximately 97% sensitive (defined as the percentage of those with disease who test positive) and approximately 90% specific (defined as the percentage of those without disease who test negative); this means that false positive and false negative results do occur. When prevalence is low, this may mean that most positives are false positives. Perhaps the most notable limitation of this test is that persons who have received the BCG vaccination at greater than one year of age may test positive regardless of whether they have been infected. Since most recent immigrants to Canada come from regions of the world that regularly implement BCG vaccination to prevent some types of TB, at least some individuals without TB will nonetheless test positive on the skin test. For these reasons, a positive skin test will usually be followed-up by other investigations.

The *chest radiograph* has long been employed by screening programs to detect patients with active, contagious TB and to identify those with inactive disease who are at high risk for reactivation (e.g., those who have evidence of scarring). However, the test characteristics are not ideal. Most individuals with positive tuberculin skin tests have normal chest radiographs. Furthermore, chest radiographs suffer from interobserver variability because there is a large subjective component to interpretation. In terms of immigration screening, chest radiographs can also be bought and sold on the black market in certain countries.

The *sputum smear* is a relatively simple diagnostic test; it involves smearing a patient's sputum on a glass slide, staining it with dyes, and examining it for the presence of suspicious bacteria. This test has limited sensitivity and specificity for all forms of pulmonary TB. The limit of detection is 10,000 bacilli per millilitre of sputum. Even if bacilli are detected on the smear, it is not fully diagnostic of TB because other nontuberculous mycobacteria and other bacteria can look morphologically similar. The sputum smear is useful in detecting the most infectious cases.

The *sputum culture* is the gold standard for the diagnosis of TB. A significant limitation of sputum culture is the often prolonged time required to obtain the final result. While positive cultures are usually reported within two weeks, it may take up to eight weeks before a sputum culture can be declared negative. Approximately 80% of Toronto TB cases are diagnosed on the basis of the sputum culture. However, in the developing world, this test is usually not available due to its relatively high cost. An advantage of this test is that organisms obtained from a culture can then undergo sensitivity testing to determine whether they are resistant to medical therapy.

### How Did CIC Screen Potential Immigrants?

At the time of the case, the CIC relied on the chest radiograph. Tuberculin skin testing was not part of the immigration screening process, which meant that people with latent TB infection would not be identified by the immigration medical exam. Should the designated medical practitioner find evidence of active (contagious) pulmonary TB, entry into Canada would be denied until the applicant had been treated for a minimum of six months and deemed to be cured. However, between the date that the medical examination was performed and the date when the applicant actually arrived in Canada, enough time could elapse that it was possible that applicants with inactive disease could reactivate and develop infectious TB. Applicants from high-risk countries for TB could also acquire a new infection or become reinfected during this interval.

**Medical Surveillance**

Since up to 5% of cases with a history of active TB will develop contagious reactivation TB, the follow-up of those with evidence of old TB on a chest radiograph is considered an important method of TB control. Therefore, if the chest radiograph from the medical exam shows evidence of inactive TB indicating prior infection, the applicant may enter Canada but his or her application would be flagged for surveillance to begin upon arrival. These persons were required to contact their local public health unit; however, there was no method of enforcement in place. It is important to note that approximately only 5% of individuals with latent TB infection will have any evidence of old TB on their chest radiograph.

Upon arriving in Canada, the name, date of birth, and Canadian address of the immigrant being placed under medical surveillance would be sent to CIC, which would notify the provincial Ministry of Health, which in turn would notify the local public health unit in the area where the new immigrant planned to live. The local public health unit would then attempt to contact the immigrant and follow his or her health status for a period of time. The length of surveillance varied across public health units: in the greater Toronto area, new immigrants might be followed for up to two years. However, because the portability conditions of the *Canada Health Act* do not require people to be insured under the provincial health insurance plan until they qualify as Canadian permanent residents and have been in a province for three months (see Chapter 1, section 7.2, *Canada Health Act*), certain provinces, including Ontario, specified that, should a new immigrant require medical care for any reason within three months of arrival, he/she would be financially responsible for that care. In theory, immigrants could buy private insurance, but such policies would usually exclude pre-existing conditions (see Chapter 1, section 5.9, Insurance, Elasticity, and Moral Hazard). Public health officials noted that one consequence was that immigrants with symptoms of active TB would often delay seeking medical attention until they had passed the three-month window period and were insured by the provincial/territorial health plan.

Refugee claimants with inactive TB were referred for surveillance through the same process as used for immigrants. At the time of the case, one difference between immigrants and refugee claimants was the federal role. Although refugee claimants, like immigrants, also would not have to be covered by the provincial health insurance plans for three months after they qualified as Canadian residents, in the event that refugees required further medical care (e.g., treatment of TB), the cost of their care was paid by the federal government under the Interim Federal Health Program. Health care providers billed the federal government directly for services provided to refugees and their dependents. As noted above, this has subsequently been modified and coverage substantially reduced.

Medical surveillance is a complicated process involving the transfer of information among three levels of government (federal, provincial, and municipal) and involves the cooperation of both the immigrant/refugee population and the health care sector. It is perhaps not surprising that approximately half of the new immigrants to Ontario who were targeted for medical surveillance never made contact with their local public health unit and only 20% of immigrants adhered to the requirements of medical surveillance. By the time of the case, the vast majority of active TB cases diagnosed in Toronto occurred in foreign-born individuals, but almost all of them were diagnosed during physician visits because of symptoms rather than because they had been under surveillance by public health. These statistics collected by public health suggested that the immigration medical screening was not identifying the majority of people who ended up developing disease once in Canada, although it may have been more effective in preventing infected individuals from being admitted to Canada at all.

APPENDIX D: REFERENCES CITED AND FURTHER READING

Citizenship & Immigration Canada. (2008). *Refugee claims in Canada: Who can apply.* http://www.cic.gc.ca/english/refugees/inside/apply-who.asp

Health Canada & Public Health Agency of Canada. (2012). *It's your health: Tuberculosis.* http://www.hc-sc.gc.ca/hl-vs/alt_formats/pacrb-dgapcr/pdf/iyh-vsv/diseases-maladies/tuberculosis-eng.pdf

Public Health Agency of Canada. (2012). *Tuberculosis in Canada 2010 –*
  *Pre-release.* Public Health Agency of Canada, Minister of Public Works
  and Government Services. http://www.phac-aspc.gc.ca/tbpc-latb/pubs/
  tbcan10pre/
World Health Organization. (2012, March). *Tuberculosis* (Fact Sheet #104).
  http://www.who.int/mediacentre/factsheets/fs104/en/index.html

The following websites may also be helpful:

The Public Health Agency of Canada TB, http://www.phac-aspc
  .gc.ca/tbpc-latb
The World Health Organization TB, http://www.who.int/topics/
  tuberculosis/en

# 3 Making Canadians Healthier

## Where Do We Start?

NURLAN ALGASHOV, PATRICIA BARANEK, SHERRY BISCOPE,
KATHRYN CLARKE, MARK DOBROW, ASMITA GILLANI, IRENE
KOO, CATHERINE L. MAH, BRANDY MCKENNA, MICHÈLE PARENT,
MIRIAM ALTON SCHARF, SHAHZAD SIDDIQUI, LOUISE SIGNAL,
RACHEL WORTZMAN, AND RAISA B. DEBER

What is health? How can government policy help to improve the health of a population?

This case addresses several policy issues, including: the determinants of health, the concept and implementation of healthy public policy, the role of health indicators, framing, public/private roles and responsibilities, policy instruments, and the roles of state/market.

**Appendices**

Appendix A: Population Health and the Determinants of Health
Appendix B: Health Indicators and Selected Data
Appendix C: Provincial Government Ministries, 2012
Appendix D: References Cited and Further Reading

**The Case**

What makes people healthy? Definitions vary (see Chapter 1, section 6.3, What Is Health?), but the focus of public policy has increasingly shifted, from defining health narrowly as the absence of disease to acceptance of a broader, socially based definition of health which recognizes that social, economic, and environmental, as well as biological and lifestyle factors, can influence a person's health (see Appendix A: Population Health and the Determinants of Health).

Using information about health to guide policy in turn evokes a number of issues. What are the appropriate roles and responsibilities for government, as opposed to the market, individuals and their families, and civil society? What policy instruments can be used? Within government, what is the responsibility of ministries of health, and what lies within the jurisdiction of other government departments? Where should policy interventions be targeted; this can range from targeting individuals to targeting the population as a whole? Who should pay for what?

Faced with continuously increasing expenditures for health care, governments have turned towards the use of indicators to monitor performance, including seeing whether they are receiving value for the money being spent. You have been asked by your provincial government to review what might make the population healthier, examine available indicators, and recommend how best to deploy resources to improve the health of the population.

## The Determinants of Health and Healthy Public Policy

Your first step was to review what was meant by health. Your review clarified that the definition of health has been somewhat contentious. Immediately after World War II, in the preamble to its Constitution, the World Health Organization (WHO) defined health as "a state of complete physical, mental and social well-being and not merely the absence of disease or infirmity" (World Health Organization, 1948). Although this definition reflected laudable objectives, it was not always clear how these goals could be achieved. Instead, the focus for health care in most industrialized nations has been on the provision of an increasingly advanced set of technologies and medical services to individuals who are ill. However, there were also a variety of different types of welfare state policies in different countries that sought to address factors that might affect health status, including social cohesion, education, and poverty.

You also discovered that Canada played a leading role in developing this new vision of health. In 1974, the federal government of Canada published a milestone document, *A New Perspective on the Health of Canadians*, commonly referred to as the Lalonde Report after the then-Minister of National Health and Welfare (Lalonde, 1974). This report suggested that the health of populations was affected by the following four categories of factors (which it termed "fields"): human biology, environment, lifestyle, and health care organization. It thus incorporated, but went beyond the traditional focus on, providing clinical services to sick people (health care organization) and understanding the biological causes of disease (human biology). It used the term "environment" to refer to both physical and social environmental factors over which individuals would have little or no control. Lifestyle referred to personal decisions that could contribute to illness or death (including smoking, diet, and exercise). The report thus was among the first government documents to recognize the importance of a broader array of what soon came to be known as "determinants of health" and to focus on how best to improve "population health."

How to act on these insights in terms of public policy, however, remained unclear. In the face of economic shocks related to oil prices in the early to mid-1970s, many jurisdictions had begun to try to reduce the size of government and pursue more fiscally conservative policies. One immediate response to the Lalonde Report was to emphasize the contribution to health of one of these fields, individual lifestyle choices, particularly since policymakers believed that these questions could be addressed at a relatively low cost to public budgets. Health promotion activities began to target the health risks associated with smoking, alcohol, nutrition, fitness, and mental health. At the federal level, in 1978, the Canadian government restructured its Department of National Health and Welfare to include a Health Promotion Directorate, the first of its kind in the world. Most provincial governments followed suit and established health promotion structures; these have had a variety of organizational homes, including public health departments, provincial ministries of health, and/or arm's length agencies. As Chapter 1, section 2.2.1 (Federalism in Canada) notes, because some questions existed as to the roles of the federal and provincial/territorial governments in dealing with these issues, the government of Canada has tended to concentrate on advocacy and generating/providing information rather than service delivery, except for the areas clearly under federal jurisdiction.

You found that the WHO has repeatedly embraced concepts associated with population health. At the World Health Assembly in 1977, WHO resolved that the main social target of governments and of WHO in the coming decades should be the attainment by all citizens of the World by the year 2000 of a level of health that would permit them to lead a socially and economically productive life. This commitment became known as the Health for All by the Year 2000 movement. In 1978, the Alma Ata Declaration emerged from an International Health Conference on Primary Health Care (PHC); it endorsed the Health for All goal, and suggested it could be attained through PHC, broadly defined as encompassing health education, health promotion, community participation, and intersectoral cooperation (World Health Organization, 1978). Another key WHO document is known as the Ottawa Charter for Health Promotion (World Health Organization, 1986). It defined health as "a resource for everyday life, not the objective of living. Health is a positive concept emphasizing social and personal resources, as well as physical capacities" and defined health promotion as "the process of enabling people to increase control over, and to improve their health." Additional information about population health and the determinants of health is noted in Appendix A.

Within Canada, at the national level, Health Canada attempted to move beyond a focus on individual risk factors and behaviours by considering the social, economic, and environmental components that determine individual behaviour and consequently affect health. A new set of strategies, including mutual aid, healthy public policy, and community developments, was added. Some of these goals were expanded on in *Achieving Health for All: A Framework for Health Promotion*, usually called the Epp Report after the then-Minister of National Health and Welfare Jake Epp (1986). These strategies stressed the importance of population health rather than just individually focused care, and of dealing with "equity" across population groups. (These key reports thus became relatively nonpartisan, since Lalonde had been a federal Liberal cabinet minister, and Epp a cabinet minister in a Progressive Conservative government.)

The term *healthy public policy* has been used to refer to ensuring that all policy actions are taken with regard to the implications for health and equity. A common definition comes from the WHO's 1988 conference in Adelaide, Australia: "Healthy public policy is characterized by an explicit concern for health and equity in all areas of policy and by an accountability for health impact. The main aim of health public policy is to create a supportive environment to enable people to lead healthy lives. Such a policy makes health choices possible or easier for citizens. It makes social and physical environments health-enhancing. In the pursuit of healthy public policy, government sectors concerned with agriculture, trade, education, industry, and communications need to take into account health as an essential factor when formulating policy. These sectors should be accountable for the health consequences of their policy decisions. They should pay as much attention to health as to economic considerations" (World Health Organization, 1988).

The healthy public policy approach has been echoed in many Canadian provinces, but it has not always been easy to operationalize. One suggestion came from Canada's Federal, Provincial and Territorial Advisory Committee on Population Health, an enthusiastic advocate for the population health approach, which broadened the Lalonde report to suggest that there were eight key determinants of health. This committee also produced two reports on the health of Canadians. Their first report found that Canadians were among the healthiest people in the world, but that health was not enjoyed equally; those who were relatively disadvantaged with regard to factors like employment and early childhood circumstances were likely to have poorer health (Federal Provincial and Territorial Advisory Committee on Population Health, 1996). Their second report provided additional data from such sources as the National Population Health Survey and the National Longitudinal Survey on Children and Youth about the health status of Canadian men and women. It related health to a wide range of factors, including: income, education and literacy, employment and working conditions, social support, violence, civic participation, child and youth development, the physical environment, personal health practices, health services, and biology and genetic endowment (Federal Provincial and Territorial Advisory Committee on Population Health, 1999). The scope for potential policy intervention broadened accordingly to include such suggestions as: create a thriving and sustainable economy with meaningful work for all; encourage lifelong learning; and foster friendship and social support networks in families and communities. Implementing these policies would require drawing in various levels of government and multiple departments, as well as workplaces, universities, urban planners, and citizens.

The Public Health Agency of Canada (PHAC) website (Public Health Agency of Canada, 2010) further expanded this list to include the following 12 determinants: (1) income and social status; (2) social support networks; (3) education and literacy; (4) employment/working conditions; (5) social environments; (6) physical environments; (7) personal health practices and coping skills; (8) healthy child development; (9) biology and genetic endowment; (10) health services; (11) gender; and (12) culture. Again, it was not clear which of these determinants should be acted on, how, or by whom. Healthy public policy, which calls for taking health consequences into account when making seemingly unrelated policies, accordingly can be viewed both as taking a broad vision of health, crossing traditional departmental and ministerial boundaries, and incorporating community participation into decision making, but also as medical imperialism (assuming that health consequences should trump other factors) and even ministerial imperialism (assuming that health ministries are more important than other government departments).

Although these findings may or may not continue to hold, you did find a 2008 study that compared the richest 20% of Canadians to the poorest 20%, and found that the poorest 20% were indeed sicker (Lightman et al., 2008). They had double the rate of diabetes and heart disease, nearly double the rate of arthritis or rheumatism, and more than three times the rate of bronchitis. They were more likely to have two or more chronic health conditions, and four times as likely to have a disability. They were much less likely to have private insurance coverage for services falling outside the *Canada Health Act* requirements (see Chapter 1, section 7.2, *Canada Health Act*), including prescription medications and dental care. However, you recognize that this study does not demonstrate the direction of causality; it was also possible that poor health contributed to poverty, particularly if those who were sick or disabled were less likely to be able to be employed full-time (and also less likely to have insurance benefits that were employment-based). There were also likely to be interactive effects if poverty made it harder to afford healthy food, or have good housing.

Attempting to implement a determinants of health framework when formulating public policy has highlighted several potential policy trade-offs. How much emphasis should be placed on the needs of the broader population, versus the needs of those requiring sickness care? How much emphasis should be placed on overall levels of health, as opposed to improving equity and paying greater attention to vulnerable populations? How much emphasis should be placed on quantity of life, as opposed to its quality?

**Indicators**

Statistics Canada and the Canadian Institute for Health Information (CIHI) have collected extensive information relating to the health status of the population. Not all information is regularly collected, but you did find some data (albeit sometimes rather old) on the burden of disease, on causes of hospitalization, and on potential years of life lost from various causes, both overall and for various age-sex groups. You also consulted data collected by the Organisation for Economic Co-operation and Development (OECD) to see how Canada compares with other industrialized nations (see also Chapter 1, section 9.2, Comparative Health Data, for what data is collected). The tables you generated are in Appendix B.

You then considered who might implement whatever initiatives you might consider, and who would be responsible for ensuring these were implemented. Your provincial government contains a wide variety of ministries and other agencies, as noted in Appendix C.

You also recognize that everyone dies of something. To what extent do cross-sectional indicators reflect the societal burden of chronic (non-communicable) disease, which is rising in many countries? Are there likely to be differences by age group? By gender? What emphasis should be placed on conditions which affect quality of life, as opposed to life expectancy? Should you focus on costs of treatment? On the likelihood of preventing adverse outcomes?

DECISION POINT

You are the chair of a healthy public policy committee. What would your priorities be? What policy initiatives would you recommend to the provincial government to make the population healthier? How might this affect how you deploy resources? Who should be responsible for designing and implementing these initiatives?

SUGGESTED QUESTIONS FOR DISCUSSION

1. How would you define/measure health? How do the various definitions of health affect the potential policies you might recommend?
2. Discuss the different indicators noted in Appendix B (including death rates, PYLL, and hospitalizations). What would each suggest as policy priorities? What might be omitted?
3. Discuss framing as it applies to how the policy problem is defined.
4. Who would be responsible for implementing these policy alternatives? Discuss the roles of government, "civil society," the market, and individuals and their families. What values/ideologies are reflected?
5. What policy instruments might you employ?
6. Discuss the campaign against smoking. What does it tell you about the strengths and weaknesses of health promotion campaigns?

APPENDIX A: POPULATION HEALTH AND
THE DETERMINANTS OF HEALTH

There is an extensive literature describing the importance of non-medical factors in affecting both individual and population health. Poverty is clearly associated with inadequacies in such necessities as housing, sanitation, and nutrition. Education is another key factor; although education is correlated with income, education is also independently associated with higher life expectancies.

Equity is also important. Wilkinson (1996) noted that there is a relation between average income and life expectancy at birth for poor countries up to a ceiling (which he placed at about US$5,000). Beyond that figure, however, he found little relation between average income and life expectancy of the citizenry. Wilkinson posited that a key factor was the distribution of wealth in the population. According to his hypothesis, an increase in average income of a nation may even be associated with a decline in overall health if most of the new wealth makes inequality worse by being concentrated in a few hands. Wilkinson also demonstrated that changes in life expectancy may be correlated with changes in income distribution. Similar results were found by Sir Michael Marmot et al. The Whitehall I and II studies followed the self-reported health and morbidity/mortality of 10,000 British civil servants over nearly two decades (Marmot et al., 1991). The participants in the Whitehall I study were male, mostly white, employed in office jobs, and living or working in the greater London area. None of the participants were subject to industrial hazards or extremes of poverty or affluence. Yet the age-standardized mortality rate of those in the highest employment grade was one-third the rate of those in the lowest employment grade, suggesting an inverse relationship between social class and mortality. Lifestyle factors as well as commonly accepted risk factors for ill health only partially explained this difference. The Whitehall II study attempted to examine the other social and behavioural factors that might contribute to differences in health status; this study also included women. Ultimately, the Whitehall studies posited that health status may be affected by such psychosocial factors as autonomy and control over decision making in addition to other known social, economic, and behavioural determinants of health. Marmot went on to chair the WHO Commission on Social Determinants of Health, founded in 2005. The commission's 2008 report, *Closing the Gap in a Generation*, called upon national governments to focus public policies on the goal of health equity. The commission argued that health inequalities arise from the range of circumstances in which people "grow, live, work, and age, and the systems put in place to deal with illness ... shaped by political, social, and economic forces" (World Health Organization, 2008).

Another widely cited document, the 1986 *Ottawa Charter for Health Promotion*, identified the prerequisites for health as peace, shelter, education, food, income, a stable ecosystem, sustainable resources, social justice, and equity (World Health Organization, 1986).

Many researchers have since pointed out that health care alone cannot counteract the effects of these factors on health. If adopted, these findings would represent a paradigm shift from a biomedical model of health to one that also focuses on broader social, economic, environmental, and physical determinants of health (Mikkonen & Raphael, 2010).

APPENDIX B: HEALTH INDICATORS AND SELECTED DATA

The indicator movement argues that "what is measured is what matters" (Bevan & Hood, 2006).

In Canada, Statistics Canada and the Canadian Institute for Health Information (CIHI), in cooperation with the Federal/Provincial/Territorial Advisory Committees on Population Health and Health Services, have divided health indicators into four types: health status (e.g., mortality rates); non-medical determinants of health (e.g., health behaviours, education, employment); health system performance (e.g., readmission rates); and community and health system indicators (e.g., population density, health provider access). CIHI has published an annual indicators report since 2002 and suggests that health indicators are useful because they can inform the public and the health sector, and be used for performance management, monitoring, quality improvement, and policy and planning (see also Chapter 1, section 9.1, Canadian Data). The WHO has also developed a series of health indicators, which it publishes yearly for all member states. Similarly, the OECD provides comparable data for its 30 member countries (see Chapter 1, section 9.2, Comparative Health Data). You note that, due to implementation of new revisions of the International Classification of

Diseases (ICD) and other coding changes, there may be breaks in some of these series, because data are considered consistent only within the same ICD revision.

You have used these sources to obtain data on a number of indicators, including: *mortality* (causes of death); *healthy life expectancy; potential years of life lost* (PYLL); *causes of hospitalization*; and selected *risk factors*. You note that there is a considerable time lag before some of this data is made available, and a tendency to make minor changes in definitions. For example, in late 2011, the most recent information about death and hospitalization by age-sex group on the PHAC website was for 2005. (There was also some data for the full population for 2008 on the Statistics Canada website, but it used similar but not directly comparable categories, so you decided to stick with the PHAC numbers.)

Table 3.1 summarizes the information you found about the top 10 causes of death for the full population of Canada in 2005. For each of these causes, you have included the number who died from that cause, the rate per 100,000 population, and the percentage that cause represented of total deaths.

You note that almost 95% of 2005 deaths were as a result of the top 10 causes; indeed, over half resulted from circulatory system diseases (31%) and cancer (30%). (This dropped to a still high 76.8% for the top 10 causes for the 2008 Statistics Canada table, which, as noted above, used slightly different categories.) You do some further analysis by age-sex group. Table 3.2 presents similar data for each age group, arranged in the same order as total deaths. In each cell, you note the rank for that age group (from #1 to #10) in parentheses, followed by the rate per 100,000 people in that age group. You add rows to Table 3.2 for those causes of death that were in the top 10 for a particular age group, but not for the full population, and for the rate and number of deaths in each age group. You further note that, if the rate was too small for one of the top 10, the exact number of deaths in the reported data is suppressed; when this occurred, you have omitted the rate from your tables.

You can see from the table that, in most age groups, the same top 10 causes did account for most of the deaths, but there were some exceptions, such as perinatal and congenital anomalies in the youngest age groups. Comparing Tables 3.1 and 3.2, you further note that 178,378 of the 230,129 total deaths (77.5%) in 2005 occurred in people over age 65.

Table 3.1. Leading Causes of Death, Canada, 2005 (all ages)

| 2005 Rank & Cause | # of Deaths | Rate per 100,000 | % of Total |
|---|---|---|---|
| 1. Circulatory system diseases | 71,749 | 222.5 | 31.18 |
| 2. Cancer | 68,790 | 213.3 | 29.89 |
| 3. Respiratory system diseases | 20,484 | 63.5 | 8.90 |
| 4. Nervous system diseases | 10,796 | 33.5 | 4.69 |
| 5. Endocrine, nutritional, and metabolic diseases | 10,266 | 31.8 | 4.46 |
| 6. Accidents (unintentional injuries) | 9,505 | 29.5 | 4.13 |
| 7. Digestive system diseases | 8,952 | 27.8 | 3.89 |
| 8. Mental disorders | 7,750 | 24.0 | 3.37 |
| 9. Genitourinary diseases | 5,200 | 16.1 | 2.26 |
| 10. Infectious & parasitic diseases | 4,154 | 12.9 | 1.81 |
| All causes | 230,129 | 713.7 | 100.00 |
| Total: Top 10 | 217,646 | | 94.58 |

Source: Adapted from Public Health Agency of Canada, Injury Prevention, Table 1, http://www.phac-aspc.gc.ca/publicat/lcd-pcd97/table1-eng.php.

Similarly, of the 71,749 deaths from circulatory system diseases, 62,122 (72%) were in this age group.

You read that life expectancy is considered to be a relatively objective indicator of a population's health in any given year, since it summarizes mortality rates from only that year and does not rely on predictions of what future mortality rates will be. The life expectancy indicator consists of the average number of years that a hypothetical group of individuals born in a specified year would live if the observed mortality rates at each age for that year were to remain constant in succeeding years. You have used data taken from OECD Health Data, November 2011. To allow international comparisons, you have used 2004 data,

Table 3.2 Leading Causes of Death in Canada 2005, Rank and Rate per 100,000 by Age Group, Ordered by Rank in Full Population

| Cause of death | < 1 | 1–4 | 5–9 | 10–14 | 15–19 | 20–24 | 25–34 | 35–44 | 45–54 | 55–64 | 65 + |
|---|---|---|---|---|---|---|---|---|---|---|---|
| Circulatory system | (#10)4.7 | (#10)0.9 | (#7)0.4 | (#5)1.0 | (#5)1.7 | (#5)2.3 | (#4)5.3 | (#4)16.5 | (#2)55.6 | (#2)159.8 | (#1)1472.1 |
| Cancer | NA | (#3)2.1 | (#2)2.6 | (#2)2.1 | (#3)3.0 | (#3)4.4 | (#3)8.3 | (#1)29.8 | (#1)111.1 | (#1)326.6 | (#2)1174.3 |
| Respiratory system | (#9)5.6 | (#7)1.0 | (#5)0.5 | (#8)0.4 | (#9)0.6 | (#8)0.9 | – | (#9)2.7 | (#8)8.2 | (#3)33.7 | (#3)441.0 |
| Nervous system | (#4)12.1 | (#4)1.6 | (#3)1.0 | (#4)1.4 | (#6)1.6 | (#6)1.8 | (#6)2.3 | (#8)3.5 | (#9)7.8 | (#7)18.5 | (#4)220.2 |
| Endocrine, nutr., & metab. | (#7)7.4 | (#5)1.5 | (#6)0.4 | (#7)0.5 | (#8)0.7 | (#7)1.2 | (#8)1.4 | (#7)3.8 | (#6)10.4 | (#5)30.2 | (#5)197.1 |
| Unintentional injuries | (#6)8.5 | (#1)5.4 | (#1)3.4 | (#1)4.5 | (#1)21.0 | (#1)25.0 | (#1)19.1 | (#2)19.0 | (#3)22.6 | (#6)23.1 | (#9)106.4 |
| Digestive system | (#8)6.8 | (#9)0.9 | (#8)0.3 | – | – | – | (#9)1.3 | (#6)14.8 | (#5)15.0 | (#4)31.7 | (#7)159.5 |
| Mental disorders | NA | – | – | – | – | – | (#10)1.2 | (#10)2.3 | (#10)4.7 | (#10)7.5 | (#6)167.4 |
| Genitourinary | NA | – | – | – | – | – | – | – | – | – | (#8)113.6 |
| Infectious & parasitic | (#5)9.1 | (#6)1.0 | (#10) | (#7)0.3 | (#10)0.4 | (#10)0.6 | (#7)1.6 | (#5)5.4 | (#7)8.7 | (#9)11.4 | (#10)68.5 |
| Blood | – | – | (#9) | – | – | – | – | – | – | – | – |
| Suicide | – | – | – | (#3)2.0 | (#2)9.8 | (#2)13.3 | (#2)11.8 | (#3)17.2 | (#4)17.9 | (#8)13.0 | – |
| Congenital anomalies | (#2)131.8 | (#2)2.6 | (#4)0.7 | (#6)0.9 | (#7)0.8 | (#9)0.7 | – | – | – | – | – |
| Homicide | – | (#8)1.0 | – | (#10)0.2 | (#4)2.3 | (#4)3.8 | (#5)3.3 | – | – | – | – |
| Perinatal | (#1)305.7 | – | – | – | – | – | – | – | – | – | – |
| SIDS | (#3)33.3 | – | – | – | – | – | – | – | – | – | – |
| All causes: Rate | 549.2 | 20.6 | 10.6 | 14.6 | 45.3 | 60.1 | 64.8 | 118.5 | 279.0 | 680.8 | 4,227.1 |
| Total number of deaths | 1863 | 282 | 198 | 311 | 986 | 1342 | 2806 | 6051 | 13765 | 24147 | 178378 |

Source: Adapted from Public Health Agency of Canada, Injury Prevention, Table 1, http://www.phac-aspc.gc.ca/publicat/lcd-pcd97/table1-eng.php.

since there is considerable missing data for subsequent years for some countries, including Canada.

OECD Health Data indicated that life expectancy at birth for Canada in 2007 was 83.0 for females and 78.3 for males, for a population average of 80.7. Both numbers were very similar to findings for other OECD countries. For those who had already reached the age of 65, additional life expectancy for females was computed to be 21.3 years, and for males 18.1 years.

*Health-adjusted life expectancy* (HALE) is defined as the average number of years that a person can expect to live in "full health" by taking into account years lived in less than full health due to disease and/or injury (World Health Organization, 2011). Although you were not able to find more recent data about this indicator for Canada, a government of Canada webpage on indicators of well-being in Canada notes that, in 2001, men were expected to spend 88.8% (68.3 years) of their life in good health, compared with 86.3% (70.8 years) for women (Human Resources and Skills Development Canada, 2012a).

*Potential years of life lost* (PYLL) is the number of years of life "lost" when a person dies prematurely before a specified age. If that value is set at age 75, then a person dying at age 25 has lost 50 years of life (75 – 25 = 50 PYLL). PYLL helps to identify causes of death which occur in younger age groups and which can, in theory, be prevented or postponed. The calculation of PYLL involves summing up deaths occurring at each age and multiplying this by the number of remaining years that would have allowed these people to live up to a selected age limit (the OECD uses 70). Anyone dying at age 40 thus represents 30 PYLL (70–40 = 30). To allow comparisons, the OECD computation also standardizes the PYLL to a reference population (in the tables you consulted, they used the total OECD population in 1980). You cannot find PYLL calculations for Canada for years after 2004; you noted that the value reported for 100,000 Canadian females aged 0–69 was 2,554; for males it was 4,168. Table 3.3 gives some OECD data comparing PYLL for Canada and selected other countries.

You also noted that the OECD reported that Canada's 2007 infant mortality rate per 1,000 live births was 5.1. While lower than that in the United States (6.8), it was higher than the rate in other developed countries (e.g., the rate in Sweden is 2.5), but you also know that there are some definitional issues about what deaths are reported (particularly in what is considered to be a live birth), and how they are classified,

Table 3.3. Potential Years of Life Lost, 2004, by Sex, Selected Countries

| 2004 | Females < 69 | Males < 69 |
|------|------|------|
| Australia | 2289 | 3946 |
| Austria | 2386 | 4619 |
| Canada | 2554 | 4168 |
| Denmark | 2818 | 4603 |
| France | 2361 | 4879 |
| Germany | 2351 | 4354 |
| Netherlands | 2500 | 3693 |
| New Zealand | 3008 | 4529 |
| Norway | 2434 | 3961 |
| Sweden | 2306 | 3535 |
| Switzerland | 2133 | 3769 |
| United Kingdom | 2723 | 4388 |
| United States | 3639 | 6228 |

Source: Organisation for Economic Co-operation and Development (2011).

which somewhat impedes the ability to use this measure for international comparisons.

You next look at the PHAC tables for leading causes of hospitalization in 2005–6, which is broken down by age group. Table 3.4 parallels Table 3.2; it provides the rank and the crude rate per 100,000 population in each age group.

You also check some government websites for risk factors. You find a page about indicators of well-being in Canada on the Human Resources and Skills Development Canada website (Human Resources and Skills Development Canada, 2012b). You do not feel it necessary to construct tables, but do note that smoking rates were down but still substantial. In 2005, 22% of Canadians reported being a smoker, compared with 29% in 1994–5. For 2008, the percentage of all females aged 15+ who were daily cigarette smokers was 15.1; for males it was 19.1. You noted that the value in 1964 had been 30% of females and 54% of males. Obesity was high and increasing; in 2005, a large proportion of Canadian adults were overweight (35%) or obese (24%), and only 39% were of normal weight. In terms of physical activity, in 2005, 47% of Canadians were considered inactive, 25% considered moderately active, and 27% considered active. You also looked at some data on risk factors. Alcohol consumption in litres per capita (for those over age 15) was 7.6 in 1964 and 8.2 in 2009.

Table 3.4 Leading Causes of Hospitalization in Canada, 2005–6, by Age Group (rank and rate per 100,000)

| Cause | All Ages | < 1 | 1–4 | 5–9 | 10–14 | 15–19 | 20–25 | 25–34 | 35–44 | 45–54 | 55–64 | 65 + |
|---|---|---|---|---|---|---|---|---|---|---|---|---|
| Circulatory system | (#1)1,196.1 | – | – | – | – | – | – | (#8)104.3 | (#6)286.4 | (#2)818.5 | (#1)1998.6 | (#1)5905.6 |
| Digestive system | (#2)926.1 | (#4)1312.4 | (#2)504.9 | (#3)269.4 | (#2)302.3 | (#3)455.0 | (#2)481.2 | (#2)562.8 | (#1)661.2 | (#1)886.6 | (#3)1253.6 | (#3)2564.1 |
| Respiratory system | (#3)742.7 | (#2)4497.3 | (#1)1966.3 | (#1)609.3 | (#3)238.9 | (#4)250.0 | (#5)182.9 | (#5)172.3 | (#8)192.9 | (#8)299.7 | (#5)678.5 | (#2)2704.2 |
| Cancer | (#4)647.8 | – | – | – | – | – | (#10)71.3 | (#7)136.9 | (#5)358.3 | (#3)695.1 | (#2)1253.6 | (#4)2361.8 |
| Unintentional injuries | (#5)600.5 | (#8)357.9 | (#4)360.0 | (#2)292.1 | (#1)348.6 | (#2)463.8 | (#3)403.0 | (#3)340.3 | (#4)368.7 | (#6)429.1 | (#7)549.3 | (#5)1919.7 |
| Mental disorders | (#6)507.7 | – | – | – | (#4)199.2 | (#1)572.9 | (#1)613.3 | (#1)623.0 | (#2)640.5 | (#4)587.7 | (#8)443.4 | (#8)663.6 |
| Genito-urinary | (#7)500.8 | (#6)852.4 | (#7)138.8 | (#6)83.1 | (#8)66.8 | (#5)142.4 | (#4)185.8 | (#4)307.7 | (#3)512.0 | (#5)533.0 | (#6)642.7 | (#7)1365.1 |
| Musculoskeletal | (#8)449.1 | – | – | (#8)66.6 | (#6)95.7 | (#6)116.7 | (#6)103.4 | (#6)148.4 | (#7)243.1 | (#7)390.5 | (#4)780.3 | (#6)1645.8 |
| Endocrine, nutr., & metab. | (#9)199.0 | (#10)168.7 | (#10)87.6 | (#9)58.7 | (#7)74.3 | (#8)92.8 | (#7)86.2 | (#9)93.9 | (#9)121.8 | (#9)171.4 | (#9)271.9 | (#9)654.7 |
| Nervous system | (#10)195.9 | (#7)420.4 | (#5)257.1 | (#5)127.3 | (#5)97.4 | (#9)81.3 | – | (#10)87.1 | (#10)115.7 | (#10)158.2 | (#10)229.1 | (#10)587.2 |
| Blood diseases | – | – | (#9)103.1 | (#7)75.7 | – | – | – | – | – | – | – | – |
| Congenital anomalies | – | (#3)1507.1 | (#6)166.3 | (#10)57.4 | (#10)45.6 | – | – | – | – | – | – | – |
| Infectious diseases | – | (#5)1012.4 | (#3)447.2 | (#4)133.7 | (#9)65.6 | (#10)79.9 | – | – | – | – | – | – |

(Continued)

Table 3.4. (Continued)

| Cause | All Ages | < 1 | 1–4 | 5–9 | 10–14 | 15–19 | 20–25 | 25–34 | 35–44 | 45–54 | 55–64 | 65 + |
|---|---|---|---|---|---|---|---|---|---|---|---|---|
| Perinatal | – | (#1)5029.4 | – | – | – | – | – | – | – | – | – | – |
| Skin/ subcutaneous tissue | – | (#9)179.1 | (#8)106.7 | – | – | – | – | – | – | – | – | – |
| Self-inflicted injuries | – | – | – | – | – | (#7)107.3 | (#8)86.0 | – | – | – | – | – |
| Assault | – | – | – | – | – | – | (#9)78.7 | – | – | – | – | – |
| All Causes | 8,696.1 | 18,202.6 | 4,948.6 | 2,224.1 | 1,993.7 | 3797.2 | 5934.4 | 8875.8 | 5669.5 | 6114.6 | 9898.6 | 24727.7 |

Source: Adapted from Public Health Agency of Canada, Injury Prevention, Table 2, http://www.phac-aspc.gc.ca/publicat/lcd-pcd97/table2-eng.php.

APPENDIX C: PROVINCIAL GOVERNMENT MINISTRIES, 2012

As of 2012, your provincial government had the following ministries:

Aboriginal Affairs
Agriculture, Food and Rural Affairs
Attorney General
Children and Youth Services
Citizenship and Immigration
Community and Social Services
Community Safety and Correctional Services
Consumer Services
Economic Development and Innovation
Education
Energy
Environment
Finance
Francophone Affairs
Government Services
Health and Long-Term Care
Infrastructure
Intergovernmental Affairs
Labour
Municipal Affairs and Housing
Natural Resources
Northern Development and Mines
Seniors' Secretariat
Tourism, Culture and Sport
Training, Colleges and Universities
Transportation
Women's Directorate

You note that most provincial/territorial governments have structures to handle similar functions, although they are not always arranged in the same way as in your province.

APPENDIX D: REFERENCES CITED AND FURTHER READING

Bevan, G., & Hood, C. (2006). What's measured is what matters: Targets and gaming in the English public health care system. *Public Administration, 84*(3), 517–38. http://dx.doi.org/10.1111/j.1467-9299.2006.00600.x

Black, D., Morris, J.N., Smith, C., Townsend, P., & Whitehead, M. (1990). *Inequalities in health: The Black report and the health divide* (2nd ed.). London: Penguin Books.

Bowen, S., & Kreindler, S.A. (2008). Indicator madness: A cautionary reflection on the use of indicators in healthcare. *Health Policy (Amsterdam), 3*(4), 41–8.

Canadian Institute for Health Information. (2005). *Select highlights on public views of the determinants of health*. Canadian Population Health Initiative. https://secure.cihi.ca/estore/productSeries.htm?pc=PCC267

Epp, J. (1986). Achieving health for all: A framework for health promotion. *Health Promotion International, 1*(4), 419–28. http://dx.doi.org/10.1093/heapro/1.4.419

Etches, V., Frank, J., Di Ruggiero, E., & Manuel, D. (2006). Measuring population health: A review of indicators. *Annual Review of Public Health, 27*(1), 29–55. http://dx.doi.org/10.1146/annurev.publhealth.27.021405.102141

Federal Provincial and Territorial Advisory Committee on Population Health. (1996). *Report on the health of Canadians*. Prepared for the Meeting of Ministers of Health. http://www.cwhn.ca/en/node/24009

Federal Provincial and Territorial Advisory Committee on Population Health. (1999). *Toward a healthy future: Second report on the health of Canadians*. Prepared for the Meeting of Ministers of Health. http://publications.gc.ca/collections/Collection/H39-468-1999E.pdf

Frankish, C.J., Casebeer, A.L., Moulton, G.E., Eyles, J.D., Quantz, D., Labonte, R., et al. (2007). Addressing the non-medical determinants of health. *Canadian Journal of Public Health, 98*(1), 41–7.

Frohlich, K.L., Ross, N., & Richmond, C. (2006). Health disparities in Canada today: Some evidence and a theoretical framework. *Health Policy (Amsterdam), 79*(2–3), 132–43. http://dx.doi.org/10.1016/j.healthpol.2005.12.010

Health Canada. (2010). *Healthy Canadians 2010: A federal report on comparable health indicators*. http://www.hc-sc.gc.ca/hcs-sss/pubs/system-regime/2010-fed-comp-indicat/index-eng.php

Human Resources and Skills Development Canada. (2012a). *Health – Life expectancy at birth*. http://www4.hrsdc.gc.ca/.3ndic.1t.4r@-eng.jsp?iid=3

Human Resources and Skills Development Canada. (2012b). *Indicators of well-being in Canada*. http://www4.rhdcc.gc.ca/h.4m.2@-eng.jsp

Lalonde, M. (1974). *A new perspective on the health of Canadians: A working document*. Minister of Supply and Services Canada. http://www.phac-aspc.gc.ca/ph-sp/pdf/perspect-eng.pdf

Lightman, E., Mitchell, A., & Wilson, B. (2008). *Poverty is making us sick: A comprehensive survey of income and health in Canada*. Wellesley Institute. http://

www.wellesleyinstitute.com/wp-content/uploads/2011/11/povertyis
makingussick.pdf

Marmot, M.G., Stansfeld, S., Patel, C., North, F., Head, J., White, I., et al. (1991). Health inequalities among British civil servants: The Whitehall II study. *Lancet, 337*(8754), 1387–93. http://dx.doi.org/10.1016/0140-6736(91)93068-K

Mikkonen, J., & Raphael, D. (2010). *Social determinants of health: The Canadian facts.* York University School of Health Policy and Management. http://www.thecanadianfacts.org/

Organisation for Economic Co-operation and Development. (2011). *Health at a glance 2011: OECD indicators.* OECD Publishing. http://dx.doi.org/10.1787/health_glance-2011-en

Public Health Agency of Canada. (2010). *What determines health?* http://www.phac-aspc.gc.ca/ph-sp/determinants/index-eng.php

Raphael, D. (2006). Social determinants of health: Present status, unanswered questions, and future directions. *International Journal of Health Services, 36*(4), 651–77. http://dx.doi.org/10.2190/3MW4-1EK3-DGRQ-2CRF

Raphael, D., & Bryant, T. (2006). The state's role in promoting population health: Public health concerns in Canada, USA, UK, and Sweden. *Health Policy (Amsterdam), 78*(1), 39–55. http://dx.doi.org/10.1016/j.healthpol.2005.09.002

Raphael, D., Curry-Stevens, A., & Bryant, T. (2008). Barriers to addressing the social determinants of health: Insights from the Canadian experience. *Health Policy (Amsterdam), 88*(2–3), 222–35. http://dx.doi.org/10.1016/j.healthpol.2008.03.015

Statistics Canada & Canadian Institute for Health Information. (2012). *Health indicators 2012.* https://secure.cihi.ca/estore/productFamily.htm?locale=en&pf=PFC1791

Tuohy, C.H., Glouberman, S., & Marmor, T. (2007). The hedgehog and the fox: Glouberman and Marmor on "healthy public policy." *Health Economics, Policy, and Law, 2*(Pt. 1), 107–15. http://dx.doi.org/10.1017/S1744133106006232

Wilkinson, R.G. (1996). *Unhealthy societies: The afflictions of inequality.* London: Routledge. http://dx.doi.org/10.4324/9780203421680

World Health Organization. (1948). *Preamble to the Constitution of the World Health Organization as adopted by the International Health Conference.* http://www.who.int/about/definition/en/print.html

World Health Organization. (1978). *Declaration of Alma-Ata.* WHO Regional Office for Europe. http://www.euro.who.int/en/who-we-are/policy-documents/declaration-of-alma-ata,-1978

World Health Organization. (1986). *Ottawa Charter for Health Promotion, 1986.* http://www.phac-aspc.gc.ca/ph-sp/docs/charter-chartre/index-eng.php

World Health Organization. (1988). *The Adelaide Recommendations: Healthy Public Policies*. http://www.who.int/healthpromotion/conferences/previous/adelaide/en/index.html

World Health Organization. (2008). *Closing the gap in a generation: Health equity through action on the social determinants of health*. Commission on Social Determinants of Health. http://whqlibdoc.who.int/publications/2008/9789241563703_eng.pdf

World Health Organization. (2011). *World health statistics 2011*. http://www.who.int/whosis/whostat/EN_WHS2011_Full.pdf

The following websites may also be helpful:

Health Data, O.E.C.D., http://www.oecd.org/health/health-systems/oecdhealthdata.htm

Human Resources and Skills Development Canada, Indicators of Well-being in Canada, http://www4.rhdcc.gc.ca/h.4m.2@-eng.jsp

Public Health Agency of Canada, What Determines Health? http://www.phac-aspc.gc.ca/ph-sp/determinants/index-eng.php; Injury Prevention, Table 1, http://www.phac-aspc.gc.ca/publicat/lcd-pcd97/table1-eng.php, and Table 2, http://www.phac-aspc.gc.ca/publicat/lcd-pcd97/table2-eng.php

Statistics Canada, Leading Causes of Death in Canada, http://www5.statcan.gc.ca/bsolc/olc-cel/olc-cel?catno=84-215-X&lang=eng

# 4 Trimming the Fat

## Dealing with Obesity

*KATERINA GAPANENKO, CATHERINE L. MAH,*
*SHAHEENA MUKHI, DAVID RUDOLER,*
*AND RAISA B. DEBER*

Rising levels of obesity have led to increasing concern that the next generation will be less healthy than their parents. The implications for health status, and health expenditures, have led to calls for remedial action. What are the alternatives, and who should be responsible for enacting them?

This case, a companion to Chapter 3 (Making Canadians Healthier), addresses several policy issues, including: the determinants of health, the concept and implementation of healthy public policy, framing, public/private roles and responsibilities, policy instruments, and the roles of state/market.

**Appendices**

Appendix A: Stakeholders and Views
Appendix B: References Cited and Further Reading

**The Case**

The proportion of people who are overweight or obese has been increasing in most countries, including Canada. The Organisation for Economic Co-operation and Development (OECD) and the World Health Organization (WHO) have both referred to obesity as a global "epidemic" (Sassi, 2010).

The rise in obesity and overweight has been closely linked to what some call the "nutrition transition," a developmental shift in global diets, food practices, and food supply chains towards greater quantity and variety of foods, accompanied by an increase in consumption of meats, fats, and processed foods (Drewnowski & Popkin, 1997). These trends have been accompanied by a shift in the burden of disease; public health successes in dealing with communicable diseases have meant that morbidity and mortality are increasingly linked to noncommunicable diseases, including cardiovascular diseases, chronic respiratory diseases, some cancers, and diabetes. Common risk factors for many of these conditions include unhealthy diets, physical inactivity, harmful use of alcohol, and tobacco use. Obesity is thus often considered both a health problem and a risk condition associated with other diseases.

In Canada, the prevalence of obesity has been rising. Precise data is often difficult to obtain, with those sources asking people to self-report their weight tending to give lower estimates of how many are overweight, but all agree that obesity is high and increasing. The Public Health Agency of Canada reported findings for 2005 based on both self-reported data and measurement of body mass index (BMI). The measurements found that a large proportion of Canadian adults were overweight (35%) or obese (24%), and only 39% were of normal weight; the remaining 2% were underweight (Human Resources and Skills Development Canada, 2012). It has been suggested that the lifespan of an obese person is approximately two to four years shorter than a person of "normal weight"; for those who are severely obese, the lifespan may be 8 to 10 years shorter (Sassi, 2010). Because childhood and youth obesity rates have also risen significantly, some have suggested that the life expectancy of this generation of children may be shorter than their parents (Olshansky et al., 2005). The rate of overweight and obesity also appears to differ across subpopulations; it appears to be more common among those already disadvantaged in terms of income and education. Obese individuals are also less likely to participate in the labour force than those with normal weights, and when they do participate, they tend to earn less (Mikkonen & Raphael, 2010). A number of public health reports have addressed how best to achieve "healthy weights" (Basrur, 2004; Canadian Institute for Health Information, 2006; Public Health Agency of Canada & Canadian Institute for Health Information, 2011).

Treating overweight, obesity, and the chronic conditions associated with them can be expensive. However, like tobacco, to the extent that obesity is associated with earlier death, the overall cost implications are less clear, particularly if "savings" through not having to pay pensions are also included. For a wide variety of reasons, prevention of obesity would appear to be a wise approach, although there is also debate about which interventions are most effective, and whether they are deemed an appropriate role for government (see Chapter 1, section 3.2, Role of the State). The outcomes of prevention initiatives are also not likely to be visible for many years.

## Background

### *Causes of Obesity*

Obesity results from a combination of biological and behavioural factors, most importantly diet and physical activity (or a lack thereof). Viewing obesity through the lens of the determinants of health, however, suggests a more complex picture. As noted in Chapter 1, section 6.3 (What Is Health?), the Lalonde report divided the factors affecting human health into four categories, which it called fields (Lalonde, 1974). In a very few cases, there are biological/genetic causes (*human biology*). Most cases are due to *lifestyle*, including too little physical activity and consuming more calories than one needs. But lifestyle is also influenced by the *environment* we live in, including a more sedentary lifestyle, communities that are oriented towards transportation by automobile rather than by foot, and the types of products being produced by the food industry. The health care system (*health care organization*) tries to deal with the resulting illnesses, but most observers agree that, in an ideal world, most attention would be paid to how to prevent these conditions from arising in the first place. (See Chapter 3, Making Canadians Healthier, for more information about the social determinants of health.)

The wide variety of factors involved in obesity points to a number of potential policy approaches. In turn, this raises questions about who is responsible for taking what actions. Different stakeholders have different interests and values (see Appendix A). In addition, one must consider issues of which level of government has jurisdiction in different areas.

A number of policy options have been suggested.

One possibility is to provide better information to people about healthy eating. Canada's Food Guide, produced by Health Canada, offers nutrition science-based guidance about what a healthy person should be eating (Health Canada, 2011). However, people do not always know the nutritional or caloric contents of various foods. Since December 2005, Canada also has had a mandatory program for labelling most pre-packaged foods. The Nutrition Facts table on the packages includes information about the caloric content and the amounts of 13 core nutrients, but these are based on the nutritional content per "serving," and there is considerable variability in how these servings are defined. Evidence suggests that many have difficulty in interpreting these labels.

Another issue is that many meals are eaten away from home, in restaurants or as takeout. Should the requirement to disclose nutritional information be extended to restaurants? This in turn, however, would require laboratory analysis of each dish, which could be expensive. Neither are the dishes always standardized; creative chefs may vary in how they make a particular dish at a particular time, and in the size of a portion. Should such requirements be extended only to chain restaurants, which attempt to serve exactly the same dish each time? And where should consumers go to obtain this information? On a website? On the menus of the restaurants? On the wall of the establishment? There are also some voluntary programs, including the Heart and Stroke Foundation's Health Check. Should these be standardized?

Others have suggested taxing less healthy foods and beverages, such as placing taxes on sugar-sweetened beverages. Another approach is to restrict how such foods are marketed, and to whom. Others have suggested outright bans on certain ingredients, such as trans fats. Others suggest limiting access to certain items from schools and other public buildings. Yet such approaches might seem overly paternalistic ("nanny state"), and interfere with people's choices about what they wish to consume (see Chapter 1, section 3.3.2, Liberty). Food also differs from tobacco, in that in most cases consuming a small (or moderate) quantity of a given food or beverage is unlikely to present any health risks.

Others have suggested that the problem is that healthier food is more expensive. A variety of proposals have been made, including subsidizing healthier meals, providing healthier products for no cost to those meeting certain criteria (e.g., through food banks, school lunches, or similar programs), or just giving increased income to the poor to allow them the option of making healthier choices. A related problem relates to transportation, and how easy it is to access stores selling healthy foods.

Others have suggested encouraging more physical activity. Some suggest informational approaches. The Canadian government also produces Canada's Physical Activity Guide. One program, Participaction, has run advertisements urging Canadians to be more physically active.

Others have suggested that local governments build more recreational facilities, which could be free or subsidized. The Canadian government provides tax credits for those enrolling their children in approved recreational activities, which differentially help those with enough income to be paying taxes.

Others have suggested changing the "built environment" within which people live. One option is to encourage bicycle lanes, hiking trails, and other mechanisms to make it easier (and less dangerous) to get more exercise. Another is to encourage good public transportation, safe and vibrant neighbourhoods, and other ways to encourage active living, including alternatives to automobiles when travelling to work or school.

Others have claimed that there is not yet good enough information to drive policy, and suggested improving the data collected to allow better disease surveillance, as well as encouraging more research.

Another option is to wait and treat individuals once they develop health problems. Various therapies are possible, including pharmaceuticals to suppress appetite, dietary counselling for lifestyle and dietary modifications, behavioural therapy, and/or surgical approaches (including gastric bypass surgery or gastric banding). These strategies place much of the onus on individuals to "eat less and be more active" in order to reduce their risk of obesity. To date, however, these efforts have yet to appear effective in decreasing rates of obesity in Canada. Those who have benefitted most are generally those who have the economic and social resources to take advantage of these interventions.

You have been asked to provide recommendations to your provincial government to help it reach its target of reducing childhood obesity by 20% over five years. You are aware that there is likely to be considerable debate about what the state can and should do (see Chapter 1, section 3.2, Role of the State). You also look at the policy instruments available (see Chapter 1, section 5.2, Policy/Governing Instruments). You also consider the views of key stakeholders.


DECISION POINT

What strategies might you consider? What would you recommend? Would focusing on childhood obesity be sufficient to address the obesity epidemic?

SUGGESTED QUESTIONS FOR DISCUSSION

1. What causes obesity? Why is it worth addressing?
2. What policy options might you recommend? What are their advantages and disadvantages? What views do they reflect concerning the appropriate role of the state in addressing obesity? Discuss trade-offs between the importance of protecting the health of the population, respecting individual liberties, and controlling health expenditures.
3. Discuss the impact of how obesity policy might be framed on what policies might be selected.
4. What criteria are you using in deciding what policy options to recommend? How might your recommendations differ if you were: the Deputy Minister of Agriculture? Of Finance? Of Economic Development? Advising the restaurant association? The food industry? The diabetes association?

APPENDIX A: STAKEHOLDERS AND VIEWS

Various policies could involve, at minimum, various *government* departments at the federal, provincial/territorial, and/or local levels with responsibility for a variety of activities, including: agriculture (can set farm policy, subsidize farmers, encourage production of healthy foods, etc.); children and youth services; community and social services; education (can encourage and/or require appropriate healthy food and physical activity standards and programs in schools); finance (can provide tax credits for fitness, etc.); health; health promotion; housing; municipal affairs; recreation and sports; and/or transportation. At the municipal/local level, municipalities, school boards, and/or public health units would often be heavily involved in the implementation of policies, particularly when they would involve transportation, urban planning, education, or public health.

Treatment-based models could also involve such *health professionals* as physicians, nurses, dietitians, and others, as well as the *pharmaceutical industry*.

*Associations* involved with key chronic diseases, including diabetes, cardiac, arthritis, and cancer, would also have an interest in policies that might help prevent these conditions (e.g., the Heart and Stroke Foundation of Canada runs a voluntary Health Check program to identify relatively healthy foods). *Individuals and their families* might also play a role (e.g., parents would presumably be concerned with the health of their children; community groups might also be mobilized).

A series of publicly funded *national agencies* exist that are formally at arm's length from government, and may be involved in collecting, analysing, and disseminating pertinent knowledge and information, and/or enforcing standards, regulations, and compliance. These include: Canadian Fitness and Lifestyle Research Institute (Funded by Health Canada, with a mandate to monitor and track physical activity levels and help promote fitness); Canadian Food Inspection Agency (enforces the regulation on mandatory nutrition labelling and advertisements set by Health Canada; produces guides to food labelling and advertising); Canadian Institute for Health Information (conducts and synthesizes data analyses on priority health issues, and disseminates its findings in a series of reports); Canadian Institutes of Health Research (could provide funding to researchers for the analysis of data generated by numerous surveillance efforts); Canadian Radio-Television and Telecommunications Commission (regulates broadcast advertising, including advertising to children); Public Health Agency of Canada (responsible for national surveillance system to report on diseases, injuries, and other preventable health risks and their determinants); and Statistics Canada (develops and implements multiple population level surveys).

The *food industry* is a major player; at the time of writing, it claimed that it was already meeting federal requirements regarding food safety, nutrition labelling, and health claims, and it opposed additional regulation as well as taxes on "junk foods." The *restaurant* industry (particularly chains) was also a key player.

*Broadcast and advertising industries* carry advertisements. They also work with the Advertising Standards Canada (self-regulatory body) to help ensure their ads meet the code.

### Voices in Favour of Anti-obesity Efforts

Toronto city councillor Paula Fletcher was quoted in the Toronto *Globe and Mail* on March 29, 2011, about her views on the sugar-sweetened beverage ban for vending machines run by the City of Toronto. She took a Mason jar filled with four cups of sugar to demonstrate how much of it a person would ingest by drinking two 500-millilitre sodas every day for a week. "It seems a little excessive to be dispensing this out of a city rec centre, a place that promotes healthy bodies," she said.

US first lady Michelle Obama, speaking on Fox News in February 2011 about her "Let's Move" initiative, said, "This is not an initiative that is about telling people what to do. It's giving people the tools to make the decisions that make sense for them."

In February 2011 Michelle Obama's anti-obesity campaign evoked support from two prominant Republicans who had struggled with weight problems. Former Arkansas governor Mike Hukabee was quoted as saying, "75% of military age youths in the United States do not qualify for military service because they're either overweight or obese and can't meet the minimum army standards. ... That's serious. ... This is no longer just a health issue, an economic issue. It is becoming an issue of national security." New Jersey governor Chris Christie said "[While] I don't want the government deciding what you can and what you can't eat ... I think Mrs. Obama being out there encouraging people in a positive way to eat well and to exercise and to be healthy, I don't have a problem with that."

Dr. David Katz, director of the Prevention Research Center at the Yale University School of Medicine, speaking to ABC News about a sweet tax, said, "When they tell us that soda, not all by itself, is the cause to the epidemic of obesity; well, duh," Katz said. "It's time for us to say that everything that isn't part of the solution is part of the problem."

The Arizona state government, led by Republican governor Jan Brewer, proposed a "Fat Fee" and "Smoke Fee" of $50 for recipients of Medicaid (a means-tested program providing medical care for the poor) if they did not follow a doctor-supervised plan to slim down.

**Voices Against**

Toronto mayor Rob Ford, speaking about the pop ban in city vending machines, told Toronto newspapers that it was "the most ludicrous idea I've ever heard. If kids want a pop, they'll cross the street, go to a plaza and buy a pop."

Paul Campos, a University of Colorado law professor, commenting on Michelle Obama's anti-obesity campaign, wrote in *The Daily Beast* on March 15, 2011, "The First Lady's 'Let's Move' campaign alienates fat children, and makes them more vulnerable to being picked on. The profound shaming and stigmatization of fat children that is an inevitable product of the campaign's absurd premise that the bodies of heavier than average children are by definition defective, and that this 'defect' can be cured through lifestyle changes ... Fat kids have enough problems without the additional burden of being subjected to government-approved pseudo-scientific garbage about how they could be thin if they just ate their vegetables and played outside more often."

Republicans Michele Bachmann and Sarah Palin were quoted as saying that Mrs Obama's campaign was a sign of government intrusion into the lives of Americans.

Coca-Cola CEO Muhtar Kent commented to ABC News about the sweet tax, "Two states that have soda taxes – West Virginia and Arkansas – also rank among the 10 worst states for obesity rates. Sugar-sweetened beverages have been singled out in spite of the fact that soft drinks, energy drinks, sports drinks and sweetened bottled water combined contribute 5.5% of the calories in the average American diet. ... It's difficult to understand why the beverages we and others provide are being targeted as the primary cause of weight gain when 94.5% of caloric intake comes from other foods and beverages."

Investigative journalist Lindsay Beyerstein blogged about the Fat Tax at Big Think that this "cruel and regressive tax" isn't about saving money or improving public health – it's about making government assistance "as degrading" as possible. "What's next, pillory stocks?"

## APPENDIX B: REFERENCES CITED AND FURTHER READING

Basrur, S. (2004). *2004 Chief Medical Officer of Health report: Healthy weights, healthy lives*: Ministry of Health and Long-Term Care. http://www.health.gov.on.ca

Canadian Institute for Health Information. (2006). *Improving the health of Canadians: Promoting healthy weights*. Canadian Population Health Initiative. https://secure.cihi.ca/estore/productSeries.htm?pc=PCC278

Drewnowski, A., & Popkin, B.M. (1997). The nutrition transition: New trends in the global diet. *Nutrition Reviews, 55*(2), 31–43. http://dx.doi.org/10.1111/j.1753-4887.1997.tb01593.x

Health Canada. (2011). *Canada's food guide*. Government of Canada. http://www.hc-sc.gc.ca/fn-an/food-guide-aliment/context/evid-fond-eng.php

Human Resources and Skills Development Canada. (2012). *Health – Obesity*. http://www4.hrsdc.gc.ca/.3ndic.1t.4r@-eng.jsp?iid=6 - M_1

Lalonde, M. (1974). *A new perspective on the health of Canadians: A working document*. Minister of Supply and Services Canada. http://www.phac-aspc.gc.ca/ph-sp/pdf/perspect-eng.pdf

Mikkonen, J., & Raphael, D. (2010). *Social determinants of health: The Canadian facts*. York University School of Health Policy and Management. http://www.thecanadianfacts.org/

Olshansky, S.J., Passaro, D.J., Hershow, R.C., Layden, J., Carnes, B.A., Brody, J., et al. (2005). A potential decline in life expectancy in the United States in the 21st century. *New England Journal of Medicine, 352*(11), 1138–1145. http://dx.doi.org/10.1056/NEJMsr043743

Public Health Agency of Canada & Canadian Institute for Health Information. (2011). *Obesity in Canada: A joint report from the Public Health Agency of Canada and the Canadian Institute for Health Information.* https://secure.cihi.ca/estore/productFamily.htm?locale=en&pf=PFC1636

Sassi, F. (2010). *Obesity and the economics of prevention: Fit not fat.* OECD. http://www.oecd.org/els/health-systems/obesityandtheeconomicsofprevention fitnotfat.htm

# 5 Trouble on Tap

## Water in Walkerton

*BRENDA GAMBLE, NANCY KRAETSCHMER,*
*KENNETH CHEAK KWAN LAM, CATHERINE L. MAH,*
*CAROLINE RAFFERTY, AND RAISA B. DEBER*

The small town of Walkerton, Ontario, earned unwanted prominence when an outbreak of waterborne disease between May and June 2000 left at least seven people dead and hundreds ill. In an effort to discover what went wrong, the provincial government set up a public judicial inquiry, under the leadership of Justice Dennis O'Connor. It was given a two-part mandate: to inquire into the circumstances that caused the illness (related to the presence of *Escherichia coli* bacteria in the town's water supply), and to focus on the issues relating to the future safety of drinking water in Ontario.

This case addresses several policy issues, including: public versus private roles in service delivery, accountability, policy instruments (particularly regulation), appropriate roles for various levels of government, and framing of issues.

### Appendices

Appendix A: Glossary
Appendix B: *E. coli* in Drinking Water
Appendix C: Timeline
Appendix D: A Brief History of Water Supply in Ontario
Appendix E: Public Private Partnerships (P3s)
Appendix F: References Cited and Further Reading

### The Case

Walkerton is a midsized rural farming community with a population of just under 5,000 people, located in Southwestern Ontario. On May 12,

2000, after four days of heavy rain, bacteria-laden cattle manure from a local farm was washed into a shallow water well (Well 5) that was part of the town's water supply. Six days later, the residents of Walkerton began to complain of bloody diarrhea, vomiting, cramps, and fever.

As required by provincial legislation, Walkerton water is routinely sampled and tested. On May 17, the private laboratory hired to do these tests reported that the water sampled on May 15 was contaminated with *E. coli* bacteria, indicating recent fecal contamination and suggesting that it might be unsafe to drink (see Appendix B for more details about *E. coli* in drinking water). As specified in its contract, the laboratory sent these results only to the Walkerton Public Utilities Commission (PUC). The general manager of the PUC, Stan Koebel, was not convinced that the results were accurate, and requested a retest. In the interim, Koebel decided not to divulge the initial test results. Within a few days, hundreds of Walkerton residents fell ill.

On May 19, Dr. Murray McQuigge, Medical Officer of Health for the Grey Bruce Health Unit (the local public health unit for that region), was notified that two patients from Walkerton had been hospitalized in the nearby town of Owen Sound for symptoms suggestive of *E. coli* O157:H7 infection; subsequent testing confirmed this. *E. coli* O157:H7 is a strain of *E. coli* that can cause severe and potentially fatal gastrointestinal infection, sometimes complicated by kidney failure. The Health Unit immediately began searching for a possible source for the infection. They called the PUC at least four times; Koebel repeatedly assured them that the water was okay. Early investigations by the Health Unit accordingly focused on a potential food-borne source for the disease, without success. By May 21, with no possible food source identified, Dr. McQuigge issued a boil water advisory for the Town of Walkerton (see Appendix A for a glossary of terms), and decided to have the Health Unit independently test the town's water. On May 23, the results of the Health Unit samples came back; they showed *E. coli* contamination throughout the water system. When confronted with these new results, Koebel finally told the Health Unit that the PUC had received earlier results showing *E. coli*, and also that the chlorinator had been operating intermittently during the first few weeks of May.

In the interim, however, a 66-year-old woman and a two-year-old girl had died, more than 150 people had sought hospital treatment, and another 500 individuals complained of symptoms. The final tally was seven deaths and about 2,300 ill (O'Connor, 2002a, 2002b). See Appendix C for a brief timeline of the events of the case.

### The Common Sense Revolution

In 1995, the Progressive Conservative (PC) party, under the leadership of Mike Harris, had won a sweeping majority in the Ontario provincial election, ousting the left-leaning New Democratic Party (NDP) government of Bob Rae. The Harris government explicitly rejected the more centrist policies that had characterized previous provincial PC governments. Their platform, termed the Common Sense Revolution, reflected the Margaret Thatcher reforms in the United Kingdom; it called for tax reductions, reducing regulatory burden, and privatization of formerly government-owned enterprises. In 1999, Harris was re-elected, again with a majority.

The PC base of support was in the rural and suburban parts of the province. Walkerton's provincial representative, Bill Murdoch, was a member of the PC party, and had represented the riding since 1990.

The provincial government's immediate reaction to the outbreak was to blame the previous NDP government for having relaxed the water standards. However, political pressure to act was high. Provincial opposition parties demanded that the government make financial aid available to Walkerton. An Australian company's offer to donate 10 million litres of bottled water to Walkerton further embarrassed the provincial government. In response, Premier Mike Harris announced a public inquiry into the Walkerton situation. The inquiry was chaired by Justice Dennis O'Connor; it was commonly referred to as the O'Connor Inquiry, or as the Walkerton Inquiry.

The search to understand what had happened soon focused on two levels – the local management of water in Walkerton and the larger issue of regulatory policy.

### Regulating Water Safety: Who Does What?

Water and sewage infrastructure are among the most fundamental public services. As has long been recognized, waterborne disease can be a major public health problem. One policy approach is to regulate. In Ontario, a variety of provincial government agencies have been involved in ensuring water safety, including the Ontario Water

Resources Commission (which no longer exists), the Ontario Ministry of the Environment (MOE), and, at the time of the case, the Ontario Clean Water Agency (OCWA).

As noted in Chapter 1, section 2.2.3 (The Roles of Local Government in Canada), municipal governments have no independent constitutional role in Canada, but fall under provincial control. Provinces are accordingly free to alter the roles and responsibilities of local governments. For the most part, water and sewage services in Ontario (as in most of Canada) are a local responsibility, with the provincial government being involved to a varying extent in regulatory oversight. (See Appendix D for a brief history of water supply in Ontario.) For many years, Ontario had directly tested drinking water in its provincial laboratories. Although reporting relationships were ambiguous, results usually went to the local agency delivering water, as well as to the provincial MOE, and to public health at both the provincial (e.g., the public health branch of the provincial Ministry of Health) and local (e.g., local health units) levels.

In the decade prior to the events in Walkerton, however, a series of shifts in federal and provincial governing priorities had led to a decentralization of services from the provincial to the municipal level, cutbacks in public funding for health and social services, and a shrinking of the government role in regulation of services, with a corresponding increase in reliance on the private sector. (See Appendix E for more information about public-private partnerships.)

In 1993, faced with large provincial deficits, Ontario's NDP government had downloaded the costs for testing drinking water onto the municipalities and downsized the provincial laboratories. Municipalities now had the choice of continuing to use the provincial labs (but paying for the testing), or using private laboratories. At least initially, many of these private laboratories were staffed by former provincial lab personnel who left government, set up their own private laboratories, and continued much as before. There were no clear provisions for quality assurance, although some labs voluntarily chose to be accredited by the Canadian Association for Environmental Analytical Laboratories and the Standards Council of Canada. That same year, the provincial government had amalgamated the Ministry of the Environment with the Ministry of Energy to form the Ministry of the Environment and Energy.

One policy of the Harris PC government was to reorient the fiscal responsibilities of the provincial and municipal levels of government.

These policies reflected a provincial preference to leave municipal issues in municipal hands, regardless of whether the municipality had the necessary resources and expertise. Following an examination of roles and responsibilities (by the provincial "Who Does What" exercise), fiscal responsibility for a number of services, including some public health activities, was downloaded from the provincial to the municipal level of government (Deber et al., 2006). These changes were highly controversial; they led, for example, to the angry resignation of Dr. Richard Schabas, Chief Medical Officer of Health for the province from 1987 to 1997, amid warnings that the new policy was likely to place public health at risk (see also Chapter 1, section 6.3.1, Public Health).

Another provincial policy introduced by the Harris government was the forced amalgamation of formerly separate communities, often over local objections, to produce fewer and larger (and presumably more cost-effective) local governments. As part of this exercise, on January 1, 1999, the town of Walkerton was amalgamated with the adjoining townships of Brant and Greenock to form the new municipality of Brockton (O'Connor, 2002a).

Among the first actions of the Harris government was to eliminate all remaining in-house provincial water testing. This was clearly in line with the emphasis of the Common Sense Revolution to lessen the size and role of government and encourage individual responsibility. In 1995, the budget of the MOE was cut by over 40% (from $287 million to $165 million). Many of the MOE staff who had been responsible for monitoring drinking water left the provincial government. After 1996, Ontario municipalities were required to hire private laboratories to test their drinking water for *E. coli* bacteria and other contamination. There was no requirement that these laboratories be accredited, and no provision requiring that the MOE or the local health authorities be notified if tainted water was found. The preferred model was self-regulation, based on the honour system. In response to concerns from the Auditor General and the MOE that the cutbacks had made it difficult for the province to monitor water quality, in 1997, the government passed Bill 57, *The Environmental Approvals Improvement Act, 1996*, which included provisions to prohibit legal action against the provincial government for failure to enforce environmental regulations.

*The Water and Sewage Services Improvement Act, 1997*, continued the effort to eliminate a provincial role in water safety. The province eliminated its Drinking Water Surveillance Program and closed four provincial laboratories. These MOE regional labs had conducted a variety of chemical analyses as requested by MOE, as well as performing water testing for municipalities; in future, private labs would perform these tests.

Some observers contended that these policy decisions around the privatization of water quality management compromised the safety of Ontario's drinking water and put profit above the health and welfare of the public. For example, both the provincial auditor's office and the MOE expressed concerns that it was now difficult for the province to monitor water quality, particularly in small communities. Proponents of privatized water testing argued, however, that private firms could more effectively and efficiently respond to water safety threats, and at little cost to the public purse. On June 13, 2000, the province announced a new plan to increase privatization of public services; municipalities were told that unless they could demonstrate that the advantages of providing a given service publicly (Direct Services) "clearly outweigh" those of providing it privately (Alternative Service Delivery), they would not be allowed to provide it publicly.

## Water Management in Walkerton

Walkerton's water management was part of the local Public Utilities Commission (PUC), which also distributed electricity to the community. Its mandate was to provide the people of Walkerton with a "continuous and abundant supply of pure and wholesome water." Their water came from seven wells, built between 1949 and 1977. Several of these were relatively shallow, and subject to contamination. One farm near Well 5 had 95 beef cattle; the farmer did not realize that his farm was so close to Well 5.

Stan Koebel was the general manager of the Walkerton PUC. He had little formal education, having only completed grade 12. He joined the water treatment operation in 1972; by 1988 he was the general manager. The foreman was his brother Frank. Neither brother had any formal training as water operators; both were "grandfathered" when such training became mandated. The subsequent Walkerton Inquiry revealed that neither knew what *E. coli* was. Indeed, Stan routinely drank untreated water from the well sites, claiming that it tasted better. Neither did they check the chlorine levels to ensure that contaminated water was not entering the water distribution system.

The Walkerton PUC had a history of customer complaints about water quality, dating back to at least 1977 (O'Connor, 2002a, 2002b).

For the most part, they involved taste rather than safety, both because the main wells serving the town contained water with a high mineral content, and because many townspeople disliked the taste of chlorine. In response, the town drilled a new well. The O'Connor report noted that it was this new well that led to some of the subsequent problems. The report noted that the surface water and "overburden" (clay, stones, and sand), including runoff from nearby agricultural land, could still flow into the new well since the shaft was not properly sealed and its aquifer was not thick enough to filter out contaminants. Without approval from the MOE and in spite of warnings from the well driller and consulting engineer, the well began pumping water to the town. Ultimately, the well was approved by the MOE on the condition that the water be chlorinated and tested frequently. However, enforcement proved spotty. The MOE also made a strong recommendation that nearby properties be purchased to ensure that contamination would not affect the groundwater; this was not acted on. Problems with the water recurred. Ten years later, testing of Walkerton water continued to show problems with the water supply. While the town told the MOE that it would meet standards to ensure water safety, there was no ministry follow-up, and hence no accountability measures (O'Connor, 2002a).

When Walkerton amalgamated with neighbouring communities in 1999, the Walkerton PUC was dissolved. Koebel now headed a new, larger PUC, which treated and distributed water and delivered electricity to the new municipality, and he also assumed operational responsibility for two smaller water systems. In mid-April 2000, the town's chlorinating equipment broke down; this was not reported to any other authority. The O'Connor Inquiry clarified that the local water operators were also in the habit of falsifying their test results. For example, they would collect samples at convenient sites (including their own homes or the PUC office), and then label them as having come from the required locations (Vicente, 2003). They also appeared to be in the habit of making fictitious entries on the daily operating sheets, rather than actually measuring the chlorine levels in the treated water. On occasion, these falsifications were detected by the MOE, including in a 1998 MOE inspection report (O'Connor, 2002a). However, the local board of the PUC accepted Stan Koebel's reassurances, and did not independently follow up to ensure that corrective action had been taken. The inquiry suggested that the board saw their role as monitoring fiscal matters, and left technical matters to the Koebel brothers. There were also suggestions that the board preferred to trust "local boys" over city-based inspectors.

## Farms

An external water consultant subsequently told the inquiry that the source of the *E. coli* O157:H7 in Walkerton's water was almost certainly cattle manure contamination of Well 5 by means of either the aquifer and/or surface run-off from the heavy rain in the period leading up to May 12, 2000. This evoked some examination of the agriculture and food industry, which is a major part of Ontario's economy. At the time of the case, Ernie Hardeman, the Ontario Minister of Agriculture, Food and Rural Affairs, had already established a task force on Intensive Agricultural Operations in Rural Ontario, which was holding public hearings in the spring and summer of 2000. Their report noted that the number of dairy farmers in Ontario had decreased from about 40,000 in 1951 to 7,200 by 1998, and that similar reductions were evident in the number of farms raising other categories of livestock. The trend was to larger farms that concentrated on one category of animal. "Factory farms" raise animals by confining them at high density; farmers often rely heavily on antibiotics, fertilizer, and pesticides to reduce the spread of disease.

Some argue that these factory farms represent greater efficiency in food production; others argue that they are harmful to the environment and cruel to animals. Certainly, there is a perception that such intensive farming operations – many of which were owned by absentee landlords and/or corporations – were less concerned with stewardship of the environment than were traditional family farmers. One goal of the agricultural task force was to develop new legislation to regulate such intensive farming practices. Among the community concerns they had identified were environmental concerns related to odour, land stewardship, and water quality. The minister noted that all livestock facilities were subject to the *Environmental Protection Act* and the *Ontario Water Resources Act, 1990* (both under the MOE). However, the environmental regulations had been written for an era of family farms; they allowed animal waste to be spread on fields. One issue being dealt with by the task force was whether rules that worked for 50–60 animals became more problematic for feedlots holding 10 to 20 times that number, with particular emphasis on whether these larger quantities would contaminate the groundwater (Ontario Ministry of Agriculture, Food and Rural Affairs, 2009).

The source of the Walkerton contamination, however, was a relatively small farm. The farmer appeared to have followed normal procedures. The consultant concluded that the contamination was an unfortunate combination of contaminated manure, a badly located well, heavy rain, and too little chlorine in the water distribution system.

## The Testing Labs

The O'Connor Inquiry noted that the Walkerton PUC had also changed testing labs on May1, 2000. Prior to that date, its testing had been done by G.A.P. EnviroMicrobial Services, Inc., but that company had decided to stop conducting routine drinking water analysis. The new company, A&L Canada Laboratories, was a private laboratory. As noted in the report, the samples being sent by the Koebel brothers were inadequate to perform the needed tests; the lab manager notified the Koebels but no one else. Similarly, when samples tested positive (on May 17), the results were sent only to the PUC; neither the MOE nor the local Medical Officer of Health was notified. Evidently, the laboratory manager had a policy of notifying only their clients unless directed otherwise, and was unaware of the relevant sections of the Ontario Drinking Water Objectives.

## Immediate Aftermath

In October 2000, even before the O'Connor Inquiry began to meet, the provincial government acted to reorganize the former MOE. Responsibilities for the Energy portfolio were moved elsewhere, and some senior officials (including the Deputy Minister) whose responsibilities had been associated with the energy portfolios moved with them. Dan Newman remained Minister of the new Ministry of the Environment, and most senior officials associated with the environment section of the former MOE remained in their jobs. New drinking water laws were also put into effect.

Within the PUC, Stan Koebel resigned with a $98,000 severance package. The water utility's secretary-treasurer told the inquiry that Stan Koebel believed that the source of the illnesses in the town was food poisoning or flu rather than contaminated water. Mayor David Thomson burst into tears at the inquiry during his testimony when he recalled learning that Stan Koebel had withheld crucial information that might have curtailed the tragedy. Frank Koebel, water foreman and Koebel's

brother, stunned the inquiry with testimony about drinking on the job
and routine falsification of safety tests and records.

On December 5, 2000, the Health Unit lifted the boil water advisory.

DECISION POINT

As a member of the Commission of Inquiry into the events in Walkerton, you have been asked to provide a series of recommendations
concerning water management at local and provincial levels. In developing these recommendations, you have been told to consider the following questions (although you are free to range beyond this list).

SUGGESTED QUESTIONS FOR DISCUSSION

1. Why did the tragedy occur? Discuss how "framing" might affect
   problem identification.
2. Discuss the concept of public goods and externalities as they apply
   to the case. Is water a public good?
3. What policy options would you suggest? Discuss the use of various policy instruments in implementing these options. What is the
   rationale for regulation? In general? For water quality? For air quality? Land use planning?
4. Discuss the advantages and disadvantages of: direct public provision; public-private partnerships; private delivery for supplying
   and testing water. How do these relate to the production characteristics of the services being provided?
5. What is the role of a municipal government? Discuss the implications of the relationships between municipal and other levels of
   government.
6. Discuss accountability. How might one ensure it?
7. Discuss street-level bureaucracy as it applies to this case.

APPENDIX A: GLOSSARY

*Aquifer*:                  A place where groundwater is natu-
                            rally stored. Aquifers typically consist
                            of sand, gravel, sandstone, or fractured
                            rock, such as limestone. The travel time

| | |
|---|---|
| | of water through an aquifer depends on the permeability of the material; the more porous the rock, the faster water travels. |
| *Boil water advisory:* | When bacterial contamination is found in drinking water, the local Medical Officer of Health can advise residents to boil drinking water for at least one minute before any kind of consumption (including not only drinking but also cooking, food preparation, or brushing teeth). |
| *Groundwater:* | When rain falls, water seeps into the ground. Groundwater is water that is found underground in cracks and spaces in soil, sand, and rocks. About 2.8 million people in Ontario rely on groundwater for their drinking supply. |
| *Groundwater contamination:* | In areas where the overburden is highly permeable, pollution from farming, sewage systems, or leakage from objects such as underground fuel storage tanks can sink quickly into the aquifer. A well in such areas will quickly pull in contaminants. |
| *Overburden:* | The top layer of earth under your feet. It typically consists of topsoil, sand, gravel, and/or clay. |
| *Well:* | A pipe sunk into the ground to tap groundwater moving through an aquifer. A deep well may tap several production zones in an aquifer. |

APPENDIX B: *E. COLI* IN DRINKING WATER

*Escherichia coli* (*E. coli*) is a type of fecal coliform bacteria commonly found in the intestines of animals and humans. Because it is easy to test for *E. coli* in drinking water, such tests are routinely carried out as part of the normal monitoring activities for any drinking water system. The presence of *E. coli* in drinking water indicates that organisms from recent sewage or animal waste contamination have entered the water supply and are not being destroyed or inhibited by disinfection processes. When drinking water test results are positive for *E. coli* the water is more likely to contain various kinds of fecal-origin pathogens, and is therefore considered unsafe for consumption.

One way for public health to deal with such microbiological contamination of the water supply is to issue a "boil water advisory" (Health Canada, 2009). Bringing water to a rolling boil for one minute will inactivate most of these pathogens. Note that all water to be consumed must be boiled, including water used for drinking, ice cubes, food preparation, and dental hygiene. Although standard boil water advisories do not require that other household water (e.g., bathing/hand-washing or laundry) be boiled, in the case of an outbreak, additional precautions regarding the use of household water use may be required.

While the majority of *E. coli* strains are harmless, including the normal strains inhabiting healthy human and animal intestines, several strains of *E. coli* are major and potentially fatal causes of food- and waterborne illness worldwide. The *E. coli* O157:H7 strain, in particular, produces a toxin that is capable of causing severe illness, including gastrointestinal infection and potentially kidney failure and death. Symptoms of *E. coli* O157:H7 infections usually appear within two to four days. Although most individuals recover without treatment within 5 to 10 days, certain groups, including children under the age of five years, the elderly, and those with chronic disease or who are immunocompromised, are at higher risk for more severe disease.

*E. coli* O157:H7 came to public prominence as a cause of illness during a 1982 outbreak in the United States that was ultimately traced to contaminated hamburger meat. Most *E. coli* O157:H7 infections in humans can be traced to food sources, although several outbreaks arising from other sources, including water, have been documented. Drinking water testing for this particular strain of *E. coli* is not normally carried out unless it is implicated in an outbreak, and drinking water is a suspected source.


APPENDIX C: TIMELINE

| | |
|---|---|
| *May 3–9, 2000*: | Chlorinator on Well 7 is removed; Well 7 is the only well operating, and is pumping unchlorinated water into the distribution system. Frank Koebel is expected to install new chlorinator, but does not. |
| *May 9, 2000*: | Well 7 is turned off and Wells 5 and 6 are activated. Well 5 is now primary source of water for the town. |

| | |
|---|---|
| *May 12, 2000:* | After heavy rain, bacteria-laden cattle manure washes into Well 5. |
| *May 15, 2000:* | Walkerton's local public utilities commission (PUC) takes routine sample of water and sends it off for testing. |
| *May 17, 2000:* | First symptoms of contaminated water appear; local doctors are treating patients with such symptoms as bloody diarrhea, vomiting, cramps, fever, and flu-like illnesses. PUC receives a fax from a lab confirming *E. coli* contamination in 15 May water sample; public health officials are not notified. |
| *May 18, 2000:* | The PUC meets; they are not told that Well 7 had been pumping unchlorinated water, or that test results had suggested possible contamination. |
| *May 19, 2000:* | Local Medical Officer of Health (MOH) is first notified by a local physician about several patients with bloody diarrhea. These include students at two local schools, a retirement home, and a long-term care facility. The PUC, run by Stan Koebel, assures health officials that the water is safe. The Health Unit begins looking for other source of contamination, such as food. |
| *May 20, 2000:* | As many as 40 more people report to hospital with bloody diarrhea. The PUC reassures officials at least twice that Walkerton's water supply is safe. |
| *May 21, 2000:* | MOH officially warns residents not to drink tap water unless it is boiled first. The Health Unit also takes independent water samples, despite being told by the PUC there is no contamination. |
| *May 23, 2000:* | Public health lab confirms results that show that water throughout Walkerton is contaminated with *E. coli*. After confronting the PUC with test results, the Health Unit is finally told about the May 17 fax. Health officials are also informed that the equipment used to put chlorine into at least one drinking well had not worked for some time. |
| *May 24, 2000:* | The first four deaths, three adults and a baby, are reported as a result of the *E. coli* outbreak. Local schools are closed. |

| | |
|---|---|
| *May 25, 2000*: | A fifth person dies after being infected with *E. coli* O157:H7. The regional police force asks the Ontario Provincial Police to conduct a criminal investigation into the origins of the outbreak. |
| *May 26, 2000*: | Ontario Premier Mike Harris visits Walkerton, saying, "We have a terrible tragedy here." The rest of his comments, including blaming the previous NDP government, anger residents. Within the week, he orders a public inquiry. |
| *May 27, 2000*: | The president of water-testing firm GAP EnviroMicrobial Services, Garry Palmateer, says that sampling done in January turned up evidence of coliform bacteria, an indication that surface water was seeping into the well water. He says his company notified the Ontario Ministry of the Environment about the problem five times. |
| *May 29, 2000*: | A clearly shaken Environment Minister Dan Newman calls a news conference to announce changes to ensure that the province's water supply remains safe. |
| *May 30, 2000*: | The deadly bacterial outbreak claims its sixth victim, an elderly patient who was being cared for at a local hospital. |
| *May 31, 2000*: | A hospital 140 kilometres south in London, Ontario, confirms that a 56-year-old woman has died, bringing the final fatality count in the contaminated-water catastrophe to seven. About 2,300 people fall ill at some point from the water. |
| *October 2000*: | The public inquiry begins. |
| *December 5, 2000*: | The Health Unit lifts the boil water advisory. |

APPENDIX D: A BRIEF HISTORY OF WATER SUPPLY IN ONTARIO

Initially, water systems in Ontario were privately owned and operated. For example, in 1837, a private company began to pipe untreated water from Lake Ontario to its customers. After 1849, when the *Baldwin Act* created a legal basis for municipalities to levy taxes, spend money, and approve regulatory by-laws over a wide variety of local matters

(Tindal & Tindal, 2008), a number of municipalities also began to own and operate water systems. This tended to be precipitated as a response to disasters, particularly fires and/or infectious diseases such as cholera. In 1882, Ontario introduced the *Municipal Waterworks Act*. This Act was permissive; it allowed, but did not compel, municipalities to operate water systems. Neither did it place responsibility with the province to provide and pay for them. (However, until 1943, municipalities were required to finance water systems through taxes, rather than through user charges.) In the 1880s, recognition of the causes of infectious disease (and the potential for transmission through unsafe food and water) was beginning, but its incorporation into practice was still relatively limited. For example, it was not uncommon for sewage to be discharged into the same sources that were being used for drinking water.

In 1884, Ontario passed the *Public Health Act*, which set up the Provincial Board of Health. Among its responsibilities was ensuring the safety of drinking water, which included legislation relating to sewage and septic systems. Municipalities were required to seek approval for water supply and sewage treatment systems from the board; in theory, the board could require them to chlorinate and/or filter their water. In practice, this took some time to become commonplace; for example, Toronto did not begin to chlorinate its water supply until 1910.

Over time, improved water quality had a significant impact on public health. As one example, typhoid fever deaths in Toronto dropped from 44.2 per 100,000 in 1910 to 0.9 per 100,000 by 1928. Recognition that the combination of increased growth and industrial development, and inadequate sewage treatment and disposal, was becoming problematic (e.g., there were large increases in the bacteria levels in the Great Lakes) prompted Ontario both to remove the ability of citizens to sue for poor water quality and to pass the *Ontario Water Resources Commission Act* in 1956. This Act encouraged construction of sewage treatment plants and water supply plants. The Ontario Water Resources Commission, an independent body that reported to the provincial Department of Health, was given complete oversight of water treatment and supply. The Commission had a staff of sanitary engineers. It conducted regular field inspections, on a random basis, and did regular testing of water samples.

Commission staff were also available to assist local operators. In 1960, the Commission began to develop courses in water and sewage treatment and operation for local operators. In the early 1970s, the Commission was amalgamated into the new Ministry of the Environment and Energy (MOE). Subsequently, the *Ontario Water Resources Commission Act* was renamed the *Ontario Water Resources Act, 1990*, and explicit provision was added to allow the MOE to regulate standards for water and sewage. They were also given the power to set qualifications for those licensed to operate water systems (albeit with grandfathering clauses to exempt many of those already on the job). Various regulations required that large waterworks must: (1) meet minimum treatment requirements; (2) have their drinking water tested by an accredited laboratory; (3) immediately notify the proper authorities of adverse test results; and (4) post notice signs to alert the public where water is untested or unsafe.

In 1990, the Liberal government of Premier David Peterson had announced plans to set up a new water and sewer corporation. It would report to the Ministry of Municipal Affairs and Housing. Responsibility for setting and enforcing environmental standards would remain with the MOE, but the new corporation would take on responsibilities for operating, maintaining, constructing, and financing facilities. This was seen as lessening conflict of interest potential for the MOE. Following the election of the Rae NDP government in 1990, these plans were somewhat modified. The new crown agency they formed in November 1993 was renamed the Ontario Clean Water Agency (OCWA); at that time, it took over the 153 water treatment plants and 77 sewage treatment facilities which the province had owned, adding these to the 116 municipally owned water and sewage facilities it was operating. By 1996, it had 800 employees and held contracts to operate 429 facilities in the province, making up 25% of Ontario's water-treatment plants and 57% of the wastewater treatment plants.

Soon after its election, the Harris PC government announced its plans to privatize OCWA. They did turn ownership of the facilities over to the municipalities. However, rather than sell the agency, they turned it into a contract services management organization. By 2000, OCWA operated and maintained more than 300 municipally owned water and sewage treatment facilities on behalf of about 200 Ontario municipalities. Indeed, in May 2000, shortly after the contamination problem was known, the provincial government directed OCWA to assume operations of the municipally operated Walkerton water system (Ontario Commission of the Walkerton Inquiry & Ontario Sewer and Watermain Construction Association, 2001; Sancton & Janik, 2001).

APPENDIX E: PUBLIC PRIVATE PARTNERSHIPS (P3S)

The terms "public" and "private" can refer to a variety of models (Deber, 2004) (see Chapter 1, section 6.1.1, Public and Private). Public can include national, state/provincial, or local governments, as well as quasi-public organizations which, although nominally private, are heavily controlled by government. Private may include not-for-profit, small business, investor-owned corporations, or individuals and their families. Different arrangements are possible for paying for services (financing) and for delivering them. A new, somewhat controversial variation has been termed public-private partnerships (P3s, or PPPs). In most of such models, much financing remains public, but delivery is the responsibility, to a varying degree, of a private entity.

The Canadian Council for Public-Private Partnerships has defined public-private partnerships as "a cooperative venture between the public and private sectors, built on the expertise of each partner, that best meets clearly defined public needs through the appropriate allocation of resources, risks and rewards" (Canadian Council for Public-Private Partnerships, 2009).

P3s are not uniform; they span a spectrum of models. One variable is ownership. Contracting-out models reject public delivery in favour of moving delivery to a private entity. (If delivery had previously been public, this process is sometimes referred to as "privatization.") Other models retain public administration, but use the private sector for various elements (including designing, building, or even operating a particular asset). The relative attractiveness of P3 models thus depends on existing rules and practices. For example, if accounting rules do not allow governments to spread the cost of a multi-year project over multiple years, governments may be reluctant to include large sums within a single year's budget. Under those circumstances, they may find it attractive to camouflage the full costs by allowing the private sector to borrow the money, and just include the annual lease payments in their budget. (In general, this will cost more in the long run, particularly if government can borrow at a lower interest rate than can the private sector.) Another element relates to "risk" and who should bear it. For example, if the costs of a project exceed those estimated, who will be responsible for meeting those additional costs? Another relates to labour relationships, particularly if public employees are unionized, and those of the private partner are not. Another relates to whether the private ownership is for-profit or not-for-profit (see Chapter 1, section 6.1.1, Public and Private).

The Canadian Council for Public-Private Partnerships, an advocacy group for such partnerships, describes a number of types of arrangements. These vary in terms of what each partner is responsible for (e.g., designing, building, operating, financing), who owns the asset (and over what time period), and who is responsible for cost overruns (Canadian Council for Public-Private Partnerships, 2001, 2009).

Another issue is profit, and whether the service can/should be provided to those who could not afford to pay for it. Advocates of P3s argue that the quest for profit will drive efficiencies, to the benefit of all. Opponents worry that corners are likely to be cut. Advocates suggest that proper regulation can minimize these risks, and that not meeting obligations can lead to fines, legal action, and damage to their reputation. Opponents note that such consequences imply that the contracts contain all necessary safeguards, that performance will be monitored, and that provisions will be enforced. Clearly, the applicability of these concerns varies across projects, dependent upon the nature of the service, and the rules in place (see Chapter 1, section 5.7, Production Characteristics).

Another issue is expertise. Government may be unwilling (or unable) to have the necessary expertise in house. P3s may enable governments to realize economies of scale, particularly for activities that may extend beyond a single jurisdiction. Paradoxically, however, researchers have suggested that the governments most in need of this sort of expertise are often the least able to monitor the activities of the outside contractors (Brubaker, 2003; Deber, 2004; Donahue, 1989; Kamerman & Kahn, 1989; Ohemeng & Grant, 2008).

Public-private partnerships for water utilities have been used in a number of US and Canadian cities, and in many countries, including the United Kingdom and France. A variety of models are used including service/management contracts, leases, concessions, build-operate-transfer, and full privatizations. The results have been controversial; governments avoided the need for the capital and operations expertise needed to improve the systems, but costs often increased.

## APPENDIX F: REFERENCES CITED AND FURTHER READING

Brubaker, E. (2003). *Revisiting water and wastewater utility privatization*. Prepared for the Government of Ontario Panel on the Role of Government Presented at "Public Goals, Private Means" Research Colloquium: Faculty of Law, University of Toronto. http://www.law-lib.utoronto.ca/investing/reports/rp39.pdf

Canadian Council for Public-Private Partnerships. (2001, January). *Benefits of water service public-private partnerships*. Paper presented to the Walkerton Inquiry, Toronto. http://www.pppcouncil.ca/bookstore/casestudies/132-water-case-studies-vol1.html

Canadian Council for Public-Private Partnerships. (2009). *About PPP (public-private partnership)*. http://www.pppcouncil.ca/resources/about-ppp/definitions.html

Deber, R. (2004). Delivering health care services: Public, not-for-profit, or private? In G.P. Marchildon, T. McIntosh, & P.-G. Forest (Eds.), *The fiscal sustainability of health care in Canada: Romanow papers* (Vol. 1, pp. 233–96). Toronto: University of Toronto Press.

Deber, R., Millan, K., Shapiro, H., & McDougall, C.W. (2006). A cautionary tale of downloading public health in Ontario: What does it say about the need for national standards for more than doctors and hospitals? *Health Policy, 2*(2), 60–75.

Donahue, J.D. (1989). *The privatization decision: Public ends, private means*. New York: Basic Books.

Health Canada. (2009). *Guidance for issuing and rescinding boil water advisories*. http://www.hc-sc.gc.ca/ewh-semt/pubs/water-eau/boil_water-eau_ebullition/index-eng.php

Kamerman, S.B., & Kahn, A.J. (1989). *Privatization and the welfare state*. Princeton, NJ: Princeton University Press.

O'Connor, D.R. (2002a). *Report of the Walkerton Inquiry: The events of May 2000 and related issues* (Pt. 1). Ontario Ministry of the Attorney General. http://www.attorneygeneral.jus.gov.on.ca/english/about/pubs/walkerton/part1/

O'Connor, D.R. (2002b). *Report of the Walkerton Inquiry: A strategy for safe drinking water* (Pt. 2). Ontario Ministry of the Attorney General. http://www.ontla.on.ca/library/repository/mon/3000/10300881.pdf

Ohemeng, F.K., & Grant, J.K. (2008). When markets fail to deliver: An examination of the privatization and de-privatization of water and wastewater services delivery in Hamilton, Canada. *Canadian Public Administration, 51*(3), 475–99. http://dx.doi.org/10.1111/j.1754-7121.2008.00034.x

Ontario Commission of the Walkerton Inquiry & Ontario Sewer and Watermain Construction Association. (2001). *Drinking water management in Ontario: A brief history*. http://www.archives.gov.on.ca/en/e_records/walkerton/part2info/publicsubmissions/pdf/drinkingwaterhistorynew.pdf

Ontario Ministry of Agriculture, Food and Rural Affairs. (2009). *Task force on intensive agricultural operations in rural Ontario consultations: Summary of consultations*. http://www.ontla.on.ca/library/repository/mon/10000/214740.pdf

Sancton, A., & Janik, T. (2001). *Provincial-local relations and drinking water in Ontario*. Walkerton Inquiry. https://ospace.scholarsportal.info/handle/1873/8281.

Tindal, C.R., & Tindal, S.N. (2008). *Local government in Canada: An introduction* (7th ed.). Scarborough, ON: Nelson Education Limited.

Vicente, K. (2003). *The human factor: Revolutionizing the way people live with technology*. New York: Routledge.

# 6 The Bite of Blood Safety

## Screening Blood for West Nile Virus

*HELEN LOOKER, DAVID REELEDER, AND RAISA B. DEBER*

In the summer of 2002, Ontario and Quebec experienced an epidemic of West Nile virus, associated with bites from mosquitoes. The public became very concerned that they were at risk of infection, and that the West Nile virus could be transmitted through the blood supply. To avoid recurrence of experiences with blood-borne transmission of human immunodeficiency virus (HIV) and hepatitis C, Canadian and US blood systems pushed for the development and implementation of a costly nucleic acid amplification testing (NAT) program to screen potential blood donors for West Nile virus.

This case addresses several policy issues, including: role of evidence, framing of issues, screening, policy trade-offs, cost-effectiveness analysis, ethics (precautionary principle), and federal-provincial roles and responsibilities.

### Appendices

Appendix A: The Canadian Blood System
Appendix B: The Tainted Blood Scandal and the Krever Commission
Appendix C: Excerpts from Minutes: Expert Advisory Committee on
    Blood Regulation
Appendix D: Cost and Cost-Effectiveness of Funding WNV Protective
    Measures
Appendix E: References Cited and Further Reading

### The Case

In the summer of 2002, Ontario and Quebec experienced several cases of West Nile virus infection in humans associated with bites from mosquitoes carrying the virus. Now, evidence suggests that this disease might be transmitted through the blood supply. What should be done?

## Background

West Nile virus (WNV) is a member of the Flaviviridae family of viruses; it is closely related to the viruses that cause St. Louis encephalitis, dengue fever, and yellow fever. The chief mode of transmission is through mosquitoes, but it can also spread through blood products.

WNV can infect and kill birds, with crows and blue jays appearing to be particularly susceptible. Mosquitoes can become infected through biting infected birds, and in turn can spread the virus to people and horses. Although the virus appears to have existed for some time, it received its name when it was first identified in the West Nile region of Uganda in 1937. The first confirmed North American outbreak of WNV infection occurred in New York City in 1999.

The US Centers for Disease Control and Prevention (CDC) has estimated that about 80% of people who are infected with WNV will show no symptoms. The remaining 20% may have flu-like symptoms, such as fever, headaches, nausea, vomiting, swollen glands, and/or rashes. However, about 1 in 150 people can develop severe illness, in the form of inflammation of the membranes around the brain and/or spinal cord (encephalitis, meningitis). This may lead to permanent neurological effects, including paralysis, coma, and convulsions. Treating WNV infection is complex. At the time of the case, no antiviral treatment existed, nor was there any vaccine that could prevent the disease. Of the small number of severe cases, 4%–14% died, with a higher fatality rate (up to 30%) for those who had to be admitted to hospital. The elderly and those on immunosuppressive drugs were at higher risk.

In August 2001, WNV was found among dead birds and in mosquitoes in southern Ontario. The first confirmed human cases in Canada occurred the following year, in both Ontario and Quebec. That summer, 325 positive human cases, 84 probable cases, and three confirmed deaths were eventually recorded. The virus was also found in birds, horses, and/or mosquitoes in Nova Scotia, Manitoba, and Saskatchewan; it has since spread to other provinces. Transmission was most likely in the warmer months when mosquitoes were common.

The immediate reaction of public health departments was to attempt to minimize transmission by stepping up mosquito control, both through application of pesticides and clearing up stagnant pools of water where mosquitoes might breed, and also by encouraging the public to use insect repellents and avoid handling dead birds.

The emergence of WNV in Canada evoked memories of previous infectious disease outbreaks that had contaminated the blood supply (see Appendix A, The Canadian Blood System). Given that 80% of those infected with WNV were asymptomatic, concerns arose that such individuals could have unknowingly donated blood infected with WNV. One study demonstrated that by 2002, 23 patients across the United States were known to have acquired West Nile virus through red blood cell transfusions, platelets, and/or fresh-frozen blood plasma, of whom 7 had died.

## Blood Safety and the Blood Supply

In the late 1970s and early 1980s, Canada's blood system had infected over 1,000 people with the HIV virus and at least another 12,000 people with hepatitis C. Those needing frequent transfusions, such as individuals with hemophilia, were particularly affected, but many cases involved people who had received tainted blood during otherwise routine surgical operations. An independent judicial inquiry led by Justice Horace Krever reported in 1997 (see Appendix B, The Tainted Blood Scandal and the Krever Commission) and concluded that one cause of what came to be known as the "tainted blood scandal" was the blood system's focus on efficiency. Krever argued that the operator's emphasis on ensuring that enough blood would be available at a reasonable cost had resulted in infected blood entering the blood supply. Krever's 50 recommendations were guided by three principles: (1) safety must transcend all other principles and policies; (2) sufficient funding should be available to ensure the safety of the blood system; and (3) the "precautionary principle" of policy behaviour should apply (see Chapter 1, section 3.6.2, The Precautionary Principle).

The tainted blood scandal had several consequences. One was a change in how the blood system was operated; the Canadian Blood Services Agency was established, along with a similar agency for Quebec. The hope was that these new agencies would do a better job of ensuring an adequate, safe, and affordable supply. Another consequence was a series of court cases brought by those who had become infected; these were settled by establishing a government program to compensate those who had become ill from receiving contaminated blood.

**Screening Blood**

Blood is a biological product that inevitably carries some risk of containing infectious agents. Transfusions may consist of "whole blood" or of blood products (including red blood cells, platelets, and plasma). On average, each whole blood transfusion requires 4.6 units of blood (where a unit represents a single donation of approximately 450 ml). In contrast, some blood products are manufactured from pooled blood donations, meaning that one infected donor can infect the entire batch. (In the case of fractionated plasma products, the number of donors pooled into a single batch may be in the hundreds. For other products, such as pooled platelets, the number of donors in a batch is typically four or five.) It is also important to ensure that the transfused blood type "matches" that of the recipient to avoid adverse reactions.

The Canadian blood system was also closely linked with the US system. At the time of writing, about two-thirds of fractionated blood product used in Canada was imported from the United States. The interdependence also means that Canada was likely to pay careful attention to safety decisions made concerning the US blood supply.

Several approaches can be used to ensure that blood transfusions are as safe as possible.

The first is to screen donors for risk factors associated with a higher likelihood of carrying transmissible infections. Such risk factors may include engaging in particular sexual activities; injection drug use; having had certain diseases such as jaundice, hepatitis, or malaria; a history of having received blood transfusions; having a recent tattoo or body piercing; and/or having travelled to high-prevalence areas. Screening can also help ensure that donors are healthy (e.g., donors are usually deferred if they are too young or too old, have a minor illness, or are pregnant). Some evidence suggested that high-risk donors were most likely to give blood in jurisdictions where blood donors were paid, and vulnerable individuals accordingly had an incentive to conceal information about their own health. In consequence, many jurisdictions, including Canada, encourage exclusive reliance on voluntary donation. Since the mid-1980s, prospective donors have been asked increasingly specific questions about their health and behaviours (including travel, but also more private matters, including sexual habits and drug use). Donors identified as potentially high-risk are designated as "permanently deferred" ("unsuitable donors" in the United States) and are not allowed to give blood. In the United States, collection sites are required by the Food and Drug Administration (FDA), the regulatory agency, to keep and disseminate lists of unsuitable donors to ensure that the blood of rejected donors will not be collected at other collection sites.

The next step is to screen the donated blood for infectious agents. As discussed in Chapter 1, section 8.2 (Screening), no screening test is perfect; both false positives and false negatives can arise. Blood that tests positive is discarded and not used for transfusions. Traditionally, the testing involved looking for antibodies, and was referred to as serological screening. However, because antibodies do not develop immediately, these tests may not detect people with recent infections. More recently, blood has been tested using nucleic acid amplification testing (NAT). These relatively expensive techniques allow the detection of genetic material (DNA or RNA) characteristic of infecting viruses even in the early stages of infection ("window period") prior to the development of antibodies. At the time of the case, before blood was issued to hospitals for use in transfusion, it was tested for the following infectious diseases: syphilis, hepatitis B and C, HIV, and human T-cell lymphotropic virus HTLV-I and II (viruses that can cause a rare form of leukemia in adults and chronic nervous system disease). In addition, Canadian Blood Services tested to determine blood groups (e.g., ABO and Rh type), to ensure that there would not be adverse transfusion reactions from incompatible matches.

With the 2003 summer mosquito season approaching, the blood system policymakers in both Canada and the United States debated whether they should add a West Nile virus blood donor screening test. This proposed test was similar to the costly nucleic acid amplification testing (referred to variously as NAAT or as NAT) screening technologies already being used for HIV and hepatitis C. Implementing this would require additional research to validate the test. Such tests also require a higher level of biosafety in the laboratories performing them; the required Level 3 laboratory facilities had not been established in all provinces (at the time of the case, they existed only in British Columbia, Manitoba, and Quebec).

Blood may also be treated before use to reduce risk of infection. For example, leukoreduction is a process that removes the white blood cells (leukocytes) from whole blood or blood products. This process, which adds approximately $30 to the cost of a unit of blood product, is said to reduce the rate of post-transfusion infection, although there is still some controversy as to the extent of benefit. Leukoreduction is universally used in Canada, Great Britain, and France, although only partially in the United States. Blood products may also undergo additional purification measures (e.g., freeze-thaw) that inactivate and/or remove many potentially infectious agents. Such processes may reduce the rate of post-transfusion infection, although they also entail added costs.

## The Stakeholders Meet

A series of consultations resulted in both Canada and the United States to determine how to deal with the possibility of WNV infection in the blood supply. Among the participants were: Canadian Blood Services, Health Canada, representatives from provincial and territorial governments, screening test manufacturers, expert advisory groups including physicians and epidemiologists, hospitals, researchers, the US FDA, the US CDC, and (in Canada) members of the public. Policies were also discussed in Health Canada's Expert Advisory Committee on Blood Regulation (see Appendix C, Excerpts from Minutes: Expert Advisory Committee on Blood Regulation).

In the autumn of 2002, the US FDA issued a request for WNV screening technologies. Requirements for screening quality (sensitivity and specificity), interoperability of the testing platform, and availability of screening kits were sufficiently stringent that only two biotechnology companies responded (GenProbe-Chiron and Roche Molecular Diagnostics). Both companies used NAT genomic technology approaches.

Other policy options were suggested. These included: collecting and stockpiling plasma during the winter months of 2003 when the blood supply would be relatively "clean" from WNV, so that this blood could be used during the summer mosquito season; quarantining and destroying potentially infected material collected during the 2002 mosquito season; and using surveillance data to collect "clean" blood from low-WNV-risk areas of the country for transfer to high-risk areas, until the first appearance of avian or human cases in the lower-risk areas. Another possibility would be to test only during the mosquito season, although this would not detect people who had travelled from areas where mosquitoes were active.

At the time of the case, the cost of a unit of blood was about $450; this had more than doubled in the past 10 years because of regulatory compliance burdens, technological advances in screening for infectious agents such as NAT and universal leukoreduction.

A number of stakeholders also raised concerns that voluntary donation was failing to meet needs, that potential donors were finding the screening process to be an invasion of their privacy, and that the costs and cost-effectiveness of advanced screening technologies were unwarranted (see Appendix D, Cost and Cost-effectiveness of Funding WNV Protective Measures).

DECISION POINT

You are a chief advisor to the provincial/territorial (P/T) Ministers of Health. They have been approached by Canadian Blood Services to fund a NAT-based genomics test for WNV in time for the upcoming 2003 mosquito season. After consulting with an expert committee, Health Canada and Canadian Blood Services have suggested that Canada use the Roche diagnostic test kit, in large part because Canadian Blood Services was already using other Roche NAT tests (for HIV and hepatitis C) and had the infrastructure in place to do so. A target was set to screen all blood donors by July 1, 2003. The estimated cost would be $10 million (approximately $10–$15 additional cost for each screened blood unit). What do you recommend?

SUGGESTED QUESTIONS FOR DISCUSSION

1. What are your options? What are the advantages and disadvantages of each?
2. What evidence would you consider relevant to assessing Canadian Blood Services' request? Discuss how different ways of framing the question might affect your response.
3. Discuss the precautionary principle as it might apply to this decision. Discuss the impact of previous policy failures (particularly, the tainted blood scandal).
4. What is cost-effectiveness analysis (CEA)? How might it apply to this decision?
5. Comment on the roles and responsibilities of: Canadian Blood Services; different levels of government, nationally and internationally; health providers; industry. How does this affect policy implementation?
6. Who pays for what? What incentives are there for industry to develop new tests, and how can governments encourage rapid technology developments on the basis of new or emerging threats?

What can governments do to protect themselves from manufacturers charging excess developmental costs? How can costs be controlled?


APPENDIX A: THE CANADIAN BLOOD SYSTEM

As noted in Chapter 1, section 2.2.1 (Federalism in Canada), health care and public health are largely a provincial responsibility, with delivery of services organized primarily at the local level. At the time of the case, the Canadian blood system was organized as follows.

Blood was provided without charge to all Canadians needing transfusions by a national not-for-profit operator operating at arm's length from government, Canadian Blood Services, except for Quebec, which is served by Héma-Québec. (In response to the recommendations of the Krever Commission, in 1998 these two agencies had replaced the Canadian Red Cross, which had been in charge of the blood supply since the 1940s. Although separate, Canadian Blood Services and Héma-Québec have a cooperative working relationship.) To reduce the need for each province to set up its own system, a 1997 Federal/Provincial/Territorial Memorandum of Understanding outlined that the provinces and territories would have full responsibility for funding Canadian Blood Services, with the contribution from each province/territory based on how much product was used by the hospitals within their jurisdictions. The federal government, through Health Canada, would retain the responsibility for ensuring that safety standards would be in place for how blood supplies would be collected, processed, and distributed.

Canadians donated blood on an unpaid volunteer basis at various clinics and blood centres throughout the country. Potential donors were screened prior to acceptance of blood into the system; once screened, blood was typed, processed, and stored, then distributed to hospitals as needed. Hospitals performing surgeries, or requiring products for medical treatment, were responsible for ensuring that recipients had their blood tested to ensure that blood transfusions would be compatible. Transfusions using donated blood are referred to as "allogenic"; patients in hospital could also request that units of their own blood, which were processed through the hospital and Canadian Blood Services, be stored for upcoming surgical procedures ("autologous" transfusion).

A 2002 Canadian Blood Services Performance Review pointed to the need for a national policy framework to assist in balancing safety and affordability. Among the issues noted was the importance of determining what level of safety is appropriate for Canadians, and at what cost. The review suggested that achieving this balance had been complicated by overlapping jurisdictional roles and concern that Canadian Blood Services not be blamed for future blood safety issues, particularly under conditions of insufficient public funding. At the time of writing, this framework was still incomplete; rather, coordination occurred at meetings of various agencies and task forces.

The main actors involved in blood policy thus included the following:

*Canadian Blood Services.* (Héma-Québec has a similar mission, but a somewhat different governance structure, and will accordingly not be analyzed in this case.) The Canadian Blood Services website described its mission as being "dedicated to giving Canadians a safe and secure blood supply system they can trust without reservation." The founding principles articulated by the federal, provincial, and territorial health ministers in 1996 included the need to: maintain/protect the voluntary donor system; pursue national self-sufficiency; encourage adequacy/security of supply; confirm safety of all blood components; ensure that blood remained free of charge to those receiving insured health services; maintain a national blood program; and achieve a cost-effective and cost-efficient system.

Canadian Blood Services estimated that it collected about 850,000 units of blood annually from voluntary, unpaid donors, and processed these units into components and products. It supplied blood to all hospitals throughout the country. Canadian Blood Services screened every blood donor and tested each unit of blood or blood product collected for a variety of transmissible diseases. Canadian Blood Services described itself as being committed to blood safety through effective screening and testing processes.

Canadian Blood Services had a two-tiered governance structure. The Board of Directors had 13 members, including the chairperson, four directors representing the provincial/territorial members, two directors representing the general public (consumers, donors, patients), and six directors providing medical/scientific/technical/business/public health expertise. In addition, the provincial/territorial Ministers of Health were designated as corporate members; their role was described as analogous to shareholders. The Canadian Blood Services Board of Directors provided initial approval for Canadian Blood Services' annual budget request, but the corporate members had to provide final budget approvals. This usually occurred at a special annual meeting of Canadian Blood Services. Canadian Blood Services' annual budget was segmented into: blood operations (collection, screening, testing, and distribution of blood); fractionated product (separation of blood into products and purchase from the United States); and Canadian Blood Services Insurance. As one reaction to the tainted blood experience, Canadian Blood Services had catastrophic insurance coverage for up to $1 billion in insurance claims.

As noted above, new safety measures, some imposed by Health Canada, and others implemented by Canadian Blood Services to be consistent with its mandate to ensure the safety of the blood system, had increased the cost of blood products in Canada. These measures included universal leukoreduction (removal of white blood cells from blood products) and nucleic acid amplification testing (NAT) for hepatitis C, HIV, and WNV. The costs associated with new donor recruitment had increased as a result of the decision to introduce donor deferral policies (temporary or permanent disqualification of individuals from donating blood based on risk of infectious disease transmission) to protect the blood system from other potential infectious agents, including variant Creutzfeldt-Jakob disease (vCJD) (Hollinger & Kleinman, 2003; Pealer et al., 2003; Wilson, 2007; Wilson et al., 2004). Such pressure was expected to continue. For example, the blood system would soon have to consider whether to adopt expensive new safety measures such as pathogen inactivation, which are techniques by which cellular products and plasma are treated to destroy known and potentially unknown infectious agents.

The budget of Canadian Blood Services had already increased over time, from $536.0 million in 1999/2000 to $828.7 million in 2003/2004 (Wilson & Hebert, 2002), based on growth in utilization as well as in the costs of screening and testing. This 55% increase was even greater than the increase in overall health care costs over the same time period, a still substantial 25%.

The *provinces and territories (P/T)* paid for the costs of the blood system, since most blood products were administered through provincially financed hospitals. As noted above, under the F/P/T Memorandum of Understanding and Canadian Blood Services By-Law, the P/T Ministers of Health also served as Canadian Blood Services corporate members; had a role in appointing the Board of Directors, including the chair; and had been involved in working with expert panels to improve blood utilization strategies. For example, a National Technical Working Task Force was established and worked in collaboration with Canadian Blood Services to develop and disseminate clinical guidelines to reduce inappropriate use of expensive fractionated product, with particular focus on intravenous immune globulin (IVIG).

*Public health* (see Chapter 1, section 6.3.1, Public Health) had a significant role in monitoring certain infectious diseases, including mosquito-transmitted WNV, but as services were organized, did not have a significant role in surveillance for transfusion-transmitted infections (see also Chapter 7, Looking for Trouble). However, public health stakeholders did work with Canadian Blood Services and Health Canada's surveillance group across the country to ensure that Canadian Blood Services was notified of the presence of WNV in humans. Canadian Blood Services in turn provided public health officials with notification of positive test results from its own donor screening testing. Information about mosquitoes, birds, and animals was also tracked by local public health units, although such information does not necessarily predict the presence of the virus in the human population.

At the federal level, *Health Canada* was responsible for protecting the safety of the blood system through the administration of an appropriate safety and regulatory framework. Blood and blood products were regulated under the *Food and Drugs Act and Regulations*, aimed at ensuring the safety of the blood supply in Canada. Specifically, Health Canada was responsible for: ensuring that laws and regulations address current safety needs; enforcing current laws and regulations applicable to blood operators; conducting regular inspections of blood establishments; licensing blood establishments; approving commercial blood products for sale in Canada; monitoring the blood system for emerging pathogens; identifying potential safety threats; assessing and managing risks related to blood safety; communicating with the public about blood safety issues; and providing leadership and coordination for all stakeholders involved in blood safety.

As noted, blood and blood products were provided at no charge from Canadian Blood Services for all services deemed "medically necessary" (see Chapter 1, section 7.2, *Canada Health Act*). That meant that *hospitals* and *physicians* could order whatever product they believed was necessary for insured services to insured persons. Canadian Blood Services attempted to meet local demand for blood product through local Canadian Blood Services operations, but would ship products across jurisdictions as required.

The *public* are also key players. As voluntary blood donors, they ensure the supply of blood and blood products. As patients, they are potential recipients of blood and blood products from Canadian Blood Services. As citizens, they also elect federal and provincial/territorial governments. As multiple surveys conducted for the national blood provider confirmed, they have multiple and potentially conflicting policy goals, including ensuring that the blood system is safe, but also that blood products are available to meet needs, and that the cost is "reasonable."

In addition, a number of *disease organizations* represent the interests of those affected by particular conditions. For example, the Canadian Hemophilia Society (CHS) represented the interests of hemophiliacs and their families. Other groups also had an interest in a safe and adequate blood supply, including the Anemia Institute for Research and Education, and a variety of groups representing cancer patients.

## APPENDIX B: THE TAINTED BLOOD SCANDAL AND THE KREVER COMMISSION

Between 1986 and 1990, the Canadian Red Cross, which had responsibility for blood services in Canada, had allowed contaminated blood into the blood supply. As noted in the case, more than 1,000 were infected with HIV and over 12,000 with hepatitis C. Certain groups were particularly affected. For example, among individuals with hemophilia, a blood disorder requiring treatment with repeated transfusions of blood components, nearly all who received blood products during that period contracted hepatitis C, and many contracted HIV/AIDS. Similar problems occurred in most other countries.

Among the responses in Canada was to set up an independent judicial inquiry into the Canadian blood system led by Justice Horace Krever; his final report was released in 1997 (Krever, 1997). As noted in the case, the basic premise taken by the Krever Commission was that the safety of blood should transcend other potential policy goals. Krever argued that most infections resulting from contaminated blood had been avoidable. One decision by the Red Cross, which attracted particular criticism, was its reluctance to adopt new screening tests, largely on grounds of perceived cost-effectiveness. One example occurred in 1986; the Red Cross did not adopt "surrogate testing" of donated blood for chemicals that might (or might not) be associated with "non-A, non-B hepatitis" (since renamed hepatitis C), although most US blood banking organizations had done so. Compounding the problem, even after a direct test for hepatitis C became available in 1989, the Red Cross had continued to use up its older untested product, evidently from a reluctance to "waste" it, for fear that blood supply might otherwise be inadequate to meet needs.

The Krever Commission's recommendations set the stage for the creation of Canadian Blood Services in 1998. One legacy of the commission was the principle that the "safety of the blood supply system is paramount." Krever called for ensuring that funding be made available to ensure safety (through newer or more sensitive tests and/or identification of pathogens, even if an impact on the number of potential donors was anticipated); and that a "precautionary principle" must apply to policy decisions (see Chapter 1, section 3.6.2, The Precautionary Principle). Adoption of this principle would imply that action should not wait for complete knowledge or evidence about potential health hazards and that cost should not be an issue; increased public trust and a lower risk of infection would ensue.

Krever also recommended enhancing the regulatory oversight role of Health Canada. He recommended that an appropriate federal bureau adopt a policy of active, not passive, regulation of the national blood supply system; that the decision-making process of the bureau be open and transparent to the public; that an active program of post-market surveillance of blood components be introduced; and that Canada harmonize internationally with many aspects of drug licensing. These recommendations continue to influence blood policy. For an excellent review of the tainted blood scandal, see Picard (1998).

APPENDIX C: EXCERPTS FROM MINUTES: EXPERT ADVISORY COMMITTEE ON BLOOD REGULATION

The Expert Advisory Committee on Blood Regulation was set up to provide Health Canada with advice on federal responsibilities related to blood. The published mandate of this committee noted that it would provide "health professional and related expertise to assist Health Canada in making appropriate risk management decisions relative to assessments of risk and benefit which have been conducted by Health Canada" concerning the regulation of the Canadian blood system, standards and procedures including prospects for international harmonization, and advice on emerging scientific issues related to quality and safety, critical events, and other matters. Members came from health professional and scientific societies, academia, and government agencies, including Health Canada. Meetings (including teleconferences) occurred quarterly, and minutes were published on its website. These minutes included brief descriptions of some discussions regarding WNV.

September 19, 2002: This meeting appears to have provided the first clear update on WNV transfusion-transmitted risk. At that time, there had not yet been any confirmed cases of WNV transmission in Canada, but the US CDC had reported that one organ donor subsequently was found to have WNV, and had infected four recipients. Canada's response was to set up a mechanism whereby local health authorities would notify blood operators when cases of WNV were suspected. A technical working group advised Health Canada that no further policy action was required at that time.

November 21, 2002: Dr. Peter Ganz, Health Canada, indicated that there was now clear evidence from the United States that WNV could indeed be transmitted through blood. Health Canada had accordingly issued a new policy directive to blood operators directing that an infected blood donor, identified based on testing and tracing from a sick recipient, must be deferred from blood donation for a period up to 56 days, including quarantining of blood already collected.

February 20, 2003: Dr. Ganz reported on a recent consultation session on WNV; stakeholders were working towards a test being available by July 1, 2003. As a contingency, Health Canada indicated that blood operators were now stockpiling plasma collected during the winter months of 2003 for use during the summer mosquito season. However, certain blood components, such as red blood cells and platelets, could not be stockpiled because of their limited shelf life (42 days and 5 days, respectively). Health Canada also indicated that blood operators had quarantined and destroyed potentially infected material collected during the 2002 mosquito season. An option of using surveillance data (e.g., birds, humans) as a proxy for WNV absence/presence to collect blood from low-risk geographic areas for transfer to high-risk areas was also discussed. Due to the urgency of the screening test, Health Canada indicated it would: (1) meet continually with the blood operators to help speed implementation of the test; (2) actively request reports from the two companies developing the test; (3) meet regularly with provincial/territorial representatives; (4) consider development of a surveillance model to predict human cases from bird cases; (5) speed turnaround from existing WNV testing at the central laboratory; and (6) adopt a proactive approach to WNV infection prevention and detection.

April 8, 2003: The committee approved (but did not require) the Roche Molecular Systems test for potential use, should the decision be taken to adopt it.

## APPENDIX D: COST AND COST-EFFECTIVENESS OF FUNDING WNV PROTECTIVE MEASURES

At the time of the case, the risk of transmission of HIV per unit of blood transfused was estimated to have fallen to approximately 1 in 1.3 million (units of blood received); the risk of transmission for hepatitis C virus was about 1 in 3.1 million. By comparison, the risk of transfusion-transmitted HIV in Canada with antibody testing for the period 1985 to 1989 was estimated to be 1 in 0.9 million. Evidence was not yet available about the risk of acquiring West Nile virus.

About 0.5% to 3% of all transfusions resulted in some adverse events, with bacterial contamination of hospital or operator equipment accounting for a large share of these events. For purposes of comparison, estimated risk of some non-transfusion-associated events was as follows. The risk of a stroke within 30 days of cardiac surgery was 1 in 60, death associated with hip replacement surgery was 1 in 100, the annual risk of death in a motor vehicle accident was 1 in 10,000, and the risk of being murdered in Canada was 1 in 60,000.

As described in Chapter 1, section 8.1, cost-effectiveness analysis is a useful way to compare the costs and consequences of various courses of action. One such analysis, using US data, compared six potential testing strategies for WNV (AuBuchon, 2005; Custer et al., 2005). The options considered incorporated the following variations: (1) testing could be done on mini-pools (of 6 to 16 donations) or individual donations, or a combination of both; (2) testing could be done year-round, or only during part of the year; and (3) strategies could also be tailored depending on whether there was an outbreak in a particular area. All the combinations they examined were compared to a baseline of no WNV testing. Their model assumed that the cost of testing, per donation, was $7 (for mini-pools) or $14 (for individual donations). Prevalence of WNV varied, with the highest rate reported for 2003, in North Dakota, being 102 per 10,000 donations. Interested readers are referred to the full paper for additional details about the model and assumptions (Custer et al., 2005).

Their analysis concluded that the least costly strategy (other than not testing at all) was mini-pool testing for half the year, which was estimated to cost $272,000 per quality-adjusted life year (QALY) gained. Even high assumptions about prevalence did not reduce the cost below $150,000 per QALY. Individual testing for everyone over the entire year was estimated to cost $897,000 per QALY. Annual national mini-pool testing followed by testing individual donations when the pool tests positive would cost $483,000 per QALY. The results were sensitive to the prevalence of WNV in the population, the costs of the tests (particularly the reagents), and treatment costs. They estimated that screening in the United States in 2003 would have prevented as many as 362 symptomatic infections and 5 severe infections with WNV. This compared to an estimated 940,000 infections estimated to have been acquired through mosquito bites in the 1999–2003 period.

For comparison, they noted the results of other cost-effectiveness analyses. In general, the rule of thumb used was that a clinical intervention should cost less than $50,000 per QALY to be deemed cost-effective. Because prevalence was relatively low, estimates from the literature place the cost-effectiveness of combined NAT for HIV and for hepatitis C virus far above that threshold, at between $5.8 million and $9.6 million per QALY.

## APPENDIX E: REFERENCES CITED AND FURTHER READING

AuBuchon, J.P. (2005). Meeting transfusion safety expectations. *Annals of Internal Medicine, 143*(7), 537–8. http://dx.doi.org/10.7326/0003-4819-143-7-200510040-00012

Canadian Blood Services. (2013). *West Nile virus (WNV)*. http://www.blood.ca/centreapps/internet/uw_v502_mainengine.nsf/9749ca80b75a038585256aa20060d703/3c83d547fcda0aef852570880058020b?OpenDocument

Canadian Broadcasting Corporation. (2007, October 1). *Canada's tainted blood scandal: A timeline*. CBC News: In Depth. http://archive.is/izSj

Custer, B., Busch, M.P., Martin, A.A., & Petersen, L.R. (2005). The cost-effectiveness of screening the U.S. blood supply for West Nile virus. *Annals of Internal Medicine, 143*(7), 486–92. http://dx.doi.org/10.7326/0003-4819-143-7-200510040-00007

Hollinger, F.B., & Kleinman, S. (2003). Transfusion transmission of West Nile virus: A merging of historical and contemporary perspectives. *Transfusion, 43*(8), 992–7. http://dx.doi.org/10.1046/j.1537-2995.2003.00501.x

Krever, H. (1997). *Commission of inquiry on the blood system in Canada: Final report*. Ottawa, ON: Public Works and Government Services Canada, Cat. No. CP32–62/3–1997E. http://publications.gc.ca/site/eng/446508/publication.html

Pealer, L.N., Marfin, A.A., Petersen, L.R., Lanciotti, R.S., Page, P.L., Stramer, S.L., et al. (2003). Transmission of West Nile virus through blood transfusion in the United States in 2002. *New England Journal of Medicine, 349*(13), 1236–45. http://dx.doi.org/10.1056/NEJMoa030969

Picard, A. (1998). *The gift of death: Confronting Canada's tainted-blood tragedy* (2nd ed.). Scarborough, ON: Harper Collins Canada.

Wilson, K. (2007). The Krever Commission: 10 years later. *Canadian Medical Association Journal, 177*(11), 1387–9. http://dx.doi.org/10.1503/cmaj.071333

Wilson, K., & Hebert, P.C. (2002). The challenge of an increasingly expensive blood system. *Canadian Medical Association Journal, 168*(9), 1149–50.

Wilson, K., McCrea-Logie, J., & Lazar, H. (2004). Understanding the impact of intergovernmental relations on public health: Lessons from reform initiatives in the blood system and health surveillance. *Canadian Public Policy, 30*(2), 177–94. http://dx.doi.org/10.2307/3552391

# 7 Looking for Trouble

## Developing and Implementing a National Network for Infectious Disease Surveillance in Canada

*CHRISTOPHER W. MCDOUGALL, DAVID KIRSCH,*
*BRIAN SCHWARTZ, AND RAISA B. DEBER*

Managing epidemics is impossible without knowing when and where they occur. Canada is obligated by international law to establish an integrated national outbreak surveillance system that will enable timely and effective public health information collection, interpretation, and sharing, as well as collaborative intervention during crises. The 2003 outbreak of SARS in Toronto and Vancouver exemplified what is at stake. What are the policy, organizational, and functional characteristics of a workable national surveillance system?

This case addresses several policy issues, including: public health, public goods, intergovernmental relations, ethical issues, privacy, and globalization.

### Appendices

Appendix A: How Public Health Is Organized in Canada
Appendix B: Surveillance, Reportable Diseases, and Outbreaks
Appendix C: Findings of Key Reports
Appendix D: International Health Regulations Reporting Requirements and Processes
Appendix E: References Cited and Further Readings

### The Case

On February 23, 2003, a woman and her husband returned from a Hong Kong vacation to their Toronto apartment, which they shared with their two sons, daughter-in-law, and infant grandson. In Hong Kong, they had stayed on the ninth floor of the Metropole Hotel. On that same floor was a physician from Guangdong province in China; despite feeling ill, he had made the trip to attend his nephew's wedding. Two days after returning to Toronto, the woman developed fever, cough, sore throat, and other flu-like symptoms. She saw her family physician on February 28. He noted a red throat but no other abnormalities, and prescribed antibiotics. On March 5, nine days after her symptoms began, she collapsed and died at home. Although the cause of death was recorded as cardiac failure, some of her symptoms were compatible with infectious illness.

Soon after, the woman's son, who had cared for her during the illness, developed similar symptoms. On March 7, he went to a local hospital emergency department (ED) and was eventually admitted to the hospital with pneumonia. In spite of intensive treatment in an isolation unit, he died on March 13. While in the ED, he unknowingly infected at least three people, including an elderly man with whom he shared a cubicle, and that man's wife. This elderly couple both eventually died as well, but not before infecting dozens more people, including members of their families, and staff at the hospitals in which they were treated. These people spread the infection to still others, including many health care workers.

At about the same time, the World Health Organization (WHO) issued a press release reporting cases of atypical pneumonia in China and Hong Kong. They subsequently traced the cases to Guangdong province; the first case appears to have been a farmer, who died in November 2002. The sick physician who had stayed at the Metropole had contracted the infection while treating atypical pneumonia patients in Guangdong. Within weeks after he had unknowingly transmitted this to other people staying at the Metropole Hotel in Hong Kong, the pathogen had spread from Hong Kong to at least 36 other countries. (Among its early victims was Dr. Carlo Urbani, the doctor who had been sent by the local WHO office to investigate the outbreak in Vietnam.)

On March 26, 2003, a provincial emergency was declared in Ontario. The largest severe acute respiratory syndrome (SARS) outbreak outside Asia was underway.

SARS claimed 44 lives in Ontario (including three nurses and a family physician), among 247 probable and 128 suspect cases. It resulted in a WHO travel advisory against non-essential travel to Toronto, over a billion dollars of lost revenue and a level of post-traumatic stress in health care workers that persisted years later. Three post-SARS commissions were convened at the national and provincial levels, and issued reports. These were usually referred to by their chairs, Naylor (National Advisory Committee on SARS & Public Health, 2003), Walker (Expert Panel on SARS & Infectious Disease Control, 2004), and Campbell (Campbell, 2004, 2005, 2006). All focused on the lack of public health preparedness and coordination in Canada and Ontario. Justice Archie Campbell articulately summarized their shared conclusion: "SARS showed that Ontario's public health system is broken and needs to be fixed. Despite the extraordinary efforts of many dedicated individuals and the strength of many local public health units (PHUs), the overall system proved woefully inadequate. SARS showed Ontario's central public health system to be unprepared, fragmented, poorly led, uncoordinated, inadequately resourced, professionally impoverished, and generally incapable of discharging its mandate."

**The Vancouver Case**

On March 7, 2003, at about the same time that the Toronto index (original) patient's son was in the ED, another man who had also stayed on the ninth floor of the Hong Kong Metropole Hotel in late February returned to Vancouver. The outcome in Vancouver was much different. The man, feeling unwell on the flight home, went directly from the airport to see his family physician, who then referred him to a Vancouver ED. He was isolated upon arrival. British Columbia ultimately reported only four probable SARS cases (only one of which was locally acquired) and no deaths.

Much of the reason Vancouver was not as badly affected was luck. Health Canada maintains an early warning system, called the Global Public Health Intelligence Network (GPHIN), which scans the Internet for reports of infectious disease outbreaks. The Network had picked up on a Chinese-language news report about a flu outbreak in mainland China from November 27, 2002. However, the report was not translated into English from Chinese, although it was reported with an English header to the WHO, which then mentioned the notice in its weekly bulletin in February 2003.

The Vancouver index patient showed symptoms of illness upon his return to Canada, and was able to provide a clear travel history to medical professionals, who may have been primed for such an appearance. One of the attending ED physicians in Vancouver had close ties to China, and was keenly aware of the atypical pneumonia cases which had been occurring there since February. In contrast, the index patient in Toronto had died at home. Her son, who spread SARS when he was hospitalized, had not travelled to Hong Kong and thus did not meet the SARS case definition. (His doctor initially suspected tuberculosis.) Indeed, the link was only discovered by an alert employee, who asked enough questions a day or two after the son's admission to discover the mother's travel history; it was confirmed by having public health workers investigate her home for travel tags on her luggage. However, that is only part of the story.

**Managing Public Health**

As noted in Chapter 1, section 2.2.1 (Federalism in Canada), much of public health has been interpreted as falling under provincial jurisdiction. This presents some issues when outbreaks cross provincial boundaries, as well as when managing an outbreak that has moved internationally and may continue to do so if not contained.

At the provincial/territorial level, responsibilities for performing public health activities are usually shared between the provincial/ territorial and regional/local authorities/units. Many functions have devolved to regional health authorities (RHAs), often with only vague provisions for reporting and accountability to other stakeholders. Critical mass is often lacking, particularly in smaller health authorities. This makes it difficult to respond to emergencies. There is considerable variation in how public health is funded and managed. In some provinces, public health activities are part of the global budgets given to RHAs. Reporting may be vague, and prevention may take a back seat when competing with short-term acute care priorities. There is also variation in how much support is available from the province. (For more information on how public health is organized in Canada, see Appendix A.)

One particular focus of attention was how to ensure surveillance.

**What Is Surveillance?**

Public health surveillance was defined by the US Centers for Disease Control and Prevention as "the ongoing systematic collection, analysis, interpretation and dissemination of data about a health-related event for use in public health action to reduce morbidity and mortality and to improve health" (Centers for Disease Control and Prevention, 2001).

Surveillance is intended to detect new or emerging threats, and it must be timely and accurate enough to allow authorities to analyze potential impacts, communicate across jurisdictions, prescribe interventions to reduce transmission, and conduct ongoing tracking to measure effectiveness. Timely information is particularly important for infectious (also called communicable) diseases, which can be transmitted from one person to another (see Chapter 1, section 6.3.1, Public Health). Because people are increasingly mobile (see Chapter 1, section 5.5, Globalization), disease surveillance systems must be integrated across geographic distances and jurisdictions, and reach all levels of the health care system.

Accomplishing this involves a broad and complex series of tasks to ensure that data flows both "up" (to and from public health bodies), and "down" (to and from providers and the public). Data must be timely, accurate, and comprehensive; it must also be securely stored with careful attention to privacy. Data can be used for a number of purposes, including: monitoring trends in patterns of disease and identifying which populations are most vulnerable; identifying emerging diseases and triggering interventions to prevent transmission (particularly critical for infectious diseases) and/or to reduce morbidity/mortality from that condition; and improving understanding of the determinants of health.

Outbreak detection is complex; it involves an array of actors (both public and private) at the local, provincial, national, and international levels. In Canada, additional complexity arises from the constitutional division of powers, which reserves for the federal government all powers not delegated to the provinces, but also gives the provinces authority over most health matters. A description of surveillance, reportable diseases, and outbreaks is found in Appendix B. Each province has its own infectious disease surveillance system, although increasingly efforts are being made to coordinate these.

For example, public health in Ontario is the responsibility of local public health units (PHUs); at the time of writing, there were 36 covering the province. Surveillance is a responsibility of these local PHUs, although they receive some support from the provincial level. At the time of the case, this rested in the office of the province's Chief Medical Officer of Health (CMOH). Ontario's *Health Protection and Promotion Act* establishes a series of "reportable diseases" that local providers must disclose to the local PHU. The list is revised regularly. Some of the diseases on the list must be reported immediately, while others can be reported on the next working day. In 2005, the province replaced its Reportable Disease Information System (RDIS) – a series of 36 stand-alone systems – with a new Integrated Public Health Information System (iPHIS), which integrated these into one central, provincially managed database. This was a clear step forward from the old system, where each week the PHUs would gather information from their local RDIS system and fax it to the province's CMOH. Nonetheless, the surveillance information would still have to be transmitted to the national level, since the federal government retained responsibility for communicating with international partners, particularly for reporting outbreaks to the WHO. Even with the new system, this meant that the province would have to fax information to Health Canada, who would then aggregate the findings. This rather cumbersome process made it difficult to respond rapidly to emerging threats. Other provinces/territories had similar problems.

**Surveillance in Canada**

The importance of developing a national network that integrates Canada's health surveillance systems had been recognized well before SARS. The ambiguity of roles and responsibilities and inconsistencies in intergovernmental relations has contributed to a series of public health crises (Wilson, 2001). (A summary of selected reports and reviews is found in Appendix C.) Action had been repeatedly recommended by various governmental audits and reports reacting to these previous public health crises, including the inquiries into the blood system (discussed in Chapter 6, The Bite of Blood Safety) and the Walkerton outbreak (discussed in Chapter 5, Trouble on Tap). In 2002, a Senate committee had recommended that the existing federal/provincial/territorial (F/P/T) infrastructure be built up with the goal of establishing a comprehensive network to link disease surveillance and control activities across all jurisdictions, eventually leading to the creation of a comprehensive national disease surveillance system (Standing Senate Committee on Social Affairs Science and Technology, 2003). Public health experts continued to argue that there were substantial gaps across the entire spectrum of surveillance functions (data collection, integration, analysis, interpretation, and dissemination). They particularly noted the gaps with regard to data sharing agreements, information technology infrastructure, uniform data quality and reporting standards, emergency response coordination, and the lack of a common list of notifiable or reportable diseases across jurisdictions. There have also been perennial disputes over who should pay for what across the levels of government. Stable funding of surveillance systems has thus been an ongoing concern, particularly because outbreaks and other potential threats that are recognized and prevented from becoming crises (through early detection, containment, and thus the avoidance of morbidity and mortality) are both difficult to quantify and hard to explain to policymakers and funding agencies, despite the fact that such crises averted clearly save significant costs in the long term.

The SARS experience highlighted these and other concerns. The national committee investigating SARS, led by David Naylor, wrote, "Long before SARS, evidence of actual and potential harm to the health of Canadians from weaknesses in public health infrastructure had been mounting but had not catalyzed a comprehensive and multi-level governmental response ... The National Advisory Committee on SARS and Public Health has found that there was much to learn from the outbreak of SARS in Canada – in large part because too many earlier lessons were ignored ... SARS is simply the latest in a series of recent bellwethers for the fragile state of Canada's federal/ provincial/ municipal public health systems. The pattern is now familiar. Public health is taken for granted until disease outbreaks occur, whereupon a brief flurry of lip service leads to minimal investments and little real change in public health infrastructure or priorities. This cycle must end" (National Advisory Committee on SARS & Public Health, 2003).

However, the cycle did not end (McDougall, 2009). Subsequent outbreaks have included contamination of processed meats with listeriosis in 2008 (22 deaths) and pandemic H1N1 in 2009 (428 deaths). Inquiries into those events have noted the continued vulnerability of Canada's overall public health response, particularly the gaps in communicating information between federal, provincial/territorial, regional, and local authorities. Sheila Weatherill, the independent investigator into the national listeriosis outbreak, noted that "there was a lack of understanding about intergovernmental protocols to deal with such emergencies, which created confusion about who should do what and when" (Weatherill, 2009). Even during the relatively mild influenza pandemic in 2009, "the Public Health Agency of Canada experienced challenges with respect to its surveillance capacity including both a lack of real-time data on key epidemiological variables and epidemiological resources to review surveillance data ... the lack of a comprehensive public health surveillance system was specifically evident in First Nation communities and represented a complex challenge for the Health Portfolio. This situation resulted in an incomplete and inconsistent national picture and therefore did not support timely decision making" (Public Health Agency of Canada, 2010b).

Despite these repeated calls, at the time of writing Canada continued to rely on a patchwork of health surveillance systems.

## Intergovernmental Relations and Health Surveillance

One key issue is the allocation of roles and responsibilities across the levels of government. Under the *Constitution Act* the majority of health care responsibilities have been interpreted as falling under provincial jurisdiction. Responsibility for health protection is less clear, with federal and provincial governments sharing responsibilities. Public health is considered primarily a provincial concern under section 92(13) of the *Constitution Act*, which gives the provinces responsibility for "property and civil rights." Further provincial authority in this field is derived from the power that provinces are given in section 92(16) over matters of a "local or private nature." Subsequent legal interpretations have stated that the provinces have jurisdiction over public health, specifically the prevention of communicable diseases, and over sanitation, although the federal government does have some limited authority through its powers over criminal law, interprovincial/international matters, and the "peace, order and good government" power.

## Federal/Provincial/Territorial Roles and Responsibilities

To the extent that protecting the health of the population is a shared federal/provincial/territorial responsibility, conflict can emerge. Among the challenges is how to manage *externalities*, *unfunded mandates*, and *data ownership*.

The issue of *externalities* (see Chapter 1, section 3.5, Public Goods and Externalities) means that policy decisions in one jurisdiction can affect others. For example, threats to health arising in one region have the potential to spread and cause harm to individuals who live in other regions. If one jurisdiction chooses not to immunize against a certain condition and a substantial number of vulnerable individuals then travel to other jurisdictions, their policy has the potential to undermine the effectiveness of immunization programs in the receiving region. Similarly, a decision by one region with respect to specific air or water quality measures may affect the health of citizens living in neighbouring regions. The potential for externalities and spillovers has been used to argue for coordinated governmental approaches. It also creates a situation in which one jurisdiction may attempt to influence others in order to protect itself.

The term *unfunded mandates* refers to costs arising from the policies/regulations passed by one level of government, which requires others to take actions to implement them (see Chapter 1, section 5.2.1, Regulation). Unsurprisingly, these other parties are often reluctant to spend their own funds, particularly if the mandated actions are not a high priority for them. For example, the Canadian government's anti-crime policies will impose costs on provincial/territorial justice systems. Unfunded mandates have also been a growing concern in provincial-local relationships.

*Data protection and ownership* is another issue of concern to provinces entering into agreements with the federal government. For large national programs to be successful, data must be shared across provinces and between the provinces and the federal government. However, data sharing may allow the federal government to create "report cards" about the performance of subnational jurisdictions, and even tie funding to meeting certain performance requirements (e.g., to achieving target levels of immunization coverage). A related issue is whether local and provincial privacy regulations create obstacles to sharing health data. A study on health surveillance identified the reluctance of provinces to share data as a potentially important barrier to the establishment of a successful national surveillance program (McDougall, 2009). At the time of writing, there was no federal legislation to compel provinces to report data. However, several less formal public health networks have been established to facilitate national (although not federal) responses to communicable diseases that have the potential to cross provincial boundaries. Such networks are also critical to the control of such foodborne illnesses as listeriosis, because food safety often affects multiple jurisdictions and multiple government departments. The nature of Canadian federalism means that these interdependent relationships would be classified as *collaborative* models of federalism (see Chapter 1, section 2.1.3, Federal vs. Unitary Models). To the extent that the federal government wishes to be involved, it may rely on signed agreement with various provinces/territories, with or without funding arrangements or other incentives to ensure their participation.

## International Health Regulations

One response to the global impact of SARS was progress on a decade-long effort to update the International Health Regulations (IHR). The negotiation process led to a substantially new agreement in 2005, whose new regulations came into effect in 2007. The IHR require countries to report certain outbreaks and events, known as Public Health Emergencies of International Concern (PHEICs), to the WHO, in order to ensure appropriate actions are taken to manage them and reduce impact within and outside the affected country. The IHR also outline various areas of technical guidance and support to help implement these new rules in developing nations. See Appendix D for more information about these regulations.

One implication is increased pressure for Canada to improve data collection and analysis (particularly to ensure timeliness). The roles of the Public Health Agency of Canada (PHAC) and of the provincial/territorial governments are still unclear. Another still unresolved issue is whether Canada should invest resources in assisting developing countries in their surveillance and containment of emerging communicable disease threats.

DECISION POINT

You are the Minister of Health of your province. A national arm's length body, Canada Health Infoway, has offered to fund a $100 million pan-Canadian surveillance project to be led by the province of British Columbia. This project will develop a pan-Canadian framework for an immunization registry, immunization management system, vaccine order and distribution system, surveillance system, and a message system to interface the provinces. Although each of the provinces will be able to be part of the requirements definition process, each province will have to fund its own implementation and the costs will be significant. Infoway may provide up to 25% of the implementation costs. What should you do? What are the principal policy issues and alternatives? What are the major factors to consider in your decision? What are the major risks in attempting to implement this system? How do you mitigate the risks?

SUGGESTED QUESTIONS FOR DISCUSSION

1. If you were building a surveillance infrastructure, how would you connect, and ensure compliance from, all sources of information (physicians and other primary care providers, hospitals, laboratories, local, provincial and federal PHUs) so as to ensure a robust, accurate, and usable system?
2. Should Canada adopt a more centralized approach to public health? What would a more centralized approach look like? What are the advantages of such an approach? What are the negative impacts of such reforms, and how would they be managed?
3. If the present system is maintained, how can Canada ensure compliance with the International Health Regulations while maintaining decentralized approaches to public health? What are the policy options? Is the reservation the government of the United States submitted to the WHO (see Appendix D) relevant to Canada? Why or why not?
4. What should Canada's foreign policy be in terms of global outbreak surveillance support? What are the issues and what is the return on investment on supporting less developed countries? What are the risks?
5. What are the ethical implications of surveillance for emerging infectious diseases such as SARS and novel strains of influenza? How do these differ from the ethics of screening and testing for other infectious diseases (e.g., HIV, tuberculosis, or syphilis) and for non-communicable diseases (such as obesity, or the various cancers and genetic disorders for which testing currently exists)?

APPENDIX A: HOW PUBLIC HEALTH IS ORGANIZED IN CANADA

As noted in the case, the federal government, for the most part, does not have direct service delivery responsibilities for health care, or for public health, except for certain specialized populations or specific functions. Instead, it relies on partnerships with provincial/territorial governments, and uses information and (to a limited extent) funding as its policy levers (see Chapter 1, section 5.2, Policy/Governing Instruments). The federal government does help to create and disseminate research findings through a variety of bodies, including the Canadian Population Health Initiatives, the Public Health Agency of Canada (PHAC) and its set of collaborating centres, the Canadian Institute for Health Information, Statistics Canada, and the Canadian Institutes for Health Research. Financing public health activities can also become problematic. Few federal transfers are targeted to public health per se; neither is it specifically mentioned in the Health Accords signed by the federal/provincial/territorial governments (see Chapter 1, section 7.1, Financing Health Care in Canada). Most public health activities do not fall within the definition of "comprehensiveness" in the *Canada Health Act* and accordingly do not form part of its national terms and conditions (Sutcliffe et al., 1997). However, several federally funded public health programs have been launched, including some funds for such activities as the National Immunization Strategy, Public Health Infrastructure Development, and the Canada Health Infoway. In general, these have been time-limited, in the form of pilot projects.

At the provincial/territorial level, responsibilities are usually shared between the provincial/territorial and regional/local authorities/ PHUs. Here, considerable use is made of the regulation and public ownership policy instruments. All provincial/territorial governments have maintained central departments with responsibility for certain public health matters, and all have the equivalent of a chief medical health officer (Shah, 2003). The statutory responsibilities of such departments vary. Most have responsibility for providing consulting/advisory services, providing policy advice, and being the spokesperson for the government on public health issues. However, some provincial/territorial governments have placed certain functions, including aspects of occupational and environmental health, with other departments within their governments. Some provinces, including Ontario and Nova Scotia, may also split health promotion off to separate ministries (although Ontario reintegrated health promotion with the Ministry of Health and Long-Term Care in 2011). Some provinces decentralized responsibility for delivering public health services to regional bodies, although the responsibilities of these bodies also varied (Sutcliffe et al., 1997). At the time of writing, BC, Nova Scotia, and New Brunswick used RHAs with close provincial oversight, Ontario used a series of local PHUs, BC supplemented the geographically based regional health authorities

with province-wide authorities with responsibility for certain specialized services (e.g., cancer care and some public health activities), and
Quebec included a third layer, assigning certain public health functions
to the Centres Local de Services Communautaires (CLSCs) (now called
Centres de Santé et de Services Sociaux, or CSSSs).

There were also differences in the management, coordination, and
delivery structures by type of public health issue, with responsibilities
often clearer for health protection issues than for other public health
responsibilities. Implementing plans can also be problematic, with
capacity and critical mass often pointed to as major issues. Epidemiologic capacity could be highly variable; many non-urban RHAs,
and even some provinces, did not have an epidemiologist on staff. At
the time of writing, electronic information systems had not yet been
implemented across the country, although Canada Health Infoway was
offering funds to help with this. In some provinces, reporting was still
monthly via paper, whereas others had implemented sophisticated and
searchable electronic databases. An additional complexity is the link-
ages to primary care (e.g., some but not all provinces had influenza
sentinel surveillance systems operating through selected primary care
settings). British Columbia has been particularly innovative. The British Columbia Centre for Disease Control (BCCDC), a provincial agency,
was given responsibility for conducting and coordinating surveillance
within the province, and helping the local public health authorities
manage outbreaks. In 1997, it had already developed a pandemic influenza plan to address the threat of H5N1 avian influenza, and outlined
specific procedures on detection and containment of novel imported
infections. BCCDC had worked for years with other parts of the health
care system in the province to ensure heightened awareness and practice of infection control in health care facilities. Enhanced surveillance
and electronic distribution systems were in place to regularly collect
and disseminate communicable disease information to and from public
health officials, health care facilities, and practitioners. At the time of
writing, at least 66 notifiable diseases were reported by the standardized Infoway IT system in BC, which was being expanded to facilitate
syndromic reporting from EDs as well as tracking of utilization of certain over-the-counter drugs in order to detect foodborne and other ID
outbreaks.

Just as delivery is complex, so is funding. Indeed, attempts to determine the level of public health funding often involve guesswork.
One BC study had suggested that "public health currently receives

approximately 2.5 to 3 per cent of the total health care budget" (British Columbia Ministry of Health, 2005), while a Nova Scotia study estimated their public health spending at 1.2 per cent (Moloughney, 2006). Provinces also varied in what was included within their public health budget (e.g., immunizations in Ontario were largely performed by physicians and thus classified in the Ontario Health Insurance Plan budget line, whereas in some other provinces they were included within the public health budget).

Public health programs are not always mandated; much falls into the "may be provided in some but not all jurisdictions" category. Dental public health is a good example. Community prevention (including fluoridation) is usually publicly financed and delivered, albeit not necessarily located within public health per se. Most clinical dental care in Canada (including individual prevention and clinical treatment) is privately financed and privately delivered. Only a very small proportion of dental care is publicly financed; the *Canada Health Act* requires coverage for medically necessary surgical-dental care only if performed in hospitals, which almost never happens.

Various levels of government may also act as third-party insurers for certain target groups, including government employees, and First Nations/Aboriginals. Governments may also directly run clinics to deliver care to defined vulnerable populations, which may include those on social assistance, and/or to some institutionalized populations (including those in long-term care). In some provinces/territories, municipalities may play a key role, although the provincial/territorial government often pays part of the cost.

Often, however, public health funding is part of a global budget that is also intended to cover other activities. Like all funding approaches, global budgets contain incentives to act in particular ways. Global budgets have the advantage of making it easier to control costs, but, from the standpoint of funders, the disadvantage of making it difficult to control how these funds are used. (From the standpoint of the fund recipients this method has the advantage of giving them flexibility in determining and reacting to local priorities.) Allocation of global budgets inevitably has political dimensions; funding is more likely to flow to the most popular and powerful programs (and their advocates). Preventive activities, in general, are less successful in such competition than immediate clinical needs. In many provinces, the RHAs are allowed to decide how much of their budget will go to public health. This has been described as downloading the acute care vs. prevention funding battle from a single battle at the provincial level to multiple battles within each community. Prevention may win, particularly in urban areas, but it often does not. Some provinces (e.g., Nova Scotia) have attempted to put "protective fences" around the public health monies, but these too are described as susceptible to being circumvented.

Global budgets also make it more difficult to "pin down" the funding for public health. As the Naylor (National Advisory Committee on SARS & Public Health, 2003) and Senate (Standing Senate Committee on Social Affairs Science and Technology, 2003) reports have noted, even provincial governments often are unaware of what public health activities are being carried out at the local level, and of the precise funding for such activities. In general, consolidated information on how these programs are delivered and funded is difficult to obtain, and has become more so as provinces have moved more functions to regional authorities. Even if numbers are provided, there are some suspicions about the data quality. For example, should a hospital-based dietitian, or a hospital infection control nurse, be considered public health or hospital funding? Ongoing policy battles about what could be managed at the local level and what requires more provincial involvement evoke the classic trade-offs between uniformity and flexibility.

Ontario, like some other provinces, was also centralizing some resources in response to stated needs for leadership and expertise that would be hard to sustain within local health units (critical mass issues), with specific mention made of epidemiology, nursing, and nutrition, the ability to allow data cleaning/preparation/analysis tasks to be performed centrally, and access to documents/resources/best practices, as well as a common communications and computer system, data quality support, software, and professional development/networking (Rush, 2005). Ontario also moved some functions into a new arm's length organization, Public Health Ontario (previously called the Ontario Agency for Health Protection and Promotion) and gave it the mandate to provide centralized support to local public health units, government, and health care providers and institutions, including "expert scientific and technical advice and support relating to: infectious diseases; infection prevention and control; surveillance and epidemiology; health promotion, chronic disease and injury prevention; environmental and occupational health; emergency preparedness and incident response." PHO also operates the public health laboratories (Public Health Ontario, 2013).

## National Networks

Two major challenges that have impeded the development of a national surveillance network were identifying what mechanisms could be used to fund surveillance infrastructure and developing data sharing agreements among governments. Although the federal government had given some funds targeted for specific initiatives, including money to the Centre for Infectious Disease Prevention and Control for blood-borne pathogens, enteric diseases (gastrointestinal illness), influenza pandemic, HIV/AIDS, and hepatitis C, and to the Centre for Chronic Disease Prevention and Control for diabetes and breast cancer, the slow progress on developing a national surveillance system was identified in both the 1999 and 2002 Canadian Auditor General reports (Office of the Auditor General of Canada, 1999, 2002). In particular, the 2002 report argued that "Health Canada should identify its health surveillance priorities and ensure that adequate and stable funding is available to develop and maintain the surveillance systems that it identifies as priorities."

The SARS outbreak had dramatically demonstrated the consequences of having poorly developed surveillance infrastructure. Several of the reports analysing what had gone wrong noted that the information flows within Toronto, from Toronto to the Ontario government, from the Ontario government to the federal government, and from the federal government to the WHO were inadequate. These information flow problems resulted from the lack of a standard system of data collection as well as the absence of data sharing agreements. Some have argued that the presence of a developed Network for Health Surveillance in Canada as originally envisioned would have contributed substantially to overcoming these obstacles and might have helped not only to avoid the issuance of a WHO travel advisory for Toronto but perhaps also to reduce the $1 billion impact the SARS outbreak had on the Ontario economy (Wilson et al., 2008b).

The Network for Health Surveillance in Canada was another attempt by federal, provincial, and territorial partners to address the deficiencies in the field of health surveillance. The objective of the project was to build capacity at all levels (regional, local, provincial/territorial, and national) to acquire and share health surveillance information with the goal of improving evidence-based decision making in the public health sector. The Network was expected to deliver better-quality surveillance information, along with easier access, timely sharing, and tools for the integration and analysis of that information. It would also provide standards for the collection of surveillance data and provide an adaptable system able to accommodate changing health surveillance needs. However, it was not intended to be a comprehensive plan for health surveillance. Individual partners could choose to operate outside of the Network if they so desired and would still remain accountable for many surveillance functions (Wilson, 2001).

Another project, National Health Surveillance Infostructure (NHSI), was expected to operationalize many of the concepts put forth by the Network project. The NHSI was a federal-provincial collaborative effort to develop Internet-based tools that would allow for national and international surveillance of diseases and other potential risks to health. Its objective was to develop an electronic infrastructure that would improve coordination of the presently fragmented health surveillance activities occurring throughout the country. Some of its key elements included: (1) integrated national public health architecture to link key public health nodes, including public health laboratories, hospitals, and physicians' offices; (2) global surveillance and early warning networks to link with international health surveillance systems to provide early information on emerging global health risks; (3) policy and program decision support systems to assist the analysis and interpretation of surveillance data and to facilitate the tracking of risk factors and diseases as well as health expenditures, the economic burden of disease, and the effectiveness of health programs and health policies; (4) integration of human health surveillance information with other determinants of health information, collection of information on such factors as socioeconomic status and level of education and assessment of their impact on health (although this was not an immediate priority); and (5) development of a comprehensive Internet-based health information resource to link health surveillance data across the country via the Internet. The NHSI core components were the Canadian Integrated Public Health System (CIPHS), Local Public Health Infrastructure Development (LoPHID), and Spatial Public Health Information Exchange (SPHINX). These were supported by the NHSI infrastructure, composed of the Public Health Intelligence Database (PHIDB), Geomatic Information System Infrastructure (GIS), and Global Public Health Intelligence (GPHIN).

One impetus towards developing surveillance systems was Canada's approval of the revisions to the International Health Regulations, which require that the national government must report within 24 hours the emergence of a public health emergency of international concern. These regulations also require countries to develop surveillance systems and conduct a capacity assessment to determine their adequacy (World Health Organization, 2005).

Some scholars have concluded that the way in which public health is organized and delivered in Canada presents some difficulties in developing a network for public health surveillance. These include the fact that the federal government does not have legislative authority in this area and thus must rely upon provincial cooperation, the comparatively low priority given to surveillance activities, and the absence of intergovernmental agreements (Wilson et al., 2008a).


APPENDIX B: SURVEILLANCE, REPORTABLE
DISEASES, AND OUTBREAKS

Surveillance may be carried out using a number of sources, including: laboratory confirmatory testing and reporting of designated or reportable diseases; testing of food or water samples; systematic reporting by selected ("sentinel") physicians or organizations of symptom complexes that may suggest patterns of diseases or conditions of interest, and real-time tracking of electronic databases for emergency department visits, 911 medical dispatch calls, and/or calls to nurse advice lines (e.g., Telehealth Ontario) to track trends of such symptom complexes.

With respect to communicable illness, an essential component to surveillance is laboratory confirmation if available; however, in an emerging infectious disease (such as SARS), laboratory testing is not possible until the novel pathogen is identified. Hence SARS cases in 2003 could be reported only as "probable" or "suspect" cases, as based on clinical findings and a history of contact with another case or travel to an affected area.

In a well-designed system, data might flow as follows for surveillance purposes.

A patient presents at a health care *facility* (e.g., hospital, long-term care home, physician's office) with symptoms of a potentially reportable disease. The patient is examined and undergoes testing. The facility sends samples to a laboratory. If the *physician* has specific concerns (e.g., a cluster of people with diarrhea who recently attended a picnic or banquet), he/she may report this directly to the PHU (by telephone or fax); indeed, the quickest and often most effective surveillance tool is an astute clinician. The *lab* sends information on reportable diseases to the local PHU; in Ontario, there are plans for the province to speed this process and provide direct access from the labs to the Integrated Public Health Information System (iPHIS). The PHU receives information from the facility, lab, and/or physician, and enters that data into a provincial dataset (e.g., iPHIS). The surveillance case worker within the PHU generates trend information and statistics and sends this information to the provincial/territorial health authority (e.g., Ontario Ministry of Health and Long-Term Care), and to PHAC if appropriate. PHAC receives information from the provinces/territories and PHUs, and forwards information to WHO as per International Health Regulations (see Appendix D). Clearly, there are many steps, and many opportunities, for information to fall through the cracks.

*Reportable diseases* are those communicable diseases designated by provincial legislation (e.g., the Ontario *Health Protection and Promotion Act*) as ones that professionals (including laboratories, physicians, and administrators of certain organizations, including hospitals and schools) are obligated to report to public health authorities. The goal of reporting is to help monitor disease, reduce transmission, and provide preventative measures. While the sharing of such clinical information is normally protected under privacy legislation, for reportable diseases such sharing is not only permitted but also obligatory, on the grounds that risks to society in the absence of reporting outweigh the breach of individual privacy. Common examples of reportable diseases include most sexually transmitted diseases, laboratory-confirmed influenza, and such vaccine-preventable diseases as measles. A full list of reportable diseases in Ontario is available on the Toronto Public Health website (Toronto Public Health, 2011).

An essential component of surveillance is determination of what constitutes a *normal* number of cases (based on historical data) and what level of increase would be sufficiently *abnormal* to be considered an *outbreak* and necessitate such control measures as removal of possible sources of foodborne illness, isolation or quarantine, mass vaccination campaigns, and/or closure of facilities such as nursing homes.

As noted in Chapter 1, section 8.2 (Screening), surveillance systems can be seen as a form of screening, by which potentially problematic cases are identified. Like other screening tests, they must balance *sensitivity* (probability of a positive test among those with the disease) and *specificity* (probability of a negative test among those without the disease) in determining the parameters of disease reporting (see Chapter 1, section 8.2.2, Assessing Screening Tests). Ideally, one would minimize the number of false positives (those testing positive who do not have the disease) and of false negatives (those with the disease who were not picked up by the test). The decision about when and who to test thus depends on such factors as the consequences of various types of error. As Chapter 1, section 8.2.3 (The Role of Prevalence) notes, the performance of tests depends heavily on the *prevalence* of the disease in the population; when there are very few cases, most positive tests will be false positives, even when the test has excellent sensitivity and specificity.

## APPENDIX C: FINDINGS OF KEY REPORTS

Health Canada is expected to track communicable diseases, chronic diseases, and injuries. In his report tabled on November 30, 1999, in the House of Commons, then–Auditor General of Canada, Denis Desautels, said that weaknesses in national surveillance of disease and injuries compromised Health Canada's ability to detect, anticipate, prevent, and control health risks associated with outbreaks of communicable diseases and with other health threats, as well as the department's ability to plan, carry out, and evaluate programs that deal with the causes and treatment of diseases. He was quoted as saying, "Health surveillance is particularly critical now, when globalization has created an environment for disease and its transmission that never existed before. Sound surveillance information can save lives" (Office of the Auditor General of Canada, 1999).

The 1999 Auditor General's Report had noted that national health surveillance was conducted mainly by Health Canada's Laboratory Centre for Disease Control (LCDC), but that LCDC depended greatly on its interaction and collaboration both with the provinces/territories and with a variety of other federal departments and non-governmental organizations. The report pointed to the absence of specific legislation, policy, or agreements to link these separate components, and noted that coordination tended to be carried out on an ad hoc basis. While work had begun on strengthening surveillance, the report concluded that key surveillance systems were not working as intended. As a result, Health Canada had difficulty in monitoring such communicable and chronic diseases as influenza, AIDS, diabetes, and foodborne disease. The report documented the attempts to manage a nationwide outbreak of a foodborne disease in the spring of 1998, and concluded that there were delays in the exchange of information to identify the scope of the outbreak, and a lack of full cooperation among the agencies in responding to it. The Auditor General was quoted as saying, "The story of how the Canadian Food Inspection Agency, Health Canada and provincial agencies handled the outbreak is disturbing. This outbreak affected hundreds of children and should raise the alarm on the urgency for the responsible authorities to work together in a comprehensive manner."

In her October 2002 report, Sheila Fraser, then–Auditor General of Canada, included a follow-up to note what actions had been taken in response to these previous Auditor General findings. She concluded that Health Canada had made some limited progress in addressing the weaknesses and gaps in national health surveillance identified in 1999, but that there were still gaps and weaknesses in the way that it tracked diseases that continued to leave Canadians vulnerable. The report found that the surveillance of certain communicable diseases, including enteric disease, influenza, and AIDS, had improved, but that Health Canada still lacked timely, accurate, and complete information for many others. She concluded that "without this information, there is a risk that actions needed to prevent illness will not be taken" (Office of the Auditor General of Canada, 2002). The Canadian Integrated Public Health Surveillance Project, which was aimed at improving the quality of information on communicable diseases, was seen as having potential, although the report noted that full implementation was still some time away.

The 2002 report also examined chronic diseases, and found that Health Canada had made significant progress in developing a national diabetes surveillance system, although gaps remained in the surveillance of most other chronic diseases, including cardiovascular disease, musculoskeletal disease, cancer (except breast cancer), chronic respiratory disease, and mental illness. Information about injuries, risk determinants, and the impact of interventions, screening, and treatment on health was also relatively lacking. The report called for Health Canada to take more leadership in improving national health surveillance, in cooperation with the provinces/territories.

In 2002, two major national reports were released on Canada's health care system: a six-volume report by the Standing Senate Committee on Social Affairs, Science and Technology, chaired by Senator Michael Kirby (referred to as the Kirby Committee), and a national commission chaired by Roy Romanow. Both included mention, in passing, of the importance of communicable disease surveillance.

In its final report, the Kirby Committee recommended that "the federal government ensure strong leadership and provide additional funding to sustain, better coordinate and integrate the public health infrastructure in Canada, as well as relevant health promotion efforts. An amount of $200 million in additional funding should be devoted to this very important undertaking" (Standing Senate Committee on Social Affairs Science and Technology, 2002). It argued that changes could be effected without legislation by using memoranda of understanding with provincial and territorial authorities on procedures and protocols to allow for greater collaboration on disease surveillance and control. In the longer term, a legislative review should be undertaken with a goal of harmonizing and improving federal and provincial health emergency legislation.

The Romanow report did not specifically address public health surveillance initiatives in Canada but did emphasize the importance of supporting international initiatives to reduce the risk of communicable diseases spreading to Canada. This requirement would necessitate ensuring appropriate reporting in Canada based on international treaties. Romanow recommended that Canada should work "with the World Health Organization to strengthen and renew the International Health Regulations on monitoring and containing communicable diseases" (Commission on the Future of Health Care in Canada, 2002).

Dr. David Naylor, in the Report of the National Advisory Committee on SARS and Public Health October 2003, noted that surveillance data did flow during SARS due to the heroic efforts of public health officials at all three levels of government, but in the face of system deficiencies, large gaps became apparent. His report recommended a $100 million per annum investment in support of provincial, territorial, and regional capacity for surveillance and outbreak containment. This would include training of personnel, enhancement of hospital-based surveillance, and development of business process agreements for collaboration (National Advisory Committee on SARS & Public Health, 2003).

Kirby's Senate committee subsequently produced another report entitled *Reforming Health Protection and Promotion in Canada: Time to Act* (Standing Senate Committee on Social Affairs Science and Technology, 2003). The report noted that, in his deposition to the committee, Dr. Naylor had stated, "First, in this imaginary and positive alternative universe, the agency would continually monitor national and international incidents, and establish and participate in comprehensive surveillance systems that would provide the ability to detect potential risk. When the next SARS begins to emerge, alerts would be sent out widely. The first time that the infectious agent turns up in Berlin or Singapore or anywhere, a series of alerts would be issued worldwide saying that virus X or bacterium B is on the move. Those alerts would then rapidly and actively be transmitted through the Canadian public health and health care systems. Medical officers of health and health care leaders would both have immediate alerts from the new agency and from the desk of the public health officer of Canada saying that there is a problem. If it were a known agent, a well-understood and agreed protocol as to what should be done would then be followed. There would also be a common set of business processes on how to respond. Therefore, instead of making it up as they went along, frontline responders would be guided by a national consensus on best practices. If it were a new agent, as soon as [a provincial government] called for help, the national agency would provide support on the ground based on already-existing protocols for collaboration." The commission's report supported Naylor's call for a national public health agency, which would use a communicable disease control fund to assist provinces and territories in building disease surveillance capacity, culminating in a national disease surveillance system.

The Expert Panel on SARS and Infectious Disease Control (Walker Commission) noted, "SARS brought to light the lack of and need for a comprehensive infectious disease surveillance infrastructure in Ontario, with the capacity to link the acute and long-term care, community, and public health sectors. The Health Surveillance Working Group agreed in 2002 that such a health surveillance infrastructure must be developed. In any effective surveillance strategy, technology plays an increasingly critical role ... Information and information technology systems ... provide the spine for effective real-time data reporting and analysis. To-date, however, efforts have been largely episodic and disease-specific" (Expert Panel on SARS & Infectious Disease Control, 2004).

APPENDIX D: INTERNATIONAL HEALTH REGULATIONS
REPORTING REQUIREMENTS AND PROCESSES

In recognition of an increasingly globalized world in which travel times are often less than the incubation period of many communicable diseases (rendering all populations vulnerable to outbreaks wherever they emerge), the World Health Assembly Member States adopted the revised International Health Regulations (IHR) in May 2005 (World Health Organization, 2005). Designed to avoid unnecessary interference in international trade and travel while protecting communities from public health threats, these rules and procedures address key elements in the prevention and control of disease spread such as: *detection*, confirmation, and assessment of events involving disease or death above expected levels for the particular time and place within a territory of a "state party" (country); *reporting* of events, if found urgent, to the national level (criteria for urgency include a serious public health impact and/or unusual or unexpected nature with high potential for spread); *assessment*, within 48 hours of reporting, of urgent events to determine the potential of becoming a public health emergency of international concern (PHEIC), with final determination of PHEIC status to be confirmed by the WHO; *notification* of the WHO, through a "national focal point," within 24 hours of this assessment, and thereafter in a timely manner informing the WHO of key detailed public health information, including, where possible: case definitions, laboratory results, source and type of the risk, number of cases and deaths, conditions affecting the spread of the disease, and the health measures employed; *reporting*, when necessary, any difficulties encountered and support required to respond to a PHEIC; and *responding* to requests from the WHO for further information to verify information received from other sources, and to collaborate and accept collaboration in response to events.

In addition, the revised IHR address measures for identification and containment of diseases at airports, marine ports, and ground crossings in people and cargoes; surveillance of travellers and migrant populations; and roles and responsibilities of carriers, authorities, state parties, and the WHO.

In Canada, PHAC has been designated as the National IHR Focal Point, and takes the lead in implementations of the IHR across F/P/T governments. In their 2010 report, PHAC noted that "the Agency complies with IHR minimum requirements that were expected by June 2009; however, some areas require attention to reach full compliance by June 2012" (Public Health Agency of Canada, 2010a).

Full compliance with the IHR requires coordination at local community, intermediate, (provincial/territorial) and national levels. Canada's legislative framework, which places responsibility of data collection and analysis at local and intermediate levels, challenges Canada's ability to be fully compliant. Similarly, the United States informed the

WHO of a reservation to the IHR, indicating its unwillingness to bind other levels of government within the United States: "The Government of the United States of America reserves the right to assume obligations under these Regulations in a manner consistent with its fundamental principles of federalism. With respect to obligations concerning the development, strengthening, and maintenance of the core capacity requirements set forth in Annex 1, these Regulations shall be implemented by the Federal Government or the state governments, as appropriate and in accordance with our Constitution, to the extent that the implementation of these obligations comes under the legal jurisdiction of the Federal Government. To the extent that such obligations come under the legal jurisdiction of the state governments, the Federal Government shall bring such obligations with a favorable recommendation to the notice of the appropriate state authorities" (World Health Organization, 2007).

## APPENDIX E: REFERENCES CITED AND FURTHER READINGS

British Columbia Ministry of Health. (2005). *A framework for core functions in public health*. Population Health and Wellness. http://www.phabc.org/pdf core/core_functions.pdf?NSNST_Flood=hrkhhdyo

Campbell, A. (2004). *SARS and public health in Ontario: The SARS commission interim report*. Ontario Ministry of Health and Long-Term Care. http://www .health.gov.on.ca/english/public/pub/ministry_reports/campbell04/camp bell04.html

Campbell, A. (2005). *The SARS Commission: Second interim report: SARS and public health legislation*. Ontario Ministry of Health and Long-Term Care. http://www.health.gov.on.ca/english/public/pub/ministry_reports/camp bell04/campbell04.html

Campbell, A. (2006). *The SARS commission – Spring of fear* (Vols. 1–3). Ontario Ministry of Health and Long-Term Care. http://www.ontla.on.ca/library/ repository/mon/16000/268478.pdf

Capacity Review Committee. (2005). *Revitalizing Ontario's public health capacity: A discussion of issues and opinions: Final report*. http://www.health.gov.on.ca/ english/public/pub/ministry_reports/capacity_review06/capacity_ review06.pdf

Centers for Disease Control and Prevention. (2001). *Updated guidelines for evaluating public health surveillance systems: Recommendations from the guidelines working group*. http://www.cdc.gov/mmwr/preview/mmwrhtml/ rr5013a1.htm

Commission on the Future of Health Care in Canada. (2002). *Building on values: The future of health care in Canada*. Final Report: Queen's Printer. http://publications.gc.ca/collections/Collection/CP32-85-2002E.pdf

Expert Panel on SARS & Infectious Disease Control. (2004, April). *For the public's health: A plan of action. Final report of the Ontario expert panel on SARS and infectious disease control*. Ministry of Health and Long-Term Care. http://www.health.gov.on.ca/english/public/pub/ministry_reports/walker04/walker04_mn.html

McDougall, C.W. (2009). *Still waiting for a comprehensive national epidemic surveillance system: A case study of how collaborative federalism has become a risk to public health*. Queen's University. http://www.queensu.ca/iigr/Working Papers/PublicHealthSeries/McDougall_Still.pdf

Moloughney, B.W. (2006). *The renewal of public health in Nova Scotia: Building a public health system to meet the needs of Nova Scotians*. Government of Nova Scotia. http://novascotia.ca/dhw/publichealth/documents/Renewal-of-Public-Health-Report.pdf

National Advisory Committee on SARS & Public Health. (2003, October). *Learning from SARS: Renewal of public health in Canada (Naylor report)*. Health Canada. http://www.phac-aspc.gc.ca/publicat/sars-sras/naylor/

Office of the Auditor General of Canada. (1999). *1999 Report of the Auditor General of Canada, Chapter 14—National Health Surveillance: Diseases and Injuries*. http://www.oag-bvg.gc.ca/internet/English/parl_oag_199909_14_e_10143.html

Office of the Auditor General of Canada. (2002, September). *A status report of the auditor general of Canada to the House of Commons, Chapter 2—Health Canada: National Health Surveillance*. Minister of Public Works and Government Services Canada. http://www.oag-bvg.gc.ca/internet/English/parl_oag_200209_02_e_12387.html

Public Health Agency of Canada. (2010a, January). *Quarantine, migration and travel health and international health regulations*. Audit Services Division. http://www.phac-aspc.gc.ca/about_apropos/asd-dsv/ar-rv/2010/qmt-qms-eng.php

Public Health Agency of Canada. (2010b, November). *Lessons learned review: Public Health Agency of Canada and Health Canada response to the 2009 H1N1 pandemic*. http://www.phac-aspc.gc.ca/about_apropos/evaluation/reports-rapports/2010-2011/h1n1/

Public Health Ontario. (2013). *About us*. http://www.publichealthontario.ca/en/About/Pages/Organization.aspx#.UqoAuqV8xFw

Rush, B. (2005, April). *Capacity mapping in public health: Results of a survey and key informant interview process with OPHA constituent societies and related associations and groups*. VIRGO Planning and Evaluation. http://opha.on.ca/getmedia/3be5c3a3-e2e3-4661-9bef-6decedab9dbb/CapacityMapping-FinalReport-2005.pdf.aspx?ext=.pdf.

Shah, C.P. (2003). *Public health and preventive medicine in Canada* (5th ed.). Toronto: Elsevier Canada.

Standing Senate Committee on Social Affairs Science and Technology. (2002). *The health of Canadians: The federal role, final report: Vol. 6. Recommendations for reform*. Parliament of Canada. http://www.parl.gc.ca/Content/SEN/Committee/372/soci/rep/repoct02vol6highlights-e.htm

Standing Senate Committee on Social Affairs Science and Technology. (2003, November). *Reforming health protection and promotion in Canada: Time to act, Ottawa, ON*. Parliament of Canada. http://www.parl.gc.ca/Content/SEN/Committee/372/soci/rep/repfinnov03-e.htm

Sutcliffe, P., Deber, R., & Pasut, G. (1997). Public health in Canada: A comparative study of six provinces. *Canadian Journal of Public Health, 88*(4), 246–9.

Toronto Public Health. (2011, June). *Communicable disease reporting*. http://www.toronto.ca/health/cdc/communicable_disease_surveillance/monitoring/pdf/reportablediseases.pdf

Weatherill, S. (2009). *Report of the independent investigator into the 2008 listeriosis outbreak: Government of Canada*. Government of Canada. http://www.cpha.ca/uploads/history/achievements/09-lirs-rpt_e.pdf

Wilson, K. (2001). The role of federalism in health surveillance: A case study of the national health surveillance "infostructure." In D. Adams (Ed.), *Federalism, democracy and health policy in Canada* (pp. 207–37). Kingston, ON: McGill-Queen's University Press.

Wilson, K., McDougall, C., Fidler, D.P., & Lazar, H. (2008a). Strategies for implementing the new international health regulations in federal countries. *Bulletin of the World Health Organization, 86*(3), 215–20. http://dx.doi.org/10.2471/BLT.07.042838

Wilson, K., von Tigerstrom, B., & McDougall, C. (2008b). Protecting global health security through the international health regulations: Requirements and challenges. *Canadian Medical Association Journal, 179*(1), 44–8. http://dx.doi.org/10.1503/cmaj.080516

World Health Organization. (2005). *Agenda item 13.1 23: Third report of Committee A*. World Health Organization 58th World Health Assembly. http://www.who.int/hdp/publications/9c.pdf

World Health Organization. (2007). *The World Health report 2007: A safer future: Global public health security in the 21st century*. http://www.who.int/whr/2007/en/index.html

The following website may also be helpful:

World Health Organization, International Health Regulations, http://www.who.int/features/qa/39/en/index.html

# 8 Filling in the Gaps

## The Decision to Utilize Agency Nursing in Tarman Hospital

KAREN ARTHURS, ANDREA BAUMANN, DOREEN DAY, SARAH DIMMOCK, LEAH LEVESQUE, ELEANOR ROSS, VERA INGRID TARMAN, AND RAISA B. DEBER

Health care is delivered by people; to operate effectively and safety, hospital units must be staffed by qualified, competent individuals. What options are available to a nurse manager and the hospital where she works to ensure that staff is available at all times to cover a hospital nursing unit?

This case addresses several policy issues, including: health human resources (HHR) shortages/surpluses, and computing the costs and consequences of alternatives, including implications for patient continuity of care and safety, and for staff nurse satisfaction and morale.

**Appendices**

Appendix A: Staffing Options
Appendix B: Cost of Agency Nurses vs. Staff Nurses
Appendix C: Nursing HHR: Shortages, Retention, and Recruitment
Appendix D: References Cited and Further Reading

**The Case**

Please note: Both Ms. Arthurs and Tarman Hospital are fictional.

Ms. Arthurs is the new nurse manager of a 23-bed unit in Tarman Hospital, a busy urban teaching hospital. Because she has to staff the unit on a 24-hours-per-day, 7-days-a-week basis, she needs to cover approximately 75 shifts per week. She must also ensure that shifts are covered when the scheduled nurse is not available due to sick time, vacation time, statutory holidays, etc. During the peak vacation times she may need to cover an additional 10 shifts per week.

Ms. Arthurs considers the following options:

1. *Increased overtime:* She can call in a nurse from her own unit's part-time/casual pool and fill remaining gaps with her own full-time staff working overtime as needed.
2. *Casual/resource pool:* She can use nurses from the hospital's central-ized pool of resource "float" nurses.
3. *Change staff/skill mix:* She can use more LPNs (licensed practical nurses) and/or PSWs (personal support workers) instead of RNs (registered nurses).
4. *Agency nurses:* She can call a nursing agency.

**Background**

To practice, nurses must be registered with their provincial/territorial regulatory body, usually referred to as the College of Nurses. There are two major categories of nurses in Canada: registered nurses (RNs) and registered/licensed practical nurses (variously called RPNs or LPNs, depending on the province). In some provinces, including Ontario, RNs must now complete a four-year degree from an accredited university-based program (although RNs who obtained their training under earlier models are "grandfathered" or "grandmothered"); LPNs must com-plete a two-year program from an accredited college. In some settings, services may also be provided by workers who are not regulated pro-fessionals, including personal support workers (PSWs).

Tarman Hospital is an acute care hospital, and its patients tend to need more intensive care, although their lengths of stay are also rela-tively short. The hospital relies heavily upon RNs, some of whom may also have specialty designations. (Appendix A provides more detail about the staffing options for Tarman Hospital.)

Tarman Hospital has three categories of staff: full-time (FT), part-time (PT), or casual (CAS). In this hospital, FT and PT staff receive ben-efits and a predictable schedule; CAS staff work on an as-needed basis, and usually do not receive benefits. The challenge for Ms. Arthurs is how to recruit and retain enough nurses to staff all the clinical areas for which she is responsible. In addition, the hospital is unionized, and the collective agreements limit how staff can be used to cover weekend and evening nursing shifts. For that reason, some hospitals use nursing agencies to fill their staffing gaps, often on a regular (even daily) basis. See Appendix B for some cost data comparing staff and agency nurses, and Appendix C for more information on nursing HHR.

In addition to filling her immediate staffing needs, Ms. Arthurs must also take into consideration some longer-term issues. For example, there is some pressure to maintain an adequate FT complement. She is aware of reports suggesting that the optimal ratio is at least 70% FT staff, and that many nurses prefer to work FT. One advantage for the hospital is that a higher proportion of FT positions appears to be associated with more effective continuity of care and lower nurse turnover rates. However, it will also be necessary to have enough PT staff to be able to cover time off, vacation, and illness for FT staff. Indeed, she knows that not having sufficient numbers of PT nurses makes it difficult to ensure adequate staffing, particularly in specialized units such as the one she now manages. Most busy acute care units require some degree of surge capacity that cannot always come from within the FT staff; overtime work is often the solution. But Ms. Arthurs is also aware of studies that have shown an association between high overtime hours and lower job satisfaction/increased nurse turnover (Baumann, 2010). One study estimated the mean turnover rate in Canadian hospitals at 19.9% – an expensive proposition given that the average cost of nursing turnover was estimated at $25,000 per nurse (Canadian Nursing Advisory Committee, 2002). Temporary staff can be used in the short term, but there are relatively high costs associated with having to hire these additional nurses.

**Factors to Consider**

There are advantages and disadvantages to each of the four options Ms. Arthurs is considering. These include:

Option 1:    *Increased overtime.* A major advantage of this option is that her FT staff already know the unit and can provide better continuity of care to the patients. However, if they are working overtime, they must be paid more. For example, an agency RN costs approximately $50/hour, while overtime for staff nurses can cost up to $70/hour, including benefits, depending on the seniority of the nurse. Appendix B gives some data about the cost of agency nursing vs. the cost of employed staff for nurses at the same seniority level (in this case, with eight years' experience). Another disadvantage to using staff nurses is that they can become burned out, resulting in an increase in sick time and injuries if they are relied upon too much.

Option 2:   *Casual/resource pool.* This strategy may also provide patient continuity, and is a cheaper alternative than overtime staff. However, relief staff are often not available on short notice. Moreover, if relief staff are centrally based in the hospital and move from unit to unit, they still may not know the patient population and/or the policies of a given unit very well.

Option 3:   *Change staff/skill mix.* This could involve hiring more LPNs and PSWs and fewer RNs. The advantages include the reduced workload for RNs if they can delegate/assign tasks to LPNs and/or PSWs. It may also be easier for management to maintain a full complement of staff. Disadvantages include the burden on the RNs to supervise the LPNs and PSWs, and the challenge in maintaining the needed standard of skill among the unregulated group of PSWs, including possible costs for training them.

Option 4:   *Agency nurses.* Major advantages of using an agency include the large numbers of staff who are usually available on short notice, and that the hospital nurse manager does not have to pay the administrative and coordinating costs of managing this pool of nurses. Disadvantages include the increased cost of hiring the agency nurse, the lack of continuity of care for patients, and the lack of accountability of the nurse to the hospital.

It is unclear to hospital management how these factors balance one another, and hence when utilization of agency nurses is a cost-effective solution. The price they pay must be high enough to cover the agency's profit; in addition, someone will have to pay for the costs assumed by the agency for administrative and clerical functions, training, insurance, and reorienting new agency staff. Most of these services are already paid for by the hospital for its FT staff. Hospital management wonders whether paying the agency for what they see as a duplication of functions plus profit for the agency is a good use of hospital resources.

The Hospital Management Committee is therefore considering its policy choices regarding agency nursing use. The CEO claims that the hospital cannot afford the services of the agency, and says that she would prefer the hospital to rely on its own PT or relief staff. However, the VP of HR and the Chief Nursing Executive note that, with nursing vacancy rates high at the hospital, they cannot afford to risk patient safety or quality of care by working short-staffed on a regular basis or negatively affecting retention rates by burning out their FT nurses.

## Arguments against Agency Nurses

Some have argued that agency nursing may have negative consequences for quality and continuity of care, patient safety and satisfaction, and accountability. They point to the landmark publication *Crossing the Quality Chasm* (Institute of Medicine, 2001), which emphasized the importance of avoiding medical error and designing processes to emphasize patient safety. One result has been increased focus on interprofessional collaboration, team communication, and patient safety incident reporting and follow-up. Many hospitals are also adopting "organizational learning" practices, which are generally implemented at the point-of-service level (Carroll & Edmondson, 2002). This approach stresses facilitating effective informal communication structures, particularly between physicians and nurses, using such mechanisms as reviews of practice, audits, problem investigations, performance appraisals, simulation, and benchmarking.

Because agency nurses are less likely to be part of the "clinical micro-systems" (individually functioning front-line teams) in hospitals, this line of argument suggests that it is challenging for short-term contract nurses from outside agencies to provide the standard of care that is now demanded for patients. (Note that the outcomes of interest may include patients' health status, patient satisfaction with care, and/or staff satisfaction.) Because they are employed by a third party and are in a given hospital intermittently, agency nurses cannot actively participate in organizational learning practices. The lack of familiarity with institutional policies and protocols, the inability to follow role models demonstrating exemplary practice, and difficulty in dealing with sensitive patient issues are all documented concerns that nurse managers have concerning agency staff. To the extent that quality improvement has focused on improving trust, communication, collaboration, and decision making within a team, use of nurses who do not usually work in that unit may affect quality of care. In addition, it is not always possible to ensure that agency nurses have a high level of knowledge of the specific patient population being served on a particular unit.

A related concern expressed about agency nursing relates to difficulties in ensuring continuity of care. Hospitals cannot benefit from the experience that workers get daily on the job if these workers are working somewhere else the next day, and patients may suffer if agency nurses are not given adequate orientation to the hospital's policies and procedures. Some worry this lack of familiarity with policy and procedures could lead to increased error rates.

Hospitals are also unable to control the total amount of time an agency nurse can work in a given week. Indeed, some agencies use nurses who are also employed FT elsewhere. This raises concerns regarding the fatigue of the nurse and his/her ability to work effectively, and the potential implications for error rates.

The extent to which these concerns are supported by data is ambiguous, particularly because units relying more heavily on agency nurses may differ in other ways from units who can retain enough permanent staff. Some studies have suggested that the float pool nurses (employed by the hospital) are most likely to document having completed selected quality indicators, and agency nurses least likely (with the unit-employed nurses in the middle). Agency nurses were indeed less likely to be communicating with physicians and patients, probably because they did not feel they knew the patients well enough.

Another dimension of quality is the effect on the workforce. Ideally, one would wish to retain a qualified, satisfied workforce. Indications of quality problems might include issues with illness / on-the-job injury, absenteeism, and recruitment/retention. Nursing can be a highly physical job, and efforts to minimize injuries and absenteeism may also be important ways to ensure that the necessary staff is available.

Another set of concerns relates to accountability. Contract nurses are accountable to their employers (the agencies), rather than to the hospital. Performance appraisals, for example, are conducted by the agencies. To some extent, accreditation may require the agencies to demonstrate the competency of their staff. However, there is a sense that agency nurses may be reluctant to report patient safety incidents or near misses to the hospital (although they may report them to the agency), or to participate in the hospital-based quality improvement protocols. This may interfere with the ability for the hospital to learn from such incidents.

## Arguments for Agency Nurses

An agency nurse can be hired as needed on a casual basis. There are many agency nurses available in urban communities such as the one where Tarman Hospital is located.

Many nursing agencies are now accredited through Accreditation Canada; its website described accreditation as an "external peer review process to assess and improve the services healthcare organizations provide to their patients and clients based on standards of excellence" (Accreditation Canada, 2012). The process of accreditation is claimed to ensure that a nursing agency is following best practices in areas such as hiring, screening, performance monitoring, and continuing education for nursing staff. From the perspective of a nursing agency, an accreditation standard is a hospital's guarantee that the agency is hiring only appropriately trained and screened nurses and that quality of care and skills training is ongoing.

From the viewpoint of the nurse, agency work may increase the flexibility and control over scheduling, place of work, and type of work held by the individual nurse. Nursing is a largely female profession. To accommodate family responsibilities, nurses may choose (at different points in their careers) to work less than FT hours. The agencies can provide maximal flexibility in terms of hours worked, place of work, and type of work. As one prominent nursing agency noted on its website, "Our agency offers you the opportunity to set your own work schedule that suits your needs and your lifestyle. You can work as much or as little as you want, in whatever field you choose (based on qualifications, of course). We believe in satisfying the needs of our personnel as well as our clients. Whether you're a Nurse or a Personal Support Worker, you set the rules that say when and where you work." Nursing agencies offer very competitive hourly rates, often above what is paid to nurses employed in hospitals. Some agencies also provide comprehensive benefits packages that include many of the same benefits afforded to staff nurses, including funding for continuing education, and extended health and dental plans. All of this appeals to a group of nurses who may enjoy a level of autonomy and control over their work schedules and environments that is not traditionally available to staff nurses.

Overall, it appears that agencies feel they are helping to deal with staffing shortages. One nursing agency stated that agencies can fill an essential need: "Nursing agencies provide hospitals with the security of knowing that we will provide competent, knowledgeable nurses to ensure that hospital units are not operating short handed or operating with exhausted nurses on overtime." The agency further noted that most hospital casual and PT pools are not large enough to support all the backfill that needs to happen, and argue that without the availability of these private sector nurses, many hospitals would be forced to close down beds and cut back on services for the public.

Nursing agencies contend that when the relationship is well managed, they are also able to provide the clinical team and the patients with high-quality staff and continuity of care. For example, one agency spokesperson highlighted its efforts to maintain specific agency staff for particular hospitals and units so that there is consistency in the nurses who work there. In addition, that agency pays its nurses to attend an orientation at the hospital where they will be working. They note that this is possible only when the hospital and agency work to form a partnership that meets the needs of the patients and serves the interests of both organizations.

Some have argued that costs of agency nurses can be less than the costs of FT personnel. Although agencies charge higher hourly rates, once benefits are calculated, the costs can be relatively equal. In addition, paying overtime to employee nurses can be much more expensive than hiring an agency nurse. (See Appendix B for sample costs.)

However, neither the hospitals nor the agencies believe that heavy reliance on agency nurses is an ideal situation. As one agency spokesperson stated, "When agency nurses become the backbone of a hospital unit's staffing, it leads to unhappiness on the part of the hospital administration and reflects badly on the agency. That isn't right, but it is the reality. The relationship works best when agencies act as the staffing safety net, not the staffing solution."

DECISION POINT

What options should Ms. Arthurs pursue? Given the advantages and disadvantages, should she utilize agency nurses on her unit? What should the Hospital Management Committee recommend? Should the committee recommend a halt to the utilization of agency nursing as a policy directive for all the inpatient units in the hospital? Should there be an overall hospital policy, or should decisions be made on a unit-by-unit basis?

SUGGESTED QUESTIONS FOR DISCUSSION

1. What would you do if you were Ms. Arthurs? What if you were a part of the Hospital Management Committee? Why?
2. What affects work satisfaction? How might this apply to nurse satisfaction in hospitals?
3. Discuss the implications of different models of nursing care, including the use of unregulated workers to perform nursing tasks. What role does professionalism play?
4. Who are agency nurses? How are they used? What are the advantages and disadvantages of using agency nursing? For nurses, unit managers and staff? What are the potential implications for: Costs? Patient safety and quality/continuity of care? Nurse morale?

APPENDIX A: STAFFING OPTIONS

*Staff nurses* are employed by the hospital, on a full-time (FT) or part-time (PT) basis. Most staff nurses are *registered nurses* (RNs). In many provinces, RNs belong to a union. Staff nurses are regularly scheduled on a shift rotation; however, if they are required to work beyond the permitted number of hours permitted by their union's collective agreement, they must be paid overtime.

The hospitals may also use *licensed practical nurses* (LPNs), who may also be called registered practical nurses (RPNs), depending on the province. LPNs work under the supervision of an RN, who delegates acts to the LPN as appropriate, based on the skills and competencies of the individual LPN. LPN training is generally through a two-year college diploma course. Staff LPNs are employed by the hospital; in many provinces, most hospital-based LPNs are members of a union, usually the Canadian Union of Public Employees (CUPE) or the Service Employees International Union (SEIU).

*Casual nurses* are also employed by the hospital and are usually unionized; however, they are not regularly scheduled on a shift rotation. They work on a casual basis and are called in as needed. They often work in a specific unit rather than as part of a float pool. Many hospitals no longer hire casual nurses, but existing FT and PT nurses can ask to move to casual status. Casual nurses are given the same orientation and training as their FT and PT counterparts. They are also offered continuing education support (according to the individual hospital's policies). As the investment in a casual nurse is similar to the investment in a FT or PT nurse, it can be costly to an organization if that nurse works only intermittently. As a result, many hospitals have instituted rules that dictate a minimum number of hours per year that a casual nurse must work as a condition of employment.

*Resource pool nurses*, also called float pool nurses, or nursing resource teams, are a pool of nurses who are trained to work on different units within the hospital to help meet the staffing needs throughout an organization. These nurses are employed by the hospital and are usually unionized. In many cases, they are not permanent FT nurses, but are PT or casual.

*Agency nurses* are employed by a third-party employer and are hired/contracted by a hospital to meet staffing needs. They may be RNs or LPNs. Agency nurses are not unionized and are accountable to their employer, not to the hospital who is hiring/contracting them. These nurses are paid a comparable hourly rate to staff nurses (sometimes they are paid a premium). Nursing agencies offer nurses a much greater degree of flexibility in terms of scheduling, where they work (e.g., hospital, home care, long-term care), and/or which population groups they serve. Most agencies now also offer a comprehensive benefits package that includes extended health and dental, malpractice insurance coverage, workers compensation coverage, and continuing education funding. The nursing agency industry (which includes both for-profit and non-profit organizations) is known to be extremely competitive and volatile. Agency administrators have described their organizations as being at the mercy of the demands of the hospitals and any shortages in the nursing labour market.

Another possibility is to make greater use of *non-regulated* workers, including personal support workers (PSWs). Many provinces, including the province where Tarman Hospital is located, have legislation that defines such matters as classifications of categories of nurses, requirements for entry to practice, scope of practice for nurses, and protection of title (i.e., who can call themselves a nurse). Another law identifies which controlled and delegated acts various health care professionals are permitted to perform (see Chapter 1, sections 6.4, Professionalism, 5.2.1, Regulation, and 7.3, Regulating Health Professionals). For example, at the time of writing, Ontario had designated 13 controlled acts, of which nurses were permitted to perform 3. Under this approach, controlled acts can be performed by more than one profession. In addition, there are provisions to allow unregulated workers (including PSWs) to perform controlled acts under specified conditions (e.g., to allow family members to assist individuals with routine activities of daily living). The legislation distinguished between *delegation* and *assignment* of controlled acts; in both cases, there is an assumption that the regulated health professional will supervise and/or teach those doing the tasks to perform them safely. In general, RNs are responsible for supervising the LPNs and PSWs on their unit.

## APPENDIX B: COST OF AGENCY NURSES VS. STAFF NURSES

Hourly rates for staff RNs are set by the Hospital Central Agreement with the union. The rates are based on nurse experience. For example, as of April 1, 2011, the starting rate was $29.36 per hour, rising with experience. The rate for an RN with 8 years' experience was $41.70; for a nurse with 25 years' experience, it was $42.44. The rates were due to increase over time; for example, as of April 1, 2013, the rate for a nurse with eight years' experience would rise to $42.85.

In addition, there were shift premiums of $1.85 for the evening shift, $2.25 for the night shift, and $2.40 for weekends, which were also due to increase over time. Holiday pay was set at 1.5 times normal hourly rate, plus a lieu day off with pay. Other premiums were payable for such activities as being a group or unit leader.

The LPN collective agreement (through CUPE) for 2009–2013 had been settled by arbitration. It did not set a common LPN wage rate for all hospitals, but did agree to use similar rates for hospitals within the same geographic area. The rate for the hospitals in the region where Tarman Hospital was located was $29.88.

Ms. Arthurs then performed some simple calculations, making the following assumptions:

- Number of RN hours needed for the unit in one month: 2,250
- Number of LPN hours needed for the unit in one month: 1,350
- Nursing salaries (RN) based on union collective agreements using the pay scale as of April 1, 2011, computed for an RN with eight years' experience
- LPN salaries based on collective agreement with the union
- Benefits in lieu for casual employees calculated at 13%

- Benefits in lieu for full-time employees calculated at 22%
- Overtime rate calculated at 1 1/2 times salary
- Agency hourly rates based on an average of four nursing agencies in the GTA (RN range: $45/hour to $56/hour)

Table 8.1. Cost Comparison for Tarman Hospital: Agency Nursing vs. Employee vs. Overtime

| Employee category | Hourly rate | Benefits (per hour) | Total (per hour) | Total (8-hr. shift) |
|---|---|---|---|---|
| **Staff nurse** | | | | |
| RN full-time (8 yrs. experience) | $41.70 | $9.17 | $50.87 | 406.96 |
| RN casual | $41.70 | $5.42 | $47.12 | 376.96 |
| RN overtime | $62.55 | n/a | $62.55 | 500.40 |
| LPN full-time | $29.88 | $6.57 | $36.45 | 291.60 |
| LPN casual | $29.88 | $3.88 | $33.76 | 270.08 |
| LPN overtime | $44.82 | | $44.82 | 358.56 |
| **Agency** | | | | |
| Hourly rate for RN | $49.50 | | $49.50 | 396.00 |
| Hourly rate for LPN | $36.50 | | $36.50 | 292.00 |

Simple calculations revealed that for one eight-hour RN shift, and taking as a baseline a FT staff nurse ($406.96), the agency nurse would cost $10.96 less ($406.96–$396). However, an RN from the casual pool would cost $30 less. On the other hand, using overtime nurses would increase costs for the shift by $93.44. For LPNs, there was a similar but not identical pattern; compared to a FT staff nurse ($291.60), the agency nurse would cost $0.40 less, a staff casual nurse $21.52 less, but a staff LPN working overtime would cost $66.96 more. Similar calculations could compute likely costs for a month or year, as a function of the vacancy rate and number of shifts that would need to be covered (as well as allowing for different costs for nurses with different seniority).

APPENDIX C: NURSING HHR: SHORTAGES, RETENTION, AND RECRUITMENT

Nursing supply refers to all registered nurses in a jurisdiction. This can be subdivided into those who are currently employed, actively seeking work, new entrants, and those who have been inactive but are rejoining the workforce. According to the Canadian Institute of Health Information (CIHI), the total number of registered nurses in Canada has steadily increased over the last decade. By 2010, there were 354,910 regulated nurses working in nursing in Canada, of whom about three-quarters were RNs. Most (about 94%) were women. Over half (58%) of RNs were working FT (Canadian Institute for Health Information, 2013).

Most analysts suggest there is still an inadequate replenishing of the nursing labour supply. Turnover is defined as the number of persons who leave/resign from a position in a given year as a percentage of the average number of employees in a given year. Labour turnover in nursing was traditionally high and affects nursing supply. The average age of nurses has increased slightly, and is in the mid-40s. According to CIHI, the highest exit rates in the country were, as expected, in the oldest age group (over 60 years). However, the age group with the second highest exit rates was in the youngest age range (under 30 years). This phenomenon was consistent across the country, although the numbers were considerably higher in some provinces than others. One possible explanation is that registration data sets are on a provincial basis, and a nurse moving from one jurisdiction to another may have been recorded as an exit (which is accurate from the viewpoint of that jurisdiction, although not from the viewpoint of nursing as a profession). Another may be that some leave temporarily to have families but may subsequently return.

Both sides of the supply/demand equation must be examined whenever there are discussions about labour shortages. The actual consumer demanding nursing services is the patient. However, the patient does not make any of the decisions regarding the quality or quantity of nursing care; the hospital is the main consumer of nursing care because it hires nurses and pays them. Thus, there is an indirect relationship between the actual recipient of nursing services and the provider. Some of the trends affecting the demand for nurses include the increasing aged population, rising patient acuity rates, and changes in the mix of RNs and LPNs. The demand for nursing services has increased in acute and long-term care facilities, and in the community.

In Canada, nursing shortages are a recurring phenomenon. Some of the literature points to seven- to eight-year cycles characterized by shortages and then followed by surpluses. Nurse retention is often affected by economic instabilities within a jurisdiction, particularly when hospitals are publicly financed. Salaries account for approximately 75% of hospital budgets, and nursing accounts for a large portion of health human resources. Layoffs tend to be a common short-term response when hospitals are forced to reduce their costs. If economic instability is not an issue, however, data shows that once nurses are employed within a sector (i.e., hospital or community) for a year, they tend to remain within that sector long-term (Alameddine et al., 2006).

A considerable literature exists on nurse satisfaction and how this relates to nurse retention. Among the factors adversely affecting satisfaction are increased workloads as well as increased patient acuity. Many hospitals have attempted to do more with less. However, understaffing may lead not only to higher total costs (often associated with overtime expenses) but also to burning out nurses.

More recently, unregulated health care workers have been introduced into the acute care settings (see also Appendix A). In response to the changes in care delivery, the provincial College of Nurses has established guidelines to assist RNs and LPNs in delegating work to these unregulated workers. This added responsibility in an environment that has nurses taking on added accountabilities has been claimed to contribute to the dissatisfaction of nurses.

Nurses' lack of control over their work schedules has historically been another cause for dissatisfaction for hospital nurses. Nurses who do not wish to work 12-hour shifts, or night shifts, or weekends, may choose to work PT or with agencies in order to control their hours. Indeed, nurses who work for agencies overwhelmingly rate flexibility as a positive aspect of their work. Some hospitals have responded to these concerns by negotiating innovative scheduling that allows nurses to work 12-hour shifts with more time off after a stretch of four shifts; however, this may also lead to exhaustion and more errors.

Registries and agencies charge "what the traffic will bear," whereas hospitals must use the union's negotiated salary scale. When demand for nurses is high, agencies can obtain hourly rates for general duty nurses that are higher than union rates, although this may exclude the costs of benefits. For example, the maximum rate charged to the hospital for both general duty and specialty nurses is up to $49.50 per hour. This is higher than the base rates, as shown in Appendix B. Agency nurses may also enjoy more flexible schedules. In addition, it is harder to staff certain units (including critical care and long-term care); some agencies are willing to pay specialty fees for nurses who work in those units, whereas union agreements makes it more difficult for hospitals to do so.

Nonetheless, the retention rate of nurses is high, and evidence suggests that most are happy with their work.

## APPENDIX D: REFERENCES CITED AND FURTHER READING

Accreditation Canada. (2012). *Home page*. http://www.accreditation.ca/

Alameddine, M., Laporte, A., Baumann, A., O'Brien-Pallas, L., Mildon, B., & Deber, R. (2006). "Stickiness" and "inflow" as proxy measures of the relative attractiveness of various sub-sectors of nursing employment. *Social Science & Medicine, 63*(9), 2310–9. http://dx.doi.org/10.1016/j .socscimed.2006.05.014

Baumann, A. (2010). *The impact of turnover and the benefit of stability in the nursing workforce*. International Centre for Human Resources in Nursing: International Council of Nurses. http://www.ichrn.com/publications/ policyresearch/Turnover_EN.pdf

Blythe, J., Baumann, A., Zeytinoglu, I., Denton, M., & Higgins, A. (2005). Full-time or part-time work in nursing: Preferences, tradeoffs and choices. *Healthcare Quarterly, 8*(3), 69–77. http://dx.doi.org/10.12927/ hcq.17157

Canadian Institute for Health Information. (2008, May). *How satisfied are nurses with being a nurse and with their current job?* National Survey of the Work and Health of Nurses. http://www.cihi.ca/cihi-ext-portal/internet/ en/document/spending+and+health+workforce/workforce/nurses/ NURSING_ZIO_2005_MAY

Canadian Institute for Health Information. (2013). *Regulated nurses: Canadian trends, 2007 to 2011*. https://secure.cihi.ca/estore/productFamily.htm?pf= PFC2016&lang=en&media=0

Canadian Nursing Advisory Committee. (2002). *Our health, our future: Creating quality workplaces for Canadian nurses*. Canadian Nursing Advisory Committee: Advisory Committee on Health Human Resources. http://www .hc-sc.gc.ca/hcs-sss/alt_formats/hpb-dgps/pdf/pubs/2002-cnac-cccsi- final/2002-cnac-cccsi-final-eng.pdf

Carroll, J.S., & Edmondson, A.C. (2002). Leading organisational learning in health care. *Quality & Safety in Health Care, 11*(1), 51–6. http://dx.doi .org/10.1136/qhc.11.1.51

Institute of Medicine. (2001). *Crossing the quality chasm: A new health system for the 21st century*. Washington, DC: National Academic Press.

Lankshear, A.J., Sheldon, T.A., & Maynard, A. (2005). Nurse staffing and healthcare outcomes: A systematic review of the international research evidence. *ANS. Advances in Nursing Science, 28*(2), 163–74.

Zeytinoglu, I.U., Denton, M., Davies, S., Baumann, A., Blythe, J., & Boos, L. (2007). Deteriorated external work environment, heavy workload and nurses' job satisfaction and turnover intention. *Canadian Public Policy, 33*(s1, Supplement), S31–47. http://dx.doi.org/10.3138/0560-6GV2-G326-76PT

# 9 Midwifery

## Special Delivery

*KAREN BORN, CAROLE-ANNE CHIASSON, SHAWNA
GUTFREUND, LISA JACKSON, ESTHER LEVY, JUDY
LITWACK-GOLDMAN, ELIZABETH MCCARTHY, WENDY
SUTTON, BETTY WU-LAWRENCE, AND RAISA B. DEBER*

A catastrophic midwife-assisted home birth resulted in pressures to incorporate midwifery into the health care system. Should midwifery be regulated, and if so, how? Who should pay for it?

This case addresses several policy issues, including: professional regulation, interest groups, policy implementation, and consumer choice in health care.

### Appendices

Appendix A: Health Providers for Birth and Delivery
Appendix B: An Overview of Midwifery across Canada
Appendix C: References Cited and Further Reading

### The Case

On October 11, 1984, two unlicensed midwives attended the home birth of a baby on Toronto's Ward Island. The house was accessible only by aircraft or ferry, and the nearest hospital was in Toronto's downtown core. At 10 p.m. the fetus's heartbeat could not be heard. Four minutes later, the child was born, and was clearly in trouble. One midwife began artificial respiration; the other called the police to help transport the baby to the Hospital for Sick Children. The harbour police did not have the key to a gate that gave access to the dock where their boat was moored. The two midwives, one of them carrying the baby and giving it mouth-to-mouth resuscitation, had to climb a fence to get to a police boat. The baby and the two midwives were taken by the Metro Police marine unit to the mainland and then by ambulance to the Hospital for

Sick Children. The baby died two days later, with the cause of death listed as asphyxiation. The resulting coroner's inquest determined that the baby would have lived had he had been brought to the hospital sooner. This finding received wide media attention, which helped to highlight the variety of ways in which babies can be delivered.

## Delivering Babies

Historically, childbirth can be risky to the mother and her baby. Indeed, in 2005, the World Health Organization estimated that the lifetime risk of maternal death in Africa was still about 1 in 16. In richer countries such as Canada, in contrast, the risk was about 1 in 2,800. Infant mortality rates have shown a similar decrease (World Health Organization, 2005). Good antenatal and perinatal care is crucial to such improved outcomes. In terms of birth and delivery, two interrelated but separate issues arise: where to give birth and who will help deliver the baby.

Although a woman can go into labour and give birth virtually anywhere, planned births usually occur at home, in a birthing centre, or in hospital. Home births can be subdivided into *freebirth* (planned births at home without the assistance of a health care professional; the woman may be assisted by a partner, family members, and/or friends) or *home birth* (planned births at home with the assistance of a health care professional, such as a midwife). Birthing centres are facilities (which can be free-standing or connected to a hospital) that provide a home-like environment. There are a limited number of birthing centres in Canada, many in the province of Quebec. At the time of writing, the most common location for giving birth in Canada was a hospital.

Births can be attended by specialist physicians (obstetricians), family doctors, nurses, midwives, doulas, and/or by family and friends. The amount of training of these individuals can also vary, as can their access to specialist care in case of an emergency. (See Appendix A for definitions of these health care providers.) In the early days, childbirth in Canada had been managed through a home-based system supported by lay midwives; by the early 20th century, this had shifted to deliveries by doctors in hospitals. Maternal and infant mortality declined. However, over time, the proportion of family physicians providing obstetrics services has decreased; it fell from 36% in 1982 to 18% in 2000 (Born, 2003). With more and more family practitioners opting out of delivering babies, obstetricians have stepped in. As giving birth has become safer, a vocal group has argued for a woman's right to select where she wishes to have her baby, and whom she wishes to assist her with that delivery. One theme was opposition to rising caesarian section rates and increasing medical intervention in childbirth. Another was for greater attention to how to manage births in rural/remote areas, and how to incorporate traditional providers (particularly for aboriginal communities). There were also increased calls for supporting alternative locations for birth, including home births and birthing centres, and for the public funding of midwifery.

### Regulating Midwifery

The debate about regulation incorporated a number of competing tensions. Some midwives sought professional self-regulation, which they hoped might lead to formal recognition of their profession, professional status, and public payment for their services. Other midwives were less enthusiastic, and expressed concerns that formal integration in the health care system would undermine their core values of community-based and personalized care. Some members of the public avidly and actively lobbied for the recognition of midwifery, while others viewed midwifery as dangerous and unproven. The views of other health professionals were also mixed; generally, family practitioners and nursing associations were supportive, while obstetricians and nursing unions were less so.

One result of the coroner's inquest was Ontario's 1993 decision to regulate midwifery as a profession. It was the first Canadian province to do so, although most others soon followed suit. Midwifery was brought in under Ontario's *Regulated Health Professions Act* and given its own professional college (see Chapter 1, section 6.4, Professionalism). By 2010, midwifery had been regulated in every province/territory other than Prince Edward Island, the Yukon, and Nunavut, and these jurisdictions were studying whether to do so (see Appendix B: An Overview of Midwifery across Canada). This approach means that midwives must be registered with their provincial/territorial college to be able to practice, although some provinces have incorporated exceptions for aboriginal midwives and healers.

### Payment Models

There are also a variety of delivery and payment models (see Chapter 1, section 6.2, Payment Mechanisms and Incentives). One issue is whether midwifery would be publicly paid for. Under the *Canada Health Act* (see Chapter 1, section 7.2, *Canada Health Act*), there is a requirement that insured services for insured persons be fully covered, without charges to the patients. However, because midwives are not physicians, there is no inherent requirement that their services be included, although provinces may choose to do so. Indeed, many provinces do pay for midwife services (see Appendix B: An Overview of Midwifery across Canada).

Another issue is how midwife practices are organized. In one model, midwives are independent practitioners, paid by the provincial medical services plan. This model resembles the way in which many physicians have practiced; variants have been used in BC, Alberta, and Ontario. Under this approach, midwives are expected to set up their own offices/clinics, and pay their own expenses, although they may choose to work in group practices/shared care arrangements. They will usually have hospital privileges in at least one local hospital, but can (and do) deliver in other settings, including the home. In some provinces, there is a cap on how many births can be billed for by a midwife in a given time period. In Ontario, midwives are provided with a provincial health provider number and are paid directly by the Ministry of Health; there is no cost to the patient. Midwives are able to set up practice independently, or in group practice with other midwives. They are eligible to apply for hospital privileges. Assuming that the facilities are available in their community, women in Ontario may choose where they want to give birth: home, birthing centre, or hospital.

Another model has midwives as paid employees, usually of regional health authorities or community health clinics. Although private practices are allowed in some of these provinces, these privately practicing midwives would not be eligible to bill the provincial health plan. Saskatchewan, Manitoba, Quebec, Nova Scotia, and the Northwest Territories use variants of this model.

Nova Scotia introduced regulated midwifery in 2009. In theory, they employed both delivery models; midwives could be employed by the regional health authority (which Nova Scotia calls a District Health Authority) or work in a private clinic. However, no such private clinics were set up, largely because the cost of malpractice insurance was seen as prohibitive. The individual health authorities were able to decide whether they wished to employ midwives. Initially, only three of the nine district health authorities chose to do so, and one (in Halifax) soon discontinued their midwifery group. By 2011 there were only four midwives practicing in the province at two sites. An external report commissioned by the Ministry of Health concluded that "in our view midwifery in NS cannot long survive in its present state. If nothing is done, the profession will collapse and the benefits of regulation will not be realized. There are too few members to meet increasing requests for midwifery care, provide services safely and effectively, and attend to the complexity of regulatory and professional association activities that are required of a newly regulated profession" (Kaufman et al., 2011, p. 10).

DECISION POINT

You are the Minister of Health of your province. You have been asked whether midwives should be regulated, whether lay (unregulated) midwives should be allowed to deliver babies, and whether midwifery should be publicly funded. You recognize that, to the extent that midwifery is seen as a challenge to the medical control of childbirth, it remains controversial. What do you recommend?

SUGGESTED QUESTIONS FOR DISCUSSION

1. Discuss the advantages and disadvantages of midwifery. What might this depend on?
2. Discuss the site of birth. Who would do the delivery? Do they need backup? What relationship should there be between midwives and family practitioners?
3. Discuss professionalism, and the advantages and disadvantages of regulation.
4. Discuss the role of interest groups in making policy, including the women's movement and the consumer movement.

APPENDIX A: HEALTH PROVIDERS FOR BIRTH AND DELIVERY

*Obstetricians* are specialist physicians with expertise in the management of pregnancy, labour, and birth. They usually work in hospital settings. In general, they will handle higher-risk pregnancies; depending on the jurisdiction and patient preference, they may also manage low-risk births.

*Family doctors* may also handle births and delivery, often in a hospital setting. They may also work in birthing centres or (uncommonly) in a home birth setting.

The criteria for *midwives* vary by jurisdiction. Many midwives are trained *nurses* (nurse-midwives); those without nursing training are often called direct-entry midwives. Some midwives have graduated from certified training programs; others (often called lay midwives) are self-trained or have trained through apprenticing with another midwife.

The Association of Midwives of Ontario used the following definition: "A midwife is a registered health care professional who provides primary care to low-risk women throughout their pregnancy, labour and birth and provides care to both mother and baby during the first six weeks following the birth. Midwives work together in group practices. A woman receives care from a small number of midwives. During regularly scheduled visits to the midwifery practice, midwives provide clinical examinations, counseling and education" (Association of Ontario Midwives, 2013).

The World Health Organization uses this definition from the International Confederation of Midwives:

A midwife is a person who has successfully completed a midwifery education programme that is duly recognized in the country where it is located and that is based on the ICM *Essential Competencies for Basic Midwifery Practice* and the framework of the ICM *Global Standards for Midwifery Education*; who has acquired the requisite qualifications to be registered and/or legally licensed to practice midwifery and use the title 'midwife'; and who demonstrates competency in the practice of midwifery.

The midwife is recognised as a responsible and accountable professional who works in partnership with women to give the necessary support, care and advice during pregnancy, labour and the postpartum period, to conduct births on the midwife's own responsibility and to provide care for the newborn and the infant. This care includes preventative measures, the promotion of normal birth, the detection of complications in mother and child, the accessing of medical care or other appropriate assistance and the carrying out of emergency measures.

The midwife has an important task in health counselling and education, not only for the woman, but also within the family and the community. This work should involve antenatal education and preparation for parenthood and may extend to women's health, sexual or reproductive health and child care.

A midwife may practise in any setting including the home, community, hospitals, clinics or health units. (International Confederation of Midwives Council, 2011)

*Doula* is a term for a woman who provides various types of support to the mother before, during, and just after childbirth, but is not expected to provide clinical services. Doulas are not regulated, and usually do not have formal training programs, although optional certification programs are available in some jurisdictions (including Canada).

APPENDIX B: AN OVERVIEW OF MIDWIFERY ACROSS CANADA

Details about midwifery are given on the website of the Canadian Midwifery Regulators Consortium (CMRC), including the legal status in each jurisdiction (Canadian Midwifery Regulators Consortium, 2013).

The CMRC website section on working conditions also gives some estimates about billing and take-home earnings. For example, for British Columbia, they estimated that a midwife could bill up to $3,042.19 for a full course of care, with a billing maximum of 60 courses of care per year, expenses between 32% and 37% of their fee (but as much as 55% for part-time practice), and a take-home income of $76,600–$124,100 for a full-time midwife; their numbers were listed as being of April 2011.

In this appendix, we briefly note the situation in each province at the time of writing and indicate: if regulated, since what date; if midwives must be registered with a provincial college; the models of practice; and who pays them and how.

*British Columbia*:
Regulated, since January 1998. Must be registered to practice, with the exception of aboriginal midwives who had already been in practice before passage of the requirements. Midwives are independent practitioners, paid by the BC Medical Services Plan for each course of care provided to a client. The payment model for midwives is similar to that for physicians, with the fees negotiated by the Midwives Association of British Columbia and the expectation that midwives must pay their expenses from these fees. The Midwives Association also manages the

Midwives Protection Plan, which provides professional liability insurance coverage. Midwives tend to work in group practices; those in solo practices usually use a registered nurse as a second birth attendant. There are some shared care models. Unlike physicians, the number of courses of care that can be provided by any midwife is capped (maximum 60 per year per midwife; most manage 40–60 per year as primary midwife, and may attend an additional 15–20 home births as second midwife). Birthing locations include hospital (midwives have hospital privileges in at least one local hospital) or home births; there were no birthing centres in the province at the time of writing.

*Alberta*:
Regulated, since July 1998. Must be registered to practice. Since 2009, services have been publicly funded by the Alberta Health Services Board. Location for birth can be hospital, home, or birthing centre.

*Saskatchewan*:
Regulated, since March 2008. Must be registered to practice. Midwives can be employed by health regions, or practice privately; only those employed by the regions are financed by government. Deliveries can be in hospital or home.

*Manitoba*:
Regulated, since 2000. Must be registered to practice. Midwives can be unionized employees of the regional health authorities (in which case their overhead is paid by the employer), or in private practice. Deliveries can be in hospital or home.

*Ontario*:
Regulated, since January 1994. Must be registered to practice, except aboriginal midwives. Midwives are independent practitioners; they are publicly funded. Deliveries can be in hospital or home, although plans were announced in 2012 to also set up two free-standing birthing centres.

*Quebec*:
Regulated, since 1999. Must be registered to practice. Midwives are autonomous professionals who work under a contract with a local Community Health Centre (CHC); equipment and supplies are provided by the employer, and professional liability insurance costs are

shared by the CHC and the midwife. Services are government-funded; deliveries can be in hospital, home, or birthing centre.

*Nova Scotia*:
Regulated, since March 2009. Must be registered to practice. Midwives are employed by one of three participating District Health Authorities as part of a primary maternity care team (where their services are government-funded); births can be in hospital or home.

*New Brunswick*:
Regulated, since August 2010. At time of writing, model of practice was private practice, with home births only, and no public funding.

*Prince Edward Island*:
Not regulated; issue was under study. Midwives are in private practice, with home births, and no public funding.

*Newfoundland and Labrador*:
Regulated, since 2010. Midwives are in private practice, with home births, and no public funding.

*Yukon Territory*:
Not regulated; issue was under study. Midwives are in private practice, with home births, and no public funding.

*Northwest Territories*:
Regulated, since 2005. Must be registered to practice. Midwives are employed by the Health and Social Services Authorities, and government-funded. Midwives do home births.

*Nunavut*:
Regulated, since 2011. Model of practice was still being established; most mothers are flown to other locations for birth. Costs are publicly funded.

APPENDIX C: REFERENCES CITED AND FURTHER READING

Association of Ontario Midwives. (2013). *Ontario midwives: Experts in normal pregnancy, birth & newborn care*. http://www.aom.on.ca

Born, K. (2003). Midwifery in Canada. *McGill Journal of Medicine, 7*(1), 1–8.

Canadian Health Services Research Foundation. (2006). *Allow midwives to participate as full members of the healthcare team.* Evidence Boost. http://www.alberta-midwives.com/EvidenceBoost_June_E.pdf

Canadian Midwifery Regulators Consortium. (2013). *Working conditions.* http://cmrc-ccosf.ca/node/60

International Confederation of Midwives Council. (2011). *Definition of the midwife.* http://www.internationalmidwives.org/assets/uploads/documents/Definition%20of%20the%20Midwife%20-%202011.pdf

Janssen, P.A., Lee, S.K., Ryan, E.M., Etches, D.J., Farquharson, D.F., Peacock, D., et al. (2002). Outcomes of planned home births versus planned hospital births after regulation of midwifery in British Columbia. *Canadian Medical Association Journal, 166*(3), 315–23.

Kaufman, K., Robinson, K., Buhler, K., & Hazlit, G. (2011). *Midwifery in Nova Scotia: Report of the external assessment team.* Government of Nova Scotia. http://novascotia.ca/dhw/publications/Midwifery-in-Nova-Scotia-Report.pdf

O'Brien-Pallas, L., Hirschfeld, M., Baumann, A., Shamian, J., Bajnok, I., Adams, O., et al. (1997). *Strengthening nursing and midwifery: A global study.* World Health Organization. http://apps.who.int/iris/handle/10665/63690

Society of Obstetricians & Gynaecologists of Canada. (2008). *A national birthing initiative for Canada.* http://sogc.org/wp-content/uploads/2012/09/BirthingStrategyVersioncJan2008.pdf

World Health Organization. (2005). *The World Health Report 2005 – Make every mother and child count.* http://www.who.int/whr/2005/en/index.html

The following website may also be helpful:

Canadian Midwifery Regulators Consortium, http://www.cmrc-ccosf.ca/node/2

# 10 The Demanding Supply

## Licensing International Doctors and Nurses in Ontario

*MOHAMAD ALAMEDDINE, CHARLES BATTERSHILL, ANDREA BAUMANN, MAUREEN BOON, KAREN BORN, ANDREA CORTINOIS, RINKU DHALIWAL, ADAM M. DUKELOW, DAVID HOFF, CAROLINA JIMENEZ, NIBAL LUBBAD, MARIA MATHEWS, GLEN RANDALL, MELISSA RAUSCH, AND RAISA B. DEBER*

A series of newspaper articles described the experiences of health care professionals who had immigrated to Ontario intending to work in their field, only to find the way blocked. How should foreign-trained professionals be handled? How many professionals were needed, and what was the fairest way to proceed?

This case addresses several policy issues, including: health human resources planning, professional self-regulation, framing, policy instruments, the impact of payment mechanisms, interest groups, and managing trade-offs across policy goals (including equity and efficiency).

### Appendices

Appendix A: Becoming a Physician
Appendix B: Becoming a Nurse
Appendix C: IMGs and Canadian Immigration Policies
Appendix D: References Cited and Further Reading

### The Case

A series of newspaper articles described the experiences of health care professionals who had immigrated to Canada intending to work in their field, only to find the way blocked. As these individuals soon discovered, their professional credentials and experience often counted for very little. According to the newspaper, many were driving cabs, delivering pizzas, or working as waiters; some even decided to leave Canada. In a story highlighting physicians who had trained outside North America, the then-Dean of the Faculty of Medicine at the University of Toronto suggested that "red tape and high barriers" faced by international candidates had excluded many qualified doctors from practice in the country.

Others quoted in the series noted that Canadian health care costs were high, and stressed the need to control the number of professionals allowed to bill for services rendered under provincial health care plans. Still others noted that admission to Canadian medical schools and post-graduate medical training programs was difficult and many potentially qualified Canadian applicants had been turned away. Other countries were less selective in their admission policies; indeed, some "offshore" medical schools were doing a thriving business training Canadian and US applicants who had been rejected by their first-choice institutions. Was it fair to admit foreign-trained students as opposed to expanding local training opportunities? How could high standards of quality be ensured?

Underlying the debate were a number of policy questions. One approach was to see the issue as related to the health care system, with an emphasis on managing health human resources (HHR). Health professionals, including physicians and nurses, are essential for providing health care, but they also generate costs. A perennial policy problem in health services planning is determining what the "right" number and mix of HHR should be. From the mid-1980s to the late 1990s, Canadian policymakers generally perceived that there were too many providers, and that reducing numbers would help curb rising health care costs. Subsequently, Canada entered an era of perceived HHR shortages. How many health care providers did we really need? If the supply of and demand for HHR was not in balance, how should this be dealt with? What were the potential roles of market forces, as opposed to planning, in determining the HHR workforce? How should policymakers balance opportunities for Canadian residents and fairness to immigrants?

Another approach, however, was to see it as a matter of justice, related to the rights of those moving into a province/territory to practice their profession. How should one deal with professionals trained in other countries? Foreign-trained physicians are often referred to as international medical graduates, or IMGs; foreign-trained nurses are often called internationally educated nurses, or IENs. Again, there were multiple ways to view this. In some cases, such professionals are recruited from abroad to fill vacancies; one might focus on the ethical issues related to "raiding" providers from jurisdictions that had paid to train them, and might still need their services. Alternatively, one might recognize that many professionals have chosen to come to Canada, a nation that often prides itself on being a nation of immigrants. In that case, how should policymakers deal with such potentially significant obstacles to enabling immigrants to practice within their profession as language proficiency requirements, cultural fluency, and professional recertification?

This case focuses on two key health professions, physicians and nurses. However, similar issues are likely to apply to the other health care professionals needed to deliver quality health care services.

## The Health Care System Approach: The Supply of HHR

In a perfect market, the principles of supply and demand operate (see Chapter 1, section 5.9, Insurance, Elasticity, and Moral Hazard). If there are too few people supplying a given service, prices for their services should rise, inducing more to enter the market. Conversely, if there are too many providers, supply should exceed demand, prices should fall, and some providers will have to find alternative ways of earning a living.

Researchers have noted some systematic reasons why these basic market principles do not fully apply to health care, and to HHR. One key difference between health care and other goods is that, ideally, care is not provided on the basis of demand, but on the basis of "need." To help minimize financial barriers, most countries meet a sizeable proportion of health costs through third-party payers, insulating individuals from the costs of care. In market terms, this often means that the "buyer" of health care is the payer, rather than the patient.

HHR are skilled professionals. As noted in Chapter 1, section 6.4 (Professionalism), professionals possess specialized knowledge, attained through established training programs, and attested to through certification procedures with the goal of ensuring quality control over those allowed to practice. The many years it takes to train them (about 4 years for a nurse, and up to 13–15 years for a physician, depending on the specialty) builds in a time lag should one wish to increase supply, unless one can attract providers from other jurisdictions who have already completed much of their training. (For the current requirements to practice in Canada, see Appendix A for physicians and Appendix B for nurses.) Once these skilled professionals have been trained, one may often wish them to continue offering their services, rather than encouraging them to exit the market whenever there is a momentary downturn in demand for their services (and hence potentially in their incomes). Quality must also be maintained; one would not want "cut-rate" surgeons offering to provide lower-quality service for a cheaper price. (A related problem is who can judge quality, and how to ensure it.)

Indeed, ensuring adequate HHR is a worldwide issue. In 2006, the World Health Organization (2006) estimated that there was a global shortage of skilled health professionals, including doctors and nurses, with poorer countries especially affected. One concern expressed by observers is that, to the extent that health care professionals are highly mobile, they will move from poorer to richer countries in search of a better lifestyle (Kabene et al., 2006). Recruiting professionals from abroad to address local HHR shortages thus presents one set of ethical issues. However, insisting that these professionals are not free to move presents another set of ethical dilemmas.

**The Stock and Flow Model**

One way of viewing the number of providers available uses the analogy of a "practice pool" or stock (see Chapter 1, section 8.4.1, Projecting Supply and Demand). One begins with a number of workers. Over time, people may enter and exit this pool; this movement is commonly referred to as a "flow." Although there are slightly different ways to describe these models, one can summarize these flows as follows. Those *entering* the stock may include new graduates, immigrants, and those returning to practice. Reasons for *exiting* may be categorized into: death, retirement, emigration, and leaving practice, either temporarily or permanently. A more nuanced view would recognize the potential for working part-time, and view the pool in terms of full-time equivalents, which could also incorporate changes in how many hours a provider was working (Bloor & Maynard, 2003). The extent to which those leaving practice could be induced to return also varies; the causes for leaving practice may be temporary (e.g., getting additional training, family leave), or more permanent (emigration, retirement, death).

Performing such calculations, however, is not simple. Note that efforts to forecast the need for HHR must capture future changes that will affect the need for care, including not only demographic factors (e.g., birth rates, death rates, immigration/emigration) but also changes in disease and treatment patterns, and in health care delivery. These changes are not always easy to predict. For example, the incidence and prevalence of diseases may change, while technological innovations can change how one might treat a particular condition. In addition, different modes of delivery may call for different configurations of health providers ("labour substitution"). In general, models have shown limited success in predicting supply and demand for HHR (Bloor & Maynard, 2003).

However, the stock and flow model does clarify that there are a number of policy levers available to manage the supply of HHR within a particular profession. These may include: changing the number of new graduates (e.g., changing enrolment in Canadian medical and nursing schools, including opening new training programs), changing the number who immigrate (e.g., either limiting or encouraging immigration of foreign-trained professionals, the training or assessment positions available to foreign-trained professionals, the postgraduate training opportunities and/or independent practice licenses), changing the number of hours worked, changing the number who emigrate, and/or affecting leaves and retirements. More complex models would also allow for substitution and cooperation across professions, including interprofessional models (e.g., supplementing physicians with nurse practitioners, using personal support workers to do some nursing work, etc.). Note that some of these levers may not take effect for many years, whereas others may produce results more quickly. For example, in contrast to training new graduates, internationally-trained professionals have already completed all or at least the largest part of their training. As such, assuming that their credentials are recognized in other jurisdictions, they may be used to "fine-tune" attempts to match the supply of health providers to the demand for them. Other possibilities that may produce more rapid results include encouraging retention of existing workers, including encouraging those currently out of the workforce to return. Distribution is another issue; there may be enough of a particular HHR in aggregate, but this may hide oversupply in some communities and undersupply in others (particularly in more rural/remote areas).

Because much of the bill for health care in most developed countries is paid from public sources, policymakers have accordingly become involved in developing mechanisms for determining how many doctors, nurses, or other professionals are needed to provide the level of care that is wanted/needed in that jurisdiction.

**Paying Providers**

Attempts to forecast costs must also recognize differences among different categories of HHR and how they are paid (see Chapter 1, sections 6.2, Payment Mechanisms and Incentives). Some HHR work for health care organizations (such as hospitals) and are paid a salary; in order to practice, they must find jobs. Most nurses would fall into this category. In contrast, independent practitioners, particularly if paid on the basis of fee-for-service (FFS), may be considered as small businesses/self-employed entrepreneurs; they can generate revenues (billings) if there is enough demand for their services. In turn, this influences who is affected by an oversupply or undersupply of HHR. If there are too few workers, it will be difficult to deliver high-quality, timely care; in addition, HHR may be able to receive higher pay since they are in demand. However, the policy implications of having too many workers will vary according to how they are paid. If they must be hired, then some will not be able to find jobs, and the pay scales may decrease. This may be "penny wise and pound foolish" if it results in the loss of highly skilled workers and generates shortages in the future, but the impact will not be immediate. However, if workers can generate their own billings, they may still be able to do well financially, even if there is an oversupply of workers with the potential for "overuse" of services. Partially for that reason, policymakers have paid particular attention to attempting to forecast and plan for physician numbers.

As noted in Chapter 1, sections 6.1 (Dimensions of Health Systems), 6.1.1 (Public and Private), and 6.1.2 (Financing and Delivery), most health care in Canada is privately delivered. Canada uses a public contracting model for paying these private providers. About 70% is publicly financed; this includes almost all physician services, as well as most hospital care. The comprehensiveness requirement of the *Canada Health Act* (see Chapter 1, section 7.2) means that provincial/territorial insurance plans must pay for any medically necessary services as long as these are provided by physicians or in hospitals. Because the public payers (provincial/territorial health insurance plans) do not directly run health care, and do not hire the people delivering health care services, considerable control rests with providers. For example, most Canadian hospitals are private, not-for-profit organizations. Although they receive most of their budget from government, hospital managers decide how to use their resources, including who (and how many) to hire of each type of HHR they employ. Physicians also act as gatekeepers to other services; for the most part, access to drugs, hospitalization, and other services require physician assent. Clearly, without the proper number and mix of physicians, health care cannot be delivered. Each physician thus represents a cost to those paying for health care services, as well as a benefit for those receiving the care.

In Canada, licensure as a physician thus often implies the ability to bill provincial health insurance plans. This means that the primary barrier faced by individuals wishing to gain entry to the practicing medical profession is entry to undergraduate medical education. Once admitted, virtually all students complete the training process, are admitted to postgraduate positions, receive their licenses, and can consequently bill for services rendered under provincial FFS insurance plans. For the most part, they are treated as independent small businesses, and, particularly if they are paid on an FFS basis, are given considerable control over what they do, and how much they will earn. In effect, many physicians in Canada can decide where they wish to practice, with some assurance that they will be paid by the publicly funded insurance plan for the services they render on the basis of a mutually negotiated fee schedule. (This differs from countries where delivery is public, and physicians must be hired; in such jurisdictions, many of which do not restrict the access to medical undergraduate education, licensed but unemployed physicians are not uncommon.) Licensure is not entirely a blank check. Some jurisdictions, including Ontario, have sought to shift physician payment from FFS to alternative payment plan arrangements that may be more susceptible to caps. In addition, those physician specialties requiring hospital resources may be affected if hospitals are working with constrained budgets (e.g., gaining access to operating room time may become problematic).

**Who Can Practice**

Under Canada's constitution (see Chapter 1, section 2.2.1, Federalism in Canada), both health and education are deemed to be largely under provincial jurisdiction. This means that each provincial/territorial government has a voice in deciding how many providers it wishes to train, rather than allowing policy to be made at the national level. Similarly, it is the provinces and territories who determine which health care professions will be regulated in their jurisdiction, although they delegate most of the details about which individuals can be registered/licensed to the health professionals through a series of self-governing provincial regulatory bodies (usually referred to as "colleges"). In addition, to the extent that health care services are publicly financed, provincial/territorial governments must consider how much they are willing to pay these workers. This is in contrast to most other regulated professions, such as law or engineering, where many professionals would be employed by and/or paid from the private sector.

The key role of all regulatory colleges is to ensure the public's health and safety, although they also may wish to further the best interests of their profession. Self-regulation means that the professions are effectively in control of their respective educational processes, professional codes of conduct, and licensing requirements. Individuals wishing to work in a regulated health profession are not allowed to practice unless they are registered with the self-governing body in their province/territory. For example, in Ontario, this is specified in the *Regulated Health Professions Act* (see Chapter 1, section 7.3, Regulating Health Professions). Ontario physicians are regulated by the College of Physicians and Surgeons of Ontario (CPSO), and nurses are regulated by the College of Nurses of Ontario (CNO). However, regulatory colleges in different provinces tend to coordinate among themselves, to set similar criteria for registration, and to make it relatively simple for those registered in one province/territory to become registered should they move elsewhere within Canada. Such mobility is relatively common; the Canadian Institute for Health Information (CIHI) looked at where physicians were practicing 10 years after first being licensed in Canada, and reported that just under two-thirds of physicians were still practicing in their first Canadian jurisdiction of practice, meaning that about one-third had moved elsewhere (Canadian Institute for Health Information, 2011). This mobility presents additional complications should a province/territory wish to ease entry of IMGs to attract providers to underserved areas, because there is little to prevent these IMGs from moving to another jurisdiction as long as they satisfy the relevant criteria.

## Training Doctors and Nurses

As noted above, clinical education is deemed to be a provincial/territorial responsibility. However, Canada's medical and nursing schools have voluntarily worked together to coordinate their efforts.

For example, clinical training for a physician involves education at an accredited medical school, followed by several years of postgraduate training (usually called *residency*; the first year of residency has sometimes been referred to as *internship*, although this term is no longer being used formally at the time of writing). This training usually (although not necessarily) occurs in a teaching hospital setting. For more details about the steps needed, see Appendix A.

Nursing does not require postgraduate training, but all provincial regulatory bodies other than Quebec have attempted to coordinate their processes, including having a common examination, administered through the Canadian Nurses Association (see Appendix B).

**Forecasting Physician Numbers**

Most countries make some attempt to forecast and plan their medical workforce, with mixed success. Planners tend to focus on the inflows, particularly the number of medical students who will be trained. However, physicians are often mobile. They may be trained in Canada, or in another country. Canadian policy has been characterized by swings between views that there were too many doctors and views that there were too few. These swings have been somewhat correlated with the state of the economy and hence with the willingness (and ability) of governments to pay for physician services.

An early influence on Canadian physician resource planning was a series of recommendations by the 1964 Royal Commission on Health Services (Hall Commission). The Hall Commission had extrapolated population growth data and argued that there would be a shortage of physicians if action were not taken. Education, including training health professionals, was under provincial jurisdiction, but many provinces then decided to expand the number of training positions they funded. By the early 1970s, four new medical schools had been opened in four provinces, Alberta (University of Calgary), Ontario (McMaster), Newfoundland (Memorial), and Quebec (Sherbrooke); the training capacity of existing schools was also increased. One consequence was that first-year enrolment more than doubled, from 817 students across 12 schools in Canada in 1965 to 1,877 students across 16 schools in 1985 (Tyrrell & Dauphinee, 1999). At the time of writing, Canada had 17 accredited faculties of medicine; their training quotas had risen to about 2,783 physicians, not counting the small number of additional students being trained for (and paid for by) foreign governments.

Both the number of physicians in practice and the number per capita increased correspondingly. The Organisation for Economic Co-operation and Development (OECD) collects standardized information for its member countries (including Canada). According to the OECD health data, in 1965, the density of practicing physicians per 1,000 population in Canada was 1.3 (which would translate into 130 practicing physicians per 100,000 population). By 1985, this had reached 2.0. In 1991, it was 2.1, and in 2010 it was 2.4, the same value as reported for the United States (Organisation for Economic Co-operation and Development, 2013).

In the early 1990s, the consensus was that the Hall Commission report had overestimated both the number of Canadian physicians who would be lost through emigration to the United States and the rate of population growth in Canada. In consequence, the ratio of physicians to population had expanded well beyond what had been expected. In 1991, the Federal/Provincial/Territorial Conference of Deputy Ministers of Health commissioned two prominent health economists, Morris Barer and Greg Stoddart, to examine physician resource policy in Canada, to develop a framework for future policy development, and to make policy recommendations (Barer & Stoddart, 1991). The report made a series of recommendations, only some of which were adopted, including recommendations relating to physician payment (Stoddart & Barer, 1992).

At a meeting in Alberta in 1991, the Provincial/Territorial Ministers of Health unanimously adopted a series of strategies to constrain the growth in numbers of physicians. Implementation was simplified because the provincial/territorial governments controlled many of the policy levers; in addition to paying for physicians and hospitals, they paid for post-secondary education, and they also financed the residency positions in hospitals used to train physicians. One part of the strategy they adopted was to reduce the number of entry positions in Canadian medical schools by 10%. In addition, a higher proportion of residency positions were assigned to specialists; since these took longer to train, the practical impact was a reduction in HHR. Family physicians were also affected because the professional colleges, who controlled registration requirements, decided to increase the mandatory residency length from one to two years for all Canadian graduates. Another element of the strategy was only partly under provincial control, since immigration was a federal responsibility. However, the provinces/territories agreed to introduce tighter controls over IMGs through decreasing the number of postgraduate positions available for IMGs living in Canada who had not been able to obtain positions through the pre-internship process. Aggravating the situation were the results of an effort by some provinces to reduce their physician costs by attempting to impose caps on their total budget for physician services (Barer et al., 1988). In that zero-sum environment, one response by physician self-regulatory bodies had been to attempt to limit licensing for IMGs so that the existing funding would not have to be spread across a larger number of physicians.

By the late 1990s, there was another shift in views about physician supply (Chan, 2002). As one example, in 1999 the Ontario government had asked Dr. Robert McKendry to prepare a report and recommendations on the physician manpower situation in Ontario; his report concluded that there was a shortage of physicians, particularly with respect to specialists in rural areas, and that immediate policy changes were required. His short-term recommendations to increase physician supply included: providing additional incentive grants to physicians working in the North; offering free tuition for students willing to relocate to the North; discounting of fees for physicians setting up new practices in overserviced areas; and increasing the annual number of IMG training positions in Ontario from 24 to 36. The provincial government quickly announced that all of these short-term recommendations would be implemented; subsequently, they also opened a new medical school in Northern Ontario, and announced the creation of an expert panel to consider long-term needs for health professionals.

Similar trends occurred nationally. By 2000, first-year medical enrolment across Canada had increased to 1,763 students, and by 2004, the number of first-year students had exceeded 2,000. In 2004, the provinces/territories reacted to perceived potential shortages by committing to planning for an increased supply, tying this to the First Ministers' Health Accord. They also increased their investment in HHR planning, hoping to avoid the classic boom/bust cycles of the past. As noted above, by 2011, there were 2,783 places available within Canadian medical schools.

### The Impact on IMGs

As noted in Appendix C, potential immigrants to Canada are evaluated on a "points" system. At the federal level, one policy alternative was to change the number of points awarded to those with medical training.

Immigration advocates suggested that this policy might send some IMGs "underground," in that they would claim their professional status on immigration applications but instead seek other routes to enter Canada (e.g., family sponsorship) and then try to gain entry to practice once they had been admitted to Canada.

Another policy was to attempt to limit training opportunities. Historically in most provinces/territories, postgraduate physician training positions had been funded from the global budgets of individual hospitals, meaning that provincial ministries of health had no direct control over either the number of graduates entering into programs or the kind of specialists generated. In 1978, Ontario's Ministry of Health had introduced the clinical education budget (CEB). The intent of the CEB was to directly fund the same number of first-year residency positions (then called internships) as the number who graduated from Ontario medical schools. This meant a firm limit on how many could complete their education in an Ontario hospital. This approach still allowed Ontario graduates to move to other provinces, but limited how many students trained elsewhere could be absorbed. To the extent that other provinces took the same approach, this "hard cap" on training slots would mean that there was little room for IMGs to be trained in Canada. Indeed, for every IMG entering the postgraduate program, one Canadian-trained student would be shut out. This hypothetical situation turned into reality in the mid-1980s when varying numbers of IMGs were admitted to postgraduate programs, displacing equal numbers of Ontario graduates and stimulating an angry reaction from Ontario's Minister of Health.

In 1986, the Joint Working Group on the Graduates of Foreign Medical Schools submitted a report to the Federal/Provincial Advisory Committee on Health Human Resources. The Joint Working Group felt that all graduates of Canadian medical schools had to be assured access to internships and that IMGs were not "entitled" to pre-registration training in Canada. The report suggested the use of improved techniques to reduce the influx of IMGs seeking licensure and supported pre-internship training for IMGs. Ontario responded to the recommendations by closing off all points of entry to graduates of foreign medical schools except for a new pre-internship program (PIP), where IMGs would be closely supervised for a year in a clinical setting. Admission to the PIP would be through competitive examination; completing the PIP would require passing written and oral examinations. To the frustrated IMGs awaiting such training positions, the PIP was seen as further reducing their opportunity to practice medicine in Canada. An added complication was that Canadian-born students who had chosen to study medicine overseas (sometimes referred to as Canadians studying abroad, or CSAs) would now have to go through the same process, rather than being able to directly gain access to Ontario postgraduate training slots. Proponents of the training and license limitations argued that these entry limitations would "even the playing field."

For IMGs, the process required to obtain a medical license in Ontario was long and complex. (See Appendix A for a brief outline and comparison between the process for Canadian and international graduates at the time of writing.) In general, the process has not recognized previous professional experience for those trained outside of Canada, and has required even those accepted to complete additional postgraduate training prior to being licensed. From the mid-1980s to the late 1990s, only 24 such positions were set aside annually for the more than 200 yearly applicants. In 2004, the Association of International Physicians and Surgeons of Ontario (AIPSO) represented over 1,100 members, and estimated that there were between 2,000 and 4,000 unlicensed IMGs living in Ontario.

Despite efforts to close off all access points except the PIP program, a small number of IMGs continued to gain the training necessary to qualify for an Ontario license by applying to the Canadian Residency Matching Service (CaRMS). The rules kept changing. IMGs in the 1990s were able to access CaRMS positions only during the second iteration of the process, competing with those Canadian graduates who had been unsuccessful during the first iteration. Given the high rate of matching in the first round, less than 10% of IMG applicants to this "second round" were successful. In 2006, the process was modified to allow IMGs to apply to the first round of the CaRMS match, but their rate of matching was still low. Indeed, the CaRMS match has become even more competitive since the number of medical graduates has increased. (The fact that only a small proportion of Canadian students are admitted into medical schools is an argument sometimes used by those who support restrictions on the ability of IMGs to access postgraduate training positions. They argue that, because this percentage is very similar to the percentage of IMGs admitted, there is no real discrimination against foreign-trained students; this ignores the fact that IMGs may have already passed through a similar selection process before being admitted to medical school in their home country.)

**Nurses**

Nurses, like physicians, must be trained in a recognized program, and must be registered by the professional regulatory body in the province where they wish to work (see Appendix B). However, as noted above, there is a key difference because of how nurses are paid. Whereas many physicians can work independently, most nurses are employed by provider organizations. Many work in hospitals, but others work in the community, long-term care settings, and physician offices. There have been periodic shortages of nurses (Canadian Institute for Health Information, 2013). When that occurs, employers have found it more and more difficult to maintain a full complement of nursing staff. In the short run, use can be made of overtime and part-time staff. In the longer run, the issues about how many nurses should be trained, and the extent to which foreign-trained nurses can be registered and employed, have many similarities to those discussed for physicians.

Because nursing is a largely female profession, many nurses may have immigrated with their spouse. To the extent that they are responsible for helping their families settle in to their new home, they may not seek employment for several years. However, this usually means that they cannot expect to be registered by the regulatory bodies without having to rewrite the national examinations. A series of studies at McMaster University have examined internationally educated nurses and their contribution to the workforce (Baumann & Blythe, 2009; Baumann et al., 2010; Blythe & Baumann, 2008; Blythe et al., 2006). The studies found that, in many communities, the increasingly diverse and multicultural Canadian population has increased the importance of ensuring that HHR can meet the multilingual and cultural demands of the population accessing health care services.

**The Equity Perspective**

However, some stakeholders viewed this issue through a very different lens. Rather than focusing on HHR planning, they focused on equity. In April 1987, a group of 50 Polish-trained IMGs challenged the introduction of the PIP program, as they felt it was unjustly restricting their access to these training positions. Some noted that IMGs had previously been welcomed in rural Ontario, where they were seen as helping to solve the problem of chronic physician shortage. The legal case became known as *Jamorski v. Ontario (Attorney General)*; it was based on sections 1, 7, and 15(1) of the Canadian *Charter of Rights and Freedoms* (see Chapter 1, section 2.2.2). The government defended the existing policy, arguing that restricting entry to 24 IMGs per year was responsible, rational, and humane, and claiming that IMG training was of poor quality when assessed against American and Canadian standards. They also suggested that Ontario already had "too many" practicing physicians, that federal immigration regulations had failed to control the number of IMGs gaining access to Ontario, and that provincial medical schools would accept cuts to their enrolment only if the influx of IMGs was stemmed. At the time, it was estimated that "surplus" physicians alone in the year 2000 would cost the government $630 million in OHIP billings.

In May 1987, Justice Hughes ruled for Ontario, stating that limits placed on IMGs to practice medicine were justifiable, given the "disastrous effects of a mushrooming health care budget" as driven by a mushrooming physician supply. Hughes felt that PIP remedied the uncertain quality of IMGs and that discriminating on the basis of original medical training was reasonable. The court ruled that the additional time and effort the IMGs had to expend to meet the requirements for licensure was justified and that the limit of 24 residency training positions per year for IMGs should be maintained.

Medicine was not alone; the provincial government had been receiving pressure from foreign-trained workers in a variety of professions and trades who were encountering similar difficulties in being licensed or certified by the self-governing regulatory bodies. One response came from the provincial Cabinet Committee on Race Relations, who in 1986 commissioned a study from a consulting group, Abt Associates, as well as establishing the Task Force on Access to Professions and Trades in Ontario the next year. Following two years of research and consultation, the Task Force filed their report in the Ontario legislature in 1989 (Cumming et al., 1989). Their report, titled *Access!*, condemned the PIP, suggesting that it did not recognize the "actual" skills of IMGs and served to reduce their opportunities for licensure in a discriminatory way. The report also suggested that increased demand for physicians in the future, as driven by factors such as the aging of the population, would make it appropriate to abolish the PIP.

With respect to nurses, the *Access!* report cited several potential barriers to the integration of foreign-trained nurses, including examinations, retraining, language testing, and equivalence assessment. It also proposed that nursing examinations be screened for cultural bias. As well, it felt that the Test of English as a Foreign Language (TOEFL) should be reviewed for its profession-specific language applicability, and that an independent agency should be established, operating under one or more ministries, to assess the skills of IMGs, nurses, and other foreign-trained individuals wishing to practice one of the Ontario-regulated professions. The proposed agency, which they suggested should be named PLAN (Prior Learning Assessment Network), would be staffed by specialists in comparative education, assisted by advisory bodies representing various occupations and ethnocultural groups, and would carry out assessments of formal and informal prior learning and provide applicants with confirmation of their educational and professional equivalents to sit licensure exams. The report, which contained various disclaimers stating that the Task Force had not been asked to assess the direct or indirect costs of its recommendations, stressed that the introduction of the element of competition and challenge between Canadian and foreign graduates was more likely to raise than to lower standards.

Responsibility for responding to the *Access!* report lay with the Ministry of Citizenship. However, the review of the report moved slowly and was further delayed by the 1990 Ontario election. The government was defeated; the social democratic New Democratic Party (NDP), led by Bob Rae, took power. Recommendations relating specifically to medicine were deferred, and government did not make a formal response. The PIP program continued unchanged, although the *Regulated Health Professions Act*, which embodied many of the "safeguards" in the report, received royal assent in 1991.

In 2004, Ontario (whose government had been led since 2003 by the Liberals, under Dalton McGuinty) did replace PIP and Ontario IMG (the organization which had been the sole route to licensure for IMGs in the province since 1992) with a new body, International Medical Graduates Ontario (IMG-Ontario), which was given responsibility for processing all IMG applications. IMG-Ontario was developed in consultation with the Royal College of Physicians and Surgeons of Canada, the College of Family Physicians of Canada, and the Medical Council of Canada and was set up as a cooperative endeavour between the Council of Ontario Faculties of Medicine, the CPSO, and the Ontario Ministry of Health and Long-Term Care (MOHLTC). The number of IMGs was determined on a specialty-by-specialty basis, but the total was set at 200. The details of the process are indicated in Appendix A.

In 2006, Ontario announced a new strategy, which it called Health-ForceOntario. This novel partnership between two provincial ministries (the MOHLTC and the Ministry of Training, Colleges and Universities) put one Assistant Deputy Minister in charge, with a mandate to report to both ministries. HealthForceOntario was expected to forecast what Ontario's HHR needs would be, based on population health needs, and then to determine how best to obtain the right supply, mix, and distribution. It was given the ability to expand training programs, including not only medical school enrolments but also programs to train such other professionals as nurses, midwives, and pharmacists. It could also encourage new roles and interprofessional models of care. The number of positions for IMGs in Ontario remained at 200.

In 2006, Ontario also passed the *Fair Access to Regulated Professions Act*. It required certain regulated professions (none of them relating to health care) to have fair registration practices, and also amended the *Regulated Health Professions Act* to require that their registration processes be "transparent, objective, impartial and fair." The *Act* also established the Office of the Fairness Commissioner, reporting to the Ministry of Citizenship and Immigration, to work with the regulatory colleges to make sure the professions comply with the law. It issued its first recommendations in 2010; issues relating to the regulated health professions were referred to HealthForceOntario.

The federal government also got involved. It funded two initiatives: the Pan-Canadian Health Human Resource Strategy (HHRS) and the Internationally Educated Health Professionals Initiative (IEHPI). The HHRS was intended to provide a means of coordinating HHR planning to help support federal/provincial/territorial, jurisdictional, and nationwide activities; its four initiatives included: Pan-Canadian Health Human Resource Planning; Interprofessional Education for Collaborative Patient-Centred Practice; Recruitment and Retention of Health Care Providers/Professionals; and Aboriginal Health Human Resource Projects (Health Canada, 2011). It also passed amendments to the Agreement on Internal Trade (AID-2009) that allow workers in regulated occupations to apply to be certified in the same occupation in another province or territory without having to undergo significant additional training, examination, or assessment. Since regulation is still on a provincial basis, the provincial/territorial professional colleges are working to clarify how these provisions will work in practice. More information is available on the Agreement of Internal Trade

(AIT) and College of Physicians & Surgeons of Alberta websites (see Appendix D).

Provinces and territories have the right to maintain specific occupational standards and can adopt exceptions to certification requirements.

However, this policy still left a large number of IMGs unable to access training slots and hence unable to practice medicine in Canada. In addition, a growing number of Canadians studying abroad (CSAs) are coming home with their MDs and hoping to be able to get a Canadian residency position.

DECISION POINT

You have been asked to advise your provincial government. What should it do about allowing foreign-trained professionals to practice?

SUGGESTED QUESTIONS FOR DISCUSSION

1. Discuss the various levers government has to control the numbers and distribution of nurses and physicians in the health care system. How is this affected by the distribution of powers between the federal and provincial/territorial governments?
2. How would your preferred policy options differ if the issue was framed in terms of:

   Costs? Efficiency? Access? Quality of care? Equity or rights of: potential providers; Canadian residents wishing to become HHR; countries from which these providers are coming? Immigration policy?
3. What are the differences between dealing with the issues of human resource supply of medical personnel and of nursing personnel?
4. What interest groups are involved here? How could the characteristics of the various groups involved influence the outcome of this dispute?
5. What are the advantages and disadvantages of self-regulation of professions in terms of public interest, as well as financial and political costs?
6. What are the strengths and weaknesses of present forecasting models used to predict supply and demand?

APPENDIX A: BECOMING A PHYSICIAN

Under Canada's constitution (see Chapter 1, section 2.2.1, Federalism in Canada), professional self-regulation is deemed to be a provincial/territorial responsibility. To practice as a physician in Canada, it is necessary to be registered by the self-regulating body in that province. In Ontario, the College of Physicians and Surgeons of Ontario (CPSO) is responsible for setting these criteria. The CPSO website lists five requirements (steps) to allow a physician to receive a certificate of registration for independent practice in Ontario, which "authorizes the holder to engage in independent, unsupervised medical practice," limited to "the areas in which he or she is educated and experienced"(College of Physicians and Surgeons of Ontario, 2013). Note that most of these steps involve national coordination. Individual provinces do not set their own qualifying examinations, but work together. However, individual providers are usually registered only in the province/territory where they are working. The five steps are as follows:

Step 1.   Hold a medical degree from an accredited Canadian or US medical school or from an acceptable medical school listed in the World Directory of Medical Schools.
Step 2.   Successfully complete Parts 1 and 2 of the Medical Council of Canada Qualifying Examination. Before being allowed to take Part 2, physicians must pass Part 1, and complete at least 12 months of postgraduate training (also referred to as "residency"); this training can be taken anywhere in the world.
Step 3.   Have a certification by examination by the national body recognizing particular specialties; this is the Royal College of Physicians and Surgeons of Canada (RCPSC) for specialists, or the College of Family Physicians of Canada (CFPC) for family physicians.
Step 4.   Have completed, in Canada, one year of postgraduate training or active medical practice, or a full clinical clerkship at an accredited Canadian medical school.
Step 5.   Hold Canadian citizenship or permanent resident status.

To maintain registration, the annual membership fee must also be paid to the provincial regulatory college (in Ontario, the CPSO).

Step 4 requires completion of a postgraduate training program in Canada. Because the number of residency positions is limited, and because people who went to medical school in one province may wish to work/train in another, Canadian training programs in the different provinces work together. To avoid restricting trainees to the province where they had attended medical school, a system of matching medical graduates to postgraduate training was organized to work at the national level. The exact model went through several iterations, beginning with a match conducted by the Canadian Association of Medical Students. In 1970, this task was formally assumed by the Canadian Association of Medical Colleges, and eventually became the responsibility of an incorporated non-profit organization currently known as the Canadian Residency Matching Service (CaRMS). The *match* is a way to centrally organize the placement of medical graduates in postgraduate training positions across the country. (Quebec francophone schools finally joined the CaRMS process in 2005.) The Canadian Resident Matching Service is a not-for-profit organization that works in close cooperation with the medical education community, medical schools and residents/students. It provides an electronic application service and a computer match for entry into postgraduate medical training throughout Canada. At the time of writing, CaRMS administers the matching process for: postgraduate Year 1 entry (R-1) residency positions; Year 3 Family Medicine – Emergency Medicine residency positions; Medicine subspecialty residency positions; Paediatric subspecialty residency positions; as well as the Canadian access to the US electronic application system for postgraduate medical training (ERAS). For more information, see the Canadian Resident Matching Service website.

All Canadian medical graduates wishing to pursue postgraduate training must accordingly apply to CaRMS and then complete a two- to five-year residency program (depending on the specialty) before applying to be certified by the appropriate national college (Step 3). A computerized algorithm matches applicants to positions. After the first iteration of the algorithm approximately 90%–93% of positions are filled. Those graduates not matched in the first round can then apply to the second round. Provinces vary in the precise process they use. For example, Ontario reserved 200 positions exclusively for IMGs.

### International Medical Graduates (IMGs)

Foreign-trained physicians had similar requirements. However, there were several different pathways for IMGs to become registered to practice in Canada, which depended in part on their postgraduate training and clinical experience and might vary somewhat from province to province, and from year to year. They had to demonstrate that they had graduated from a medical school (Step 1), passed the Medical Council of Canada's Evaluating Examination and Part 1 of the Medical Council of Canada Qualifying Examination (similar to Step 2), and be a Canadian citizen, permanent resident, or intend to immigrate to Canada (similar to Step 5). Ontario also required physicians to be certified by the RCPSC or the CFPC (Step 3).

However, there were additional differences. Step 4 was the main hurdle. A number of different processes were used at various times. For example, at one time, after successfully demonstrating graduation from an accredited medical school, immigration to Canada, and passing the examinations, applicants would have to apply to an assessment centre (Centre for the Evaluation of Health Professionals Educated Abroad), and then apply for a residency position through CaRMS. At the time of the case, Ontario had attempted to simplify matters by setting up IMG-Ontario. It maintained two separate application streams (for family medicine or for specialists), and four possible entry levels. The clerkship level applied only to the specialist stream, and was deemed similar to the final year of undergraduate medical school. The Postgraduate Year 1 (PGY1) level applied to both streams, and allowed entrance into the first year of a residency training program. The Postgraduate Year 2 (PGY2) level applied only to specialists, and allowed entrance into the second year of a specialty residency. One minor difference was that all family medicine candidates had to complete a four-month pre-residency program before they could begin the actual residency. Another was that the first 8–12 weeks of the PGY1 or PGY2 would be an Assessment Verification Period, which involved evaluating the candidates to ensure that they would be able to perform at the expected level. The final possibility, for those with substantial prior training, would be the Practice Ready Assessment; this involved a six-month assessment in a supervised clinical setting. Candidates might pass unconditionally, conditionally (in which case they would be prescribed further training), or fail and be dismissed from the program.

Depending on prior experience, these foreign-trained physicians might be able to apply at the clerkship or PGY1 entry levels. In that case, they would not require prior postgraduate training, but would be treated similarly to graduates of Canadian medical schools. With a minimum of one year of postgraduate training in their specialty, they could apply to the PGY2 entry level. If they had completed a postgraduate medical education program, they could apply to the Practice Ready Assessment entry level; this would also be considered their independent professional practice experience.

In addition, it was necessary that IMGs demonstrate fluency in English or French; there were a number of different ways to satisfy this requirement, including passing such tests as the Test of English as a Foreign Language (TOEFL), and the Test of Spoken English (TSE), or the French examination offered by the Office Québécois de la Langue Française. Reference letters were mandatory. Some but not all provinces (including the IMG-Ontario programs), at some but not all times, required participants to sign a return of service agreement and serve for a specified number of years in a community designated as underserviced; this was sometimes described as being an exchange for having received government funding for the assessment and/or the training programs.

As of December 1, 2008, four new pathways to registration in Ontario were added: (1) Physicians with a Canadian Medical Degree and Postgraduate Training without RCPSC or CFPC Certification; (2) IMG with Canadian Postgraduate Training without RCPSC or CFPC Certification and Practicing Independently in Canada; (3) Canadian or US Medical Degree with US Postgraduate Training and Certification; and (4) IMG with US Postgraduate Training and Certification. The details of the process were very similar to those noted previously, with the assumption that the IMG would have successfully immigrated to Canada between Step 1 (graduation from an acceptable medical school) and Step 2 (passing the Medical Council of Canada Evaluating Exam). The applicant would also be required to pass the two English proficiency tests noted previously (the TOEFL and the TSE). At that stage, the IMG could apply to IMG-Ontario or its successor. Prior to applying, applicants had to choose which program stream they were applying to (specialty vs. family medicine) and which of the four levels of entry.

Adding to the complexity, there were a number of ways in which the IMG could demonstrate medical knowledge. In most provinces, the candidate had to pass the Medical Council of Canada Evaluating Examination (MCCEE) to demonstrate equivalent general medical knowledge, and to apply for a residency position through the Canadian Resident Matching Service (CaRMS). Although it was not mandatory to write the Medical Council of Canada Qualifying Examination (MCCQE) Part I and the National Assessment Collaboration (NAC) Objective Structured Clinical Examination (OSCE) (launched in March

2011), IMGs applying for entry-level postgraduate training positions (PGY1) were encouraged to write them; it was felt that these tests could provide information about candidates' clinical skills, and priority might accordingly be given to those who had successfully completed them. The selection process might incorporate a clinical skills examination and/or personal interview, in addition to the review of their dossier. However, British Columbia was the only province where passing NAC OSCE or the BC OSCE was a mandatory requirement.

After the assessment period, successful candidates would write the Medical Council of Canada Eval. Exam Part II. Should they pass, they would be licensed by the Medical Council of Canada, and could then apply to be certified by the appropriate national body (RCPSC for specialists, or CFPC for family physicians). The final step was registration by the provincial regulatory body; in Ontario, this is the CPSO.

In some cases, specialists are permitted to take the certification examinations without additional postgraduate training, through special assessments of equivalency of training by the Royal College of Physicians and Surgeons of Canada. For example, IMGs with independent licenses (restricted or unrestricted) are ineligible to apply to CaRMS, but may be able to apply to the Ontario MOHLC's Re-Entry program or the Centre for Evaluation of Health Professionals Educated Abroad's (CEPHEA) assessment for PGY2.

At the time of writing, certain provinces (including Newfoundland, Nova Scotia, New Brunswick, Prince Edward Island, and Ontario) required all those receiving IMG stream residency positions to commit to a Return of Service and practice for a given period in that province.

**Medical School Accreditation**

As noted above, Step 1 requires that an applicant hold a medical degree from an accredited medical school. It is difficult to compare the educational standards and the selectivity of the more than 200 countries where IMGs may have studied. For example, in many countries, virtually everyone who applies to a medical school is accepted. Canadian schools, on the other hand, admit only 10%–20% of the students who apply. For example, in 2011, the Ontario medical schools accepted 952 of 5,297 applicants; the University of Toronto accepted 259 of 2,956 applications (Ontario Universities' Application Centre, 2013).

The accepted solution is accreditation. The Council on Accreditation of Canadian Medical Schools, a body established in association with the Canadian Medical Association, accredits all medical schools in Canada.

US medical schools are accredited by the Liaison Committee on Medical Education. The two groups work closely together, including cross appointments. For the purposes of licensure, an accredited medical school in another province or in the United States is deemed equivalent to an accredited medical school in that province. Therefore, students graduating from any Canadian or American medical school can apply for postgraduate training positions and licensing on essentially the same basis (although they may need to be citizens/residents of the country where they wish to study). An unaccredited medical school – that is, a medical school outside Canada or the United States – may be considered "acceptable" for the purpose of licensure only if it is listed in the appropriate directory. For many years, this was World Health Organization's (WHO) World Directory of Medical Schools, which listed schools, in 157 countries, which required a bachelor's degree and/or an entrance examination for admission. However, WHO had no authority to grant any form of recognition or accreditation to the medical schools in its directory, and inclusion in the directory did not necessarily reflect the quality of medical programs at those schools. At the time of writing, the WHO had transferred responsibility for maintaining this list to the AVICENNA Directory, maintained by the University of Copenhagen in collaboration with the World Health Organization and the World Federation for Medical Education (WFME) (World Federation for Medical Education, 2013).

In 2005, in response to the Report of the Canadian Task Force on Licensure of International Medical Graduates from 2004, the Medical Council of Canada (MCC), in partnership with the Federation of Medical Regulatory Authorities of Canada (FMRAC) and supported by Human Resources and Social Development Canada (HRSDC), established the Physician Credentials Registry of Canada (PCRC) to provide a centralized repository for physicians' core medical credentials. PCRC verified a physician's medical credential documents and stored the information in an online repository that can be shared with provincial and territorial medical regulatory authorities and certifying and qualifying bodies in Canada. As of 2012, the following medical regulatory authorities and other stakeholders were accepting the documents in PCRC's files: Centre for the Evaluation of Health Professionals Educated Abroad, Collège des Médecins du Québec, College of Family Physicians of Canada, College of Physicians and Surgeons of Alberta, College of Physicians and Surgeons of British Columbia, College of Physicians and Surgeons of Manitoba, College of Physicians and Surgeons of Newfoundland and Labrador, College of Physicians and Surgeons of Nova Scotia, College of Physicians and Surgeons of Ontario, College of Physicians and Surgeons of Prince Edward Island, College of Physicians and Surgeons of Saskatchewan, Health Match BC, the Canadian Resident Matching Service (CaRMS), the Royal College of Physicians and Surgeons of Canada, and the Yukon Medical Council.

Once PCRC has approved his/her credentials, the IMG may proceed to write the licensing exams.

APPENDIX B: BECOMING A NURSE

Nurses must be licensed or registered in the province/territory where they will be working. Potential nurses must graduate from a recognized training program. They must write the Canadian Registered Nurses Examination (except in Quebec, which has its own exam). On its website, the College of Nurses of Ontario (the provincial regulatory body) lists the following criteria which must be met.

All nurses who wish to practice as an RN or RPN in Ontario must hold a current General Certificate of Registration with the College. To obtain one, applicants must first meet a series of requirements: completion of an acceptable nursing or practical nursing program (or equivalent); evidence of recent safe nursing practice; successful completion of national nursing registration examination; evidence of fluency in written and spoken English or French; registration or eligibility for registration in the jurisdiction where the applicant completed his/her nursing program; proof of Canadian Citizenship, Permanent Residency, or authorization under the *Immigration and Refugee Protection Act* (Canada) to engage in the practice of nursing; and good character and suitability to practice, as indicated by a Declaration of Registration Requirements and a Canadian Criminal Record Synopsis (College of Nurses of Ontario, 2013).

Several programs have been set up to help internationally educated nurses become licensed. For example, in Ontario, they include the Post-RN BScN for Internationally Educated Nurses at York University and the Post-Diploma Degree Program at Ryerson University.

APPENDIX C: IMGS AND CANADIAN IMMIGRATION POLICIES

IMGs have long contributed to Canada's physician supply (Canadian Institute for Health Information, 2009). For example, almost half of the almost 7,000 new physicians and surgeons added to Canada's total supply between 1951 and 1961 were foreign-trained. In certain provinces such as Manitoba, Saskatchewan, and Newfoundland and Labrador, IMGs have made up a substantial percentage of the total number of physicians. Many IMGs have practiced in Canada's northern and other underserviced areas; they are also overrepresented in certain specialties, such as psychiatry and pathology. CIHI estimated that, in 2007, internationally educated physicians were 22.3% of the total physician workforce in Canada, ranging from a high of 36.9% in Newfoundland and Labrador to a low of 10.9% in Quebec. In contrast, internationally educated nurses accounted for only 7.4% of the RN nursing workforce, and tended to be clustered in the larger communities, particularly in Ontario, Alberta, and British Columbia (Canadian Institute for Health Information, 2007).

In the 1970s and the first half of 1980s, specialist physicians were allowed easy access to Canadian practice, because the Royal College of Physicians and Surgeons of Canada had an "open policy" to examinees. If IMGs could meet Canadian standards for their specialty, they were often exempted from additional residencies. Exemptions were also granted to the "specially" qualified. For example, exemptions were often given to physicians with international research reputations. Exemptions could also be granted to specialists willing to serve in certain areas (e.g., northern Ontario) for a specified time period (e.g., at least three years). Specialist IMGs who had been certified in the 1970s accounted for one-third of Canada's specialists practicing in 1980.

Until 1985, Ontario deemed training obtained in most Commonwealth English-speaking countries as being equivalent to Canadian training. An Ontario license would be issued if the candidate had served a one-year residency in such Commonwealth countries as Australia, Ireland, or South Africa. For the vast majority of IMGs, however, the only route to licensure was to first win a residency position through competitive processes in a Canadian teaching hospital.

In 1986, the CPSO changed eligibility rules for IMGs to require two postgraduate training years in a Canadian hospital. A specialist's certificate from the Royal College of Physicians and Surgeons was no longer sufficient to exempt the IMGs from these two years. At that time, immigration rules had already been changed to make it more difficult for IMGs to gain admission into Canada.

In 2002, the *Immigration and Refugee Protection Act* replaced the 1976 *Immigration Act*. The new legislation concentrated on skills, training, and potential for integration into the Canadian workforce and was intended to choose workers with transferable skill sets rather than specific occupational backgrounds. While the policy no longer limited entry to certain professional groups, it still left room for refusing entry to IMGs based on their ability to integrate with the current workforce.

Canada's admissible categories of immigrants are divided into: *economic class* (which in turn includes a number of categories of skilled workers, professionals, and investors); *family class* (which includes the spouse, common-law partner, dependent children, and parents of Canadians); and *refugees and persons in need of protection class*. Over time, the precise categories, and numbers allowed in each, have varied (see also Chapter 2, Danger at the Gates, Appendix B). The economic class, also called the independent category, is based on a *points* system that takes into account education, experience, arranged employment, age, language, and adaptability (which includes existing ties to Canada). In 2010, the government capped the number who could be admitted under the Federal Skilled Worker (FSW) program without an offer of arranged employment at 20,000 and further reduced this to 10,000 in 2011. To be admissible, FSW applicants must also be one of 29 listed National Occupational Classifications (NOC) professions (which do include specialist physicians, family physicians, registered nurses, and licensed practical nurses); there are yearly subcaps of 1,000 (reduced to 500 in 2011) for each NOC category. These criteria are stricter than in previous years, and further changes are likely.

APPENDIX D: REFERENCES CITED AND FURTHER READING

Barer, M.L., Evans, R.G., & Labelle, R.J. (1988). Fee controls as cost control: Tales from the frozen north. *Milbank Quarterly, 66*(1), 1–64. http://dx.doi.org/10.2307/3349985

Barer, M. L., & Stoddart, G. L. (1991). *Toward integrated medical resource policies for Canada: Background document*. Federal/Provincial/Territorial Conference of Deputy Ministers of Health, Centre for Health Services and Policy Research.

Baumann, A., & Blythe, J. (2009). *Integrating internationally educated health care professionals into the Ontario workforce* (Report No. 20). Ontario Hospital Association, Nursing Health Services Research Unit, and McMaster University. http://www.hrhresourcecenter.org/node/2932

Baumann, A., Blythe, J., & Ross, D. (2010). Internationally Educated Health Professionals: Workforce Integration and Retention. *Healthcare Papers, 10*(2), 8–20.

Bloor, K., & Maynard, A. (2003). *Planning human resources in health care: Towards an economic approach, an international comparative review.* Canadian Health Services Research Foundation. http://www.hrhresourcecenter.org/node/274

Blythe, J., & Baumann, A. (2008). *Supply of internationally educated nurses in Ontario: Recent developments and future scenarios* (No. 9). Health Human Resources Series. Nursing Health Services Research Unit, McMaster University. http://nhsru.com/publications/supply-of-internationally-educated-nurses-in-ontario-recent-developments-and-future-scenarios

Blythe, J., Baumann, A., McIntosh, K., & Rheaume, A. (2006). *Internationally educated nurses in Ontario: Maximizing the brain gain* (No. 3). Human Health Resources Series. Nursing Health Services Research Unit, McMaster University. http://nhsru.com/publications/internationally-educated-nurses-in-ontario-maximizing-the-brain-gain-2

Canadian Institute for Health Information. (2007). *Internationally educated physicians and nurses in Canada.* http://www.cihi.ca/CIHI-ext-portal/pdf/internet/CCIH_CONFERENCEPOSTER_2007_EN

Canadian Institute for Health Information. (2009). *International medical graduates in Canada: 1972 to 2007.* https://secure.cihi.ca/estore/productSeries.htm?pc=PCC499

Canadian Institute for Health Information. (2011). *Supply, distribution and migration of Canadian physicians, 2010.* https://secure.cihi.ca/estore/productFamily.htm?locale=en&pf=PFC1680

Canadian Institute for Health Information. (2013). *Regulated nurses: Canadian trends, 2007 to 2011.* https://secure.cihi.ca/estore/productFamily.htm?pf=PFC2016

Chan, B.T.B. (2002). *From perceived surplus to perceived shortage: What happened to Canada's physician workforce in the 1990s?* Canadian Institute for Health Information. https://secure.cihi.ca/estore/productSeries.htm?pc=PCC161

College of Nurses of Ontario. (2013). *Requirements for becoming a nurse in Ontario.* http://www.cno.org/become-a-nurse/

College of Physicians and Surgeons of Ontario. (2013). *Independent practice certificate of registration.* http://www.cpso.on.ca/Registering-to-Practise-Medicine-in-Ontario/Registration-Requirements/Independent-Practice-Certificate-of-Registration

Cumming, P. A., Lee, E., & Oreopoulos, D. G. (1989). *Access! Task force on access to professions and trades in Ontario.* Ontario Ministry of Citizenship. http://regulatorsforaccess.ca/resources/guideothersrc.aspx.

Health Canada. (2011). *Health human resource strategy.* http://www.hc-sc
.gc.ca/hcs-sss/hhr-rhs/strateg/index-eng.php

Kabene, S.M., Orchard, C., Howard, J.M., Soriano, M.A., & Leduc, R. (2006).
The importance of human resources management in health care: A global
context. *Human Resources for Health, 4*(20), 1–17.

Ontario Universities' Application Centre. (2013). *Medical school application
statistics.* http://www.ouac.on.ca/statistics/med_app_stats/

Organisation for Economic Co-operation and Development. (2013). *OECD
health data 2012.* http://www.oecd.org/health/health-systems/oecdhealth
data.htm

Stoddart, G.L., & Barer, M.L. (1992). Toward integrated medical resource
policies for Canada: 6. Remuneration of physicians and global expenditure
policy. *Canadian Medical Association Journal, 147*(1), 33–8.

Tyrrell, L., & Dauphinee, D. (1999). *Task force on physician supply in Canada.*
Canadian Medical Forum Task Force. http://effectifsmedicaux.ca/reports/
PhysicianSupplyInCanada-Final1999.pdf

World Federation for Medical Education. (2012). *Avicenna.* http://www.wfme
.org/projects/directories/avicenna

World Health Organization. (2006). *The World Health Report 2006 – Working
together for health.* http://www.who.int/whr/2006/en/index.html

The following websites may also be helpful:

Agreement on Internal Trade, Table of Contents, http://www.ait-aci
.ca/index_en/labour.htm

Association of Faculties of Medicine of Canada (AFMC), http://www
.afmc.ca/about-e.php

Canadian Association of Schools of Nursing, http://www.casn.ca/en/

Canadian Nurses Association – Becoming an RN-Education, http://
www.cna-aiic.ca/en/becoming-an-rn/education

Canadian Resident Matching Service, https://www.carms.ca/en/
about

College of Physicians & Surgeons of Alberta, Alberta Medical Practice
Permit, Labour Mobility Agreements, http://www.cpsa.ab.ca/
services/Registration_Department/Alberta_medical_licence/
AIT_TILMA.aspx

Foundation for the Advancement of International Medical Education
and Research (FAIMER), http://www.faimer.org/resources/imed
.html

HealthForceOntario, http://www.healthforceontario.ca/en/Home

Nursing Health Services Research Unit, http://nhsru.com; Publications http://nhsru.com/publications; see in particular http://nhsru.com/category/publications/international-nursing

Ontario Hospital Association (OHA), http://www.oha.com/ien

Ontario Ministry of Health and Long-Term Care: International Medical Graduates, http://www.health.gov.on.ca/english/providers/project/img/img_mn.html

Pan Canadian Health Human Resource Strategy, http://www.hc-sc.gc.ca/hcs-sss/hhr-rhs/strateg/index-eng.php

# 11 Primary Health Care in Ontario

## Inching towards Reform

MONICA AGGARWAL, MUNAZA CHAUDHRY, STEPHANIE
GAN, NADA VICTORIA GHANDOUR, WILLIAM KOU,
LESLIE MACMILLAN, CATHERINE L. MAH, MEGHAN
MCMAHON, LUCINDA MONTIZAMBERT, ALLIE PECKHAM,
DAVID RUDOLER, RENA SINGER-GORDON, DEBRA ZELISKO,
AND RAISA B. DEBER

Over the past several decades in Canada, academics, health professionals, and provincial and national commissions have indicated that reform of primary care is key to sustaining a high-performing health care system. Yet despite considerable investment, primary care reform has proven difficult to achieve. What are the implications of different ways of organizing and financing primary care, and why has reform proved to be so difficult?

This case addresses several policy issues, including: primary care delivery models, implications of different modes of reimbursement, and the factors involved in achieving reform, with particular emphasis on the role of institutions and interest groups.

### Appendices

Appendix A: Paying Doctors
Appendix B: Selected Ontario Primary Care Reform Models
Appendix C: PHC Goals as Cited in National Reform Documents
Appendix D: References Cited and Further Reading

### The Case

*Primary care* (PC) has been defined as the first point of contact with the health system, where (ideally) services are provided comprehensively, continuously, and in a consistent manner, undifferentiated by physical, social, or cultural characteristics (Starfield, 1994). A related term, *primary health care* (PHC) has been defined by the World Health

Organization (1978) as "the first level of contact of individuals, the family and community with the national health system bringing health care as close as possible to where people live and work, and constitutes the first element of a continuing health care process." Although the terms can overlap, PC and PHC have somewhat different meanings. PC focuses on individual patients, while PHC is expected to focus on the population as well as on individuals. PC focuses on the provider, while PHC focuses on the community. PC focuses on physician-based care, while PHC focuses on health care teams. Primary care reform efforts in Canada and abroad have attempted to shift from a model of PC to some form of PHC (Aggarwal, 2009).

Health reformers argue that PHC should be at the centre of any high-performing health care system. A number of issues evoke attention. One is access, and ensuring that every resident has a regular source of PHC. Statistics Canada (2012) reported that, for 2011, about 15% of Canadians over the age of 15 did not have a regular medical doctor. Although many of these people could still obtain care (albeit from walk-in clinics or hospital emergency rooms), continuity of care was likely to suffer. In Ontario, the proportion was smaller (about 9%) and diminishing, but still worrying. In particular, solo practice often meant problems for patients when their doctors retired. Another issue was quality of care, with particular attention to integration with other areas of the health care system. Critics of the existing system have noted that each sector is funded independently; these "silos" are seen as encouraging a fragmented system that often stresses shifting costs to other payers rather than encouraging cost-effectiveness and integrated care. Reformers have called for improving quality of care, encouraging health promotion and disease prevention, and integrating other health professionals into integrated care models. A third issue was cost; the proportion of health expenditures being devoted to physician services had jumped, and critics wondered whether, particularly in times of fiscal crisis, there was sufficient value for the money being spent. At the time of the case, physician services accounted for about 13% of total health expenditures (the third-largest category); almost all of the costs for physicians were paid through public expenditures, and those costs were growing by approximately 6% per year (see Chapter 1, section 9.1, Canadian Data).

**About Primary Health Care**

PHC can be defined in terms of where care is provided, which usually is in physician offices and/or outpatient clinics. Alternatively, it can be defined in terms of its key features, which include its place in the continuum of care (first contact), continuity of care (as opposed to episodic visits), comprehensiveness, gatekeeping (with referral to more specialized care when required), and coordination of a variety of health professionals involved in treating the "whole patient" (and/or his/her family). We will use the term PHC in this case study, recognizing that many of the models employed would be better described as PC.

A series of international, national, and provincial reports has emphasized the potential for improving how PHC is financed and delivered, and noted the potential for it to improve the quality and cost-effectiveness of health care.

PHC can be funded and delivered in a number of different ways. PHC models vary both across and within jurisdictions. Key distinctions among these models include the following: who is cared for and where; what types of services are available and when; who is providing the care; how care is paid for; and how PHC interfaces with other sectors of the health care system.

## Who Is Cared for and Where?

Patients vary considerably in how much care they need (see also Chapter 1, section 5.9, Insurance, Elasticity, and Moral Hazard). PHC models differ in the extent to which they try to serve a general population, and in how they integrate PHC with specialist care. In some models, PHC focuses on those who are relatively healthy, and sends those with greater needs to specialists. Some models allow PHC practices to focus on a defined population (where the population can be defined in multiple ways, including by ethnocultural group or socioeconomic status). Models may also vary in terms of whether individuals and families are permitted to choose their own PHC provider or are assigned to providers who are made responsible for caring for all individuals within a specified population (usually defined in geographic terms).

## What Types of Services Are Available and When?

The basket of services can also vary by practice model and/or patient need. In one set of models, PHC includes only first-line or "gatekeeper" services. In others, the practice may deliver a more comprehensive or continuous type of care (e.g., chronic disease management, social support, coordination of specialist services, follow-up services, and/or after-hours care). Patients may also be referred to specialists for assistance in proposing a disease management strategy, with the PHC provider expected to provide much of the actual care. There is also variability in whether emergency services (episodic care) are offered in PHC practices, or whether the PHC practices focus on scheduled services and expect those needing episodic care to go to walk-in clinics and/or hospital emergency rooms (particularly if such emergencies occur after regular office hours). Some PHC providers provide obstetrics care; most do not. The extent to which they provide chronic disease prevention and management also varies. PHC providers are typically a patient's first point of access to the health care system and are the providers patients see most often to obtain care for chronic diseases (Macinko et al., 2003). Ideally, PHC also adopts a patient-centred approach to care; since people may have more than one disease, PHC providers may be better suited to managing the whole patient than would occur if care were fragmented among a series of specialists. However, providing such care can be time-consuming, and PHC providers would also need to liaise with specialists, and to keep up with current evidence-based treatment guidelines. A number of shared care models can be used, but these are most feasible when the practice has enough patients with such conditions, and thus work best for larger PHC practices, and/or practices specializing in a particular patient category.

## Who Is Providing the Care?

Some models are physician-based, while other, more complex models are based on multidisciplinary teams working within an integrated model of care. Different health professionals are regulated differently in different jurisdictions (see Chapter 1, section 6.4, Professionalism). There are also variations in what care is covered by insurers in the various jurisdictions. Including a range of interdisciplinary providers in PHC raises issues about teamwork, overlapping responsibilities and scopes of practice, payment models, and how to ensure quality of care.

## How Is Care Paid For?

As noted in Chapter 1, section 6.2 (Payment Mechanisms and Incentives), there are various ways of paying for health care (Deber et al., 2008; Leger, 2011). Most systems pay for PHC using various combinations of payments on the basis of the services provided (*fee-for-service*, also called FFS), the population served (*capitation*), the time spent (*salary*), and/or the *outcomes* achieved. Note that different payment mechanisms may require that certain organizational mechanisms be in place. For example, paying salaries presumes the existence of a larger organization that will employ the providers, which may not be compatible with models where individual providers run their own practices. Capitation requires some mechanism for determining which population will be served by that organization. For geographically based capitation models, one can compute how many live in that jurisdiction and fund practices on that basis. Where people are able to select their own providers, however, as is usually true for PHC, payment models are often associated with the practice of *rostering*. Rostering is the term used for forcing (or encouraging, depending on the model) each patient to enrol with a particular provider (which may either be an individual physician or a group of PHC providers). That provider agrees to provide an agreed-upon basket of PHC services for its rostered patients in return for an agreed-upon payment (which may be *risk-adjusted* to account for differences in the likely costs; these adjustments are generally made on the basis of age and sex, although some models do attempt to incorporate some measures of health status). In general, the current state of risk adjustment is relatively poor at accounting for the variability in likely expenditures for individual patients, although the differences may average out if the providers are not "cream-skimming" their patients and selectively rostering only healthy patients. More recently, pay-for-performance (P4P) schemes that pay for desired outcomes have been implemented in several jurisdictions, including the United Kingdom and the United States.

Each type of payment model embodies particular economic incentives. Some encourage providers to deliver more services, while others encourage them to do less. Some encourage them to select which patients they wish to see. For example, capitation has been criticized for promoting cream-skimming (risk selection), where providers make more money if they choose only the healthiest patients in order to avoid the costs associated with caring for those with complex or continuing care needs. For more information about physician payment and how it relates to these PHC models, see Appendix A.

### How Does PHC Interface with Other Parts of the Health Care System?

There is also considerable variation in how primary health care interfaces with other parts of the health care system. In some models, different subsectors may function as silos. Other models may seek to coordinate care (e.g., using electronic health records to facilitate transfer of information from one provider to another); the PHC provider may then take on the role of gatekeeper to more specialized services. Other models may integrate various care systems into a common organization. Variants include giving certain organizations budgets with which to purchase a specified basket of care for their rostered patients. This can vary in how extensive the basket is (e.g., some UK models set up primary care physician-led organizations, which in turn were expected to purchase hospital services for their patients), as well as in what, if any, penalties exist for patients seeking care outside of their network (and who pays these penalties).

### The Impact of Policy Legacies on PHC Reform in Canada

PHC in Canada has been influenced by a number of policy legacies (see Chapter 1, section 2.3, Historical Institutionalism, Path Dependency, and Policy Legacies). Among these are Canadian federalism and how this affected the rules of the game in financing health care (see Chapter 1, section 7.2, *Canada Health Act*). Indeed, Hutchison et al. (2001) argue that these legacies have been major barriers to reforming PHC in Canada.

Under the *British North America (Constitution) Act, 1867*, Canadian provinces have jurisdiction over much of health care (see Chapter 1, section 2.2.1, Federalism in Canada). As a result, the federal government has had few policy levers to implement health care policy and set national standards. Historically, the policy lever most often used by federal governments has been fiscal, including various forms of transfer payments to the provinces. These have included both cash and "tax points" (reducing federal tax rates and allowing provinces to fill the "tax room"), and include both unspecified payments (often termed "equalization") along with transfers for specific purposes (see Chapter 1, section 7.1, Financing Health Care in Canada). Health insurance was introduced gradually, and focused on the most expensive segments of the system – initially hospitals, and then physicians. This focus on hospital and physician services was entrenched within the comprehensiveness definition of the *Canada Health Act* (see Chapter 1, section 7.2, *Canada Health Act*). The system did not seek to change the way in which health services were being delivered; instead, it implemented a public contracting model of public payment for private delivery (see Chapter 1, sections 6.1.1, Public and Private, and 6.1.2,

Financing and Delivery). PHC physicians thus retained their status as private business owners, but instead of obtaining payments from patients and private insurers on an FFS basis, most received FFS payments from the provincial insurance plan (see Chapter 1, section 6.2, Payment Mechanisms and Incentives). In most cases, the fee schedule is negotiated between the provincial medical association and the provincial government. However, there has been a significant change in how providers are paid; although there are still many solo practitioners working on an FFS basis, an increasing number of family physicians are involved in alternative models. Ontario has set up a plethora of models (see Appendix B for a brief description of some of them).

**Barriers and Facilitators**

Historically physicians have been the dominant profession in health care. This historical distribution of power has sometimes presented problems when trying to implement models that involve collaboration between physicians and other providers because physicians have often viewed such collaboration as a potential threat to their professional autonomy. Similarly, efforts to increase accountability have challenged the relationship between the government and physicians. Traditionally this relationship was one based on trust; government would compensate physicians, trusting that their professional obligations would ensure ethical practices, and physicians would in turn be able to provide health care services without much government interference.

Interprofessional models present another set of challenges. Health professions legislation in most jurisdictions is based on distinct professions, each with their own educational requirements, practice standards, and regulatory colleges. There is no common approach to governance or accountability across professions, and there can be overlapping scopes of practice. Traditionally, professional liability models are focused on individuals rather than teams, and are legally based within each profession rather than on shared accountability. This has presented some problems in trying to make quality improvement a standard cultural element of primary health care practice, rather than a solo activity driven by individual providers.

**What Remains to Be Done?**

The main changes in PHC in Canada have focused on revisions to physician remuneration models, using varying mixes of incentives and payment structures. As such, they have been described as being relatively modest reforms, although one goal has been an attempt to speed the adoption of electronic medical records (Hutchison, 2008). As Hutchison and colleagues (2001) suggested, "Despite their wide variety and substantial numbers, innovations in the organization, funding, and delivery of primary care in Canada have been at the margins of primary care rather than at its core" (p. 122). Almost all Canadian provinces have moved to regional governance models for the local planning, funding, and coordination of health care services. However, regionalization activities in most provinces have not included physician services or PHC, which has made it difficult to integrate PHC services with other sectors of health care delivery.

Despite the reforms, differences appear to have persisted in access to PHC services, particularly for those with high burden of disease, and for vulnerable populations (Glazier et al., 2008). One Ontario study found that the capitated models appear to have enrolled healthier and wealthier patients, and saw fewer patients than did physicians in the FFS models (Glazier et al., 2009).

## Key Actors and Interests

Regardless of jurisdiction, the medical profession has a strong and influential voice in this debate (Ham & Alberti, 2002). Hutchison (2008) states that "system level innovation in primary healthcare is only possible with the support, or, at a minimum, the acquiescence of organized medicine" (p. 12). In Ontario, for example, the Ontario Medical Association (OMA) has had exclusive bargaining rights for physician services in Ontario since 1997; representatives of the OMA and the Ontario Ministry of Health and Long-Term Care (MOHLTC) negotiate the multi-year physician services agreements. Under these arrangements, PHC reform would require "new money" and could not be drawn from the existing budget for physician services. These arrangements also exclude other health care providers from these negotiations (Fooks, 2004).

A number of other physician groups are careful observers of this policy field, including bodies representing family physicians (in Ontario, the Ontario College of Family Physicians). The provincial regulatory bodies (e.g., the College of Physicians and Surgeons of Ontario) must ensure that professional standards are met. The OMA is also a member of the Canadian Medical Association (CMA), a national body composed of the provincial physician associations. The CMA carefully watches activities in each province/territory. Nationally, family practitioners must meet the standards of the College of Family Physicians of

Canada. A group of reform-minded providers have formed the Canadian Doctors for Medicare to argue for a strong publicly funded system and have also joined the debate.

The other providers who may work on interdisciplinary teams also have a keen interest in PHC. Note that some such providers, including nurse practitioners and midwives, may also be paid on an FFS basis. Some are pushing for the ability to directly bill the Ontario Health Insurance Plan (OHIP) rather than have to be paid by provider organizations. Others are attracted by opportunities for shared overhead by working in certain PHC models, as well as by the potential for improving patient care. However, they are reluctant to move from a position of autonomous practice to a situation that can be perceived as working for a physician boss. Other professionals are attracted by the ability to provide comprehensive PHC.

Some hospitals have indicated an interest in providing space, management services, information technology assistance, and/or expertise for PHC practices, particularly if this can reduce demand on the hospitals to provide care (both through emergency department visits and/or inpatient visits) that could have been delivered on an outpatient/community basis.

There has been little political demand from the public for PHC reform as long as people feel that they have access to care. Public attention has been focused on services that involve waiting lists and acute care services. To date, there has been little public pressure to change how PHC is delivered.

DECISION POINT

You are a senior government official in the provincial government and are responsible for primary health care policy in your province. You have been asked to develop a strategy for the next steps for primary care reform. You can build on existing initiatives and infrastructure within your province, or take primary care reform in new directions. What directions would you recommend?

SUGGESTED QUESTIONS FOR DISCUSSION

1. What do you think have been the key objectives of primary
   care reform? Why do you think the Ontario government has

implemented so many different types of primary care models? Do these models represent innovations or variations on a theme?

2. What explains policy stasis and policy change in the primary care reform context?
3. What do you think are the most important elements of primary care reform and why? Discuss the implications of: different payment mechanisms; use of different health care providers; health promotion, illness prevention and chronic disease management; and integration with other parts of the health care system.
4. If you were to implement or expand on some of these elements, what barriers might you encounter? Which elements would involve the most resistance from key actors and stakeholders?
5. How should government involve key stakeholders in primary health care reform efforts?

APPENDIX A: PAYING DOCTORS

At the time of writing, most family physicians in Canada were paid through one of six compensation schemes: (1) fee-for-service; (2) blended fee-for-service; (3) blended capitation; (4) blended salary; (5) salary; and/or (6) blended complement. The Ontario PHC models described in Appendix B use all of these approaches.

In *fee-for-service* (FFS) payment, physicians are compensated for each individual procedure that they perform. The list of insured procedures is contained within the provincial fee schedule (in Ontario, Ontario Schedule of Benefits for Physician Services). In most provinces, the fees for each procedure are negotiated between the provincial ministry of health and the provincial medical association. Up until the early 2000s, FFS was the most common form of compensation for physicians in most of Canada, including Ontario.

In *blended fee-for-service* payment (also called enhanced FFS), physicians are compensated primarily through FFS, but also enrol patients and agree to provide them with a small basket of primary care services. For this, physicians receive a small incentive for enrolling each patient, rather than billing FFS for those activities in that basket. In addition, they are eligible to receive other bonuses and premiums for performing specific procedures or delivering particular services to enrolled patients. In Ontario, the size and contents of the basket of services and the incentives provided are determined through negotiations between the provincial ministry of health (MOHLTC) and the Ontario Medical Association (OMA).

*Blended capitation* provides physicians with an age- and sex-adjusted base payment for each patient they enrol. To receive this payment, physicians agree to provide a basket of comprehensive primary care services (much larger than the basket in the blended FFS model) to these patients. As in the blended FFS model, physicians can no longer receive the full FFS payment for services in the basket that are provided to enrolled patients. However, they can still receive FFS payments for patients that are not enrolled (up to a maximum amount per year) and/ or for services that are not in the designated basket. In addition, physicians are eligible to receive a range of premiums and incentives for providing particular services. Again, in Ontario, the size and contents of this basket of services and the type of incentives provided are determined through negotiations between the MOHLTC and the OMA.

*Blended salary* payment provides physicians with a base salary for the provision of comprehensive primary care services to a roster of enrolled patients, as well as a similar range of premiums and incentives as are provided to physicians in the blended capitation scheme. The basket of services in this model is larger than in any other model, meaning it is more unlikely physicians in this model will be able to bill FFS, except for non-enrolled patients (up to a maximum amount per year).

Pure *salary* payment for physicians is rare in the Ontario context. The only primary care model to adopt this scheme was the Community Health Centre (CHCs). In CHCs, physicians do not enrol patients and are not permitted to bill FFS (more information on CHCs can be found in Appendix B: Selected Ontario Primary Care Reform Models). However, there have been some efforts to make some of the incentive payments available in other models available to CHC physicians.

*Blended complement* provides physicians with compensation based on the number of physicians that are participating in the group (rather than the number of patients). Physicians are also eligible to receive incentives and premiums for the provision of particular services to patients enrolled with that group of physicians. In Ontario, this model was available only to primary care practices located in particular areas of the province (typically in rural communities) and to a few specialized practices.

In addition to receiving a base payment for the delivery of primary care services, family physicians in Ontario are also eligible to receive a variety of *incentives* and *premiums* for the delivery of specific services to enrolled patients. Examples include incentives for providing such services as obstetrical deliveries, hospital service, palliative care, vaccinations, cancer screening, participating in continuing medical education, after-hours care, newborn care, chronic disease management, smoking cessation counselling, and ensuring continuity of care.

Note that most non-physician team members are paid on a salaried basis from the funds made available to the practice.

## APPENDIX B: SELECTED ONTARIO PRIMARY CARE REFORM MODELS

Ontario has introduced a wide variety of PHC models; they are sometimes referred to as the "alphabet soup." Key ones are briefly described below, recognizing that similar models can be found in most jurisdictions.

*Community Health Centres (CHCs)* are primary care organizations that provide first access primary care services and social services to patients in communities ranging from 5,000 to 30,000 people. They are community-led; an elected Board of Directors governs CHCs and includes representatives from the community. The Board ensures that delivered programs are compatible with the needs of the community and accountable to their funding agencies. CHCs are funded through global budgets. The first Ontario example of this model was in 1963, before the province had universal insurance for physician services, when local community groups (led by several local unions) had set up the Group Health Centre (GHC) in the northern community of Sault Ste. Marie. Similar models were set up in the 1980s, and were termed Community Health Centres (CHCs). All featured rostered patients, salaried physicians, and multidisciplinary teams. Governance varied, but this category of models hired salaried physicians to provide a comprehensive array of services to its members. CHCs provide health advice and deliver various programs within a population health framework (e.g., smoking cessation, diabetes, family planning, and treatment of sexually transmitted diseases). Health care providers are paid on salary and provide prevention and primary care services in a collaborative, multidisciplinary team environment. They also coordinate an array of social services for their clients and the local community agencies.

The GHC was born from a trade union's desire for a better community and concern over inaccessible health care and rising costs. The physician shortage and rising health care costs in that community in the late 1950s had raised concern among the unionists over the future of the local health care system. In direct opposition to the local physicians, the GHC was established, although it had little support from the local medical community and the provincial government.

The excitement generated by the CHCs waned in the 1970s. In 1975, the Ministry put a halt to further expansion of CHCs and Health Services Organizations (discussed below), citing the OMA position that there was inadequate evidence and evaluation of their effectiveness. However, in 1982 Larry Grossman, the Conservative Minister of Health, took an interest in CHCs, and convened a task force (chaired by Fraser Mustard) to examine primary care in Ontario. Armed with the task force's recommendation, Grossman acknowledged the distinct and unique role of CHCs by globally funding the CHC program. The era of CHCs being considered "experimental pilot projects" had come to an end.

In 1987, David Peterson's Liberal government announced the intent to double the number of CHCs, and by November 1989, 90% of this target had been achieved. In 1994, subsequent to questions raised by the Auditor General, the CHC program suffered another setback when funding for the maintenance and establishment of new CHCs was frozen pending further assessment. The Ministry lifted the funding freeze in 1999, resulting in the creation of two additional CHCs and a satellite clinic. By December 2000, there were 56 CHCs in Ontario, located in urban and rural areas, serving approximately 294,000 active registered patients or about 2.5% of the Ontario population. Their overall annual budget was $133.5 million, of which about $120 million came from the Ontario government.

A government review of the CHC program found that they provided valuable care to disadvantaged higher-risk populations; the number of CHCs thus grew considerably. At the time of writing, CHCs primarily served patients who had difficulty in accessing primary care and were at higher risk of developing illness. This disadvantaged population tended to involve certain ethnocultural groups, the less educated, single-family parents, and/or low-income earners.

Physicians have, in general, not been comfortable with models where physicians are not in charge. Indeed, another early model, *Health Services Organizations (HSO)*, introduced in 1973, also involved having the patients rostered, but was physician-led. Physicians were paid a standard capitated rate for each enrolled patient based on the age and sex of the patient. The government's goal was to promote a new method of delivery that would reduce the per capita costs of health care, while maintaining or improving the quality of care. The objective was to shift care from the hospital into the community, change utilization by patients and establish accessible, coordinated, and efficient health care at the primary care level. Like the GHC experience, it was believed that the HSO approach would be cost-effective through such mechanisms as decreasing the use of institutional care and increasing the use of non-physician health care providers. By 1987, there were 27 HSOs, and then-Premier David Peterson pledged to double the number of people served by HSOs within five years. However, physicians proved reluctant to participate in a model involving an alternative payment system that they saw as threatening their professional autonomy, financial independence, and conditions of work, and as undermining the continuity and closeness of their relationship with patients. In 1990, the Ministry evaluated the HSO program; they concluded that it had "serious shortcomings" and that it had increased health care costs without demonstrating improvements in quality or comprehensiveness of services. Although the NDP provincial government did not eliminate the HSO program, it made structural changes, including reducing capitation rates by 13.5%, eliminating incentive funding for reducing hospital utilization, and capping roster size at 2,500 patients. Physicians who were once a part of these HSOs left for other alternatives. At the time of writing, HSOs had largely been abandoned, although there were still 49 HSOs in existence, with the majority located in the Waterloo and Hamilton areas. The approximately168 full-time equivalent HSO physicians managed about 265,000 rostered patients, with an annual capitation budget of about $39 million, although physicians could bill additional FFS for a certain number of procedures.

At the time of writing, Ontario physicians could choose from an alphabet soup of PHC models. Most of these require patients to be rostered, but vary in how providers are paid (see Appendix A), and in which non-physician providers are parts of the team.

In their 2004 provincial budget, the Ontario government announced the implementation of 150 *Family Health Teams* (FHTs), which would include not only physicians but also nurse practitioners and other health care providers, and which would provide comprehensive primary health care on a 24/7 basis. This target was not only met but exceeded; about 170 were established. FHTs are composed of interprofessional teams of family physicians, plus such other interdisciplinary health providers (IHPs) as nurse practitioners, registered nurses (RNs), registered practical nurses (RPNs), mental health and social workers, dietitians, pharmacists, and others who provide comprehensive primary care to their enrolled patients. FHTs are governed by a Board of Directors. They differ from CHCs in that the operational funding and the funding for the IHPs are established through agreements between the FHT Board and the MOHLTC, while the physician funding proceeds through separate agreements. Physicians in FHTs are compensated through mixed capitation or salary. FHTs also include provisions for shared care and collaborative care models between family doctors and consulting specialists. By January 2009, FHTs had funding approved for over 1,300 IHPs and had over 1,500 participating family physicians. FHTs were still mostly owned and operated by physicians. However, despite the Ontario government's focus on FHTs, most Ontarians did not receive their primary care services in one of these centres. (Note that patients enrolled with FHTs received a more comprehensive array of services, whereas most Ontarians enrolled in other models would have to rely on private insurance or out-of-pocket payment to receive many of the non-physician services offered in the FHTs, unless they received them within a hospital setting.)

The most widely used set of models remains physician-focused. The *Comprehensive Care Model* (CCM) is built on solo physicians, but has them enrol at least some of their patients, with an expectation that these physicians will provide comprehensive PHC to their enrolled patients and some after-hours care. The *Family Health Groups* (FHG) are similar, but are based on groups of at least three physicians. They are expected to provide comprehensive primary care to their enrolled patients on a 24/7 basis, although some of this can be accomplished through the use of Telephone Health Advisory Services. Organizations using these models are paid through a blended funding model weighted towards FFS.

*Family Health Networks* (FHN) and *Family Health Organizations* (FHO) resemble FHGs in that they are composed of groups of three or more physicians, and are expected to provide comprehensive care to their enrolled patients. However, they are paid on blended funding models weighted towards capitation payments, and are expected to put more emphasis on chronic disease management, disease prevention, and health promotion. FHOs were implemented in 2004 to replace the former HSOs. They have a larger basket of services and a higher base rate payment than do FHNs. By 2010, a majority of Ontario family physicians had moved into the FHO model.

In 2007, the Ontario government made a small step away from exclusively physician-led models when it announced the implementation of 25 *nurse practitioner–led clinics*. This model hired nurse practitioners (NPs) to lead teams consisting of RNs, RPNs, collaborating physicians, and others to provide primary care services to unattached patients and other vulnerable populations that are relatively hard to serve. These clinics are similar to FHTs in that they comprise teams of interdisciplinary providers; however, they are operated and led by NPs rather than by physicians. The implementation of nurse practitioner–led clinics has been targeted to what have been referred to as "underserved communities" in order to improve access to PHC. Such clinics are governed by a Board of Directors, and receive their funding through an agreement with the Nursing Secretariat of the MOHLTC. The clinicians are salaried. Similarly, a number of community-led *Aboriginal Health Access Centres* have been set up to provide a combination of traditional healing, primary care, cultural programs, health promotion programs, community development initiatives, and social support services to First Nations, Metis, and Inuit communities both on- and off-reserve. By 2011, about 3% of Ontario residents were being served by these non-physician-led models.

## APPENDIX C: PHC GOALS AS CITED IN NATIONAL REFORM DOCUMENTS

On September 11, 2000, the Canadian First Ministers agreed that "improvements to primary health care are crucial to the renewal of health services" and highlighted the importance of multidisciplinary teams. In response to this agreement, the Government of Canada established the $800-million Primary Health Care Transition Fund (PHCTF), which provided funds, over a six-year period, to the provinces/territories for primary care reform initiatives. All of these initiatives were expected to meet the following five common objectives:

1. To increase the proportion of the population with access to primary health care organizations which are accountable for the planned provision of comprehensive services to a defined population;

2. To increase the emphasis on health promotion, disease and injury prevention, and chronic disease management;
3. To expand 24/7 access to essential services;
4. To establish multidisciplinary teams so that the most appropriate care is provided by the most appropriate provider; and
5. To facilitate coordination with other health services (such as specialists and hospitals).

Funds were one-time and have not been renewed (Health Canada, 2007).

Two national commissions reported in 2002. The Romanow Commission (Commission on the Future of Health Care in Canada, 2002) viewed primary care reform as a move from an emphasis on PC to PHC. To achieve this transition the Commission set out the following priorities:

1. Continuity and coordination of care: to reduce system fragmentation for patients.
2. Early detection and action: This includes a focus on risk factors for chronic disease.
3. Better information on needs and outcomes: This includes the implementation of electronic health records.
4. New and stronger incentives: This includes financial incentives, better funding schemes for primary care practices, recognition of work-life conditions for primary care staff, and a focus on incentivizing improvements in quality of care.

The Senate Committee, under Senator Kirby (Standing Senate Committee on Social Affairs Science and Technology, 2002), supported the continued federal role in promoting the following objectives: A continued federal role in promoting the implementation of multidisciplinary primary health care teams that: are working to provide a broad range of services, 24 hours a day, 7 days a week; strive to ensure that services are delivered by the most appropriately qualified health care professional; utilise to the fullest the skills and competencies of a diversity of health care professionals; adopt alternative methods of funding to fee-for-service, such as capitation, either exclusively or as part of blended funding formulae; seek to integrate health promotion and illness prevention strategies in their day-to-day work; and progressively assume a greater degree of responsibility for all the health and wellness needs of the population they serve.

APPENDIX D: REFERENCES CITED AND FURTHER READING

Aggarwal, M. (2009). *Primary care reform: A case study of Ontario.* Toronto: University of Toronto.

Commission on the Future of Health Care in Canada. (2002). *Building on values: The future of health care in Canada.* http://publications.gc.ca/collections/Collection/CP32-85-2002E.pdf

Deber, R., Hollander, M.J., & Jacobs, P. (2008). Models of funding and reimbursement in health care: A conceptual framework. *Canadian Public Administration, 51*(3), 381–405. http://dx.doi.org/10.1111/j.1754-7121.2008.00030.x

Fooks, C. (2004). Implementing primary care reform in Canada: Barriers and facilitators. In R. Wilson, S.E.D. Shortt, & J. Dorland (Eds.), *Implementing primary care reform: Barriers and facilitators* (pp. 129–37). Montreal: McGill-Queen's University Press.

Glazier, R.H., Klein-Geltink, J., Kopp, A., & Sibley, L.M. (2009). Capitation and enhanced fee-for-service models for primacy care reform: A population-based evaluation. *Canadian Medical Association Journal, 180*(11), E72–81. http://dx.doi.org/10.1503/cmaj.081316

Glazier, R.H., Moineddin, R., Agha, M.M., Zagorski, B., Hall, R., Manuel, D.G., et al. (2008, July). *The impact of not having a primary care physician among people with chronic conditions.* Institute for Evaluative Clinical Sciences. http://www.ices.on.ca/file/Impact_no%20physician_July14-08.pdf

Glazier, R.H., Zagorski, B.M., & Rayner, J. (2012, March). *Comparison of primary care models in Ontario by demographics, case mix and emergency department use, 2008/09 to 2009/10.* Institute for Clinical Evaluative Sciences. http://www.ices.on.ca/file/ICES_Primary%20Care%20Models%20English.pdf%7D

Ham, C., & Alberti, K.G.M.M. (2002). The medical profession, the public, and the government. *British Medical Journal, 324*(7341), 838–42. http://dx.doi.org/10.1136/bmj.324.7341.838

Health Canada. (2007). *Primary health care transition fund.* http://www.hc-sc.gc.ca/hcs-sss/prim/phctf-fassp/index-eng.php

Hutchison, B. (2008). A long time coming: Primary healthcare renewal in Canada. *Healthcare Papers, 8*(2), 10–24. http://dx.doi.org/10.12927/hcpap.2008.19704

Hutchison, B., Abelson, J., & Lavis, J. (2001). Primary care in Canada: So much innovation, so little change. *Health Affairs, 20*(3), 116–31. http://dx.doi.org/10.1377/hlthaff.20.3.116

Katz, A., Glazier, R.H., & Vijayaraghavan, J. (2009, February). *The health and economic consequences of achieving a high-quality primary healthcare system in Canada: Applying what works in Canada: Closing the gap.* Canadian Health

Services Research Foundation (CHSRF). http://www.cfhi-fcass.ca/Libraries/Primary_Healthcare/11498_PHC_Katz_ENG_FINAL.sflb.ashx

Leger, P.T. (2011, March). *Physician payment mechanisms: An overview of policy options for Canada* (Paper No. 3). CHSRF Series of Reports on Cost Drivers and Health System Efficiency. http://www.cfhi-fcass.ca/Publications AndResources/ResearchReports/CommissionedResearch/11-03-15/f24f57b9-aa81-4ab2-a539-d85746d36789.aspx

Macinko, J., Starfield, B., & Shi, L. (2003). The contribution of primary care systems to health outcomes within Organization for Economic Cooperation and Development (OECD) countries, 1970–1998. *Health Services Research,* *38*(3), 831–65. http://dx.doi.org/10.1111/1475-6773.00149

Standing Senate Committee on Social Affairs Science and Technology. (2002). *The health of Canadians: The federal role, final report: Volume 6. Recommendations for reform.* Parliament of Canada. http://www.parl.gc.ca/37/2/parlbus/commbus/senate/com-e/SOCI-E/rep-e/repoct02vol6-e.htm

Starfield, B. (1994). Is primary care essential? *Lancet, 344*(8930), 1129–33. http://dx.doi.org/10.1016/S0140-6736(94)90634-3

Statistics Canada. (2012, June). *Access to a regular medical doctor, 2011.* http://www.statcan.gc.ca/pub/82-625-x/2012001/article/11656-eng.htm

World Health Organization. (1978). *Declaration of Alma-Ata.* WHO Regional Office for Europe. http://www.euro.who.int/en/who-we-are/policy-documents/declaration-of-alma-ata,-1978

# 12 At Any Price?

## Paying for New Cancer Drugs

*LAURIE BOURNE, RACHNA CHAUDHARY, DAVID FORD, OLIVIA
HAGEMEYER, CHRISTOPHER J. LONGO, ELAINE MEERTENS, AND
RAISA B. DEBER*

How much is it worth paying for how much benefit? Both practical
(e.g., what does it mean to say a treatment works) and ethical issues
have become particularly pronounced in dealing with new pharmaceutical treatments, such as the use of Avastin for people with colorectal
cancer.

This case addresses several policy issues, including: cost-effectiveness
analysis and the role of technology assessment, resource allocation ethics
and rationing, the role of patients in decision making, and the implications of the public-private mix, with a focus on pharmaceutical pricing.

### Appendices

Appendix A: Colorectal Cancer and Its Treatment
Appendix B: Drug Approval Processes in Selected Jurisdictions
Appendix C: Stakeholder Views
Appendix D: Cost-effectiveness Analysis
Appendix E: Modelling the Cost-effectiveness of Avastin
Appendix F: References Cited and Further Reading

### Treating Colorectal Cancer

Colorectal cancer (CRC) is a leading cause of cancer deaths in many
countries, including Canada. CRC refers to tumours in the colon, rectum, or appendix. The incidence of CRC increases with age. In the
United Kingdom, for example, the median age of patients at diagnosis
was over 70 years (Tappenden et al., 2007b). (See Appendix A for additional information about CRC and its treatment.)

If detected early, CRC is highly treatable. However, it may spread to nearby lymph nodes, and then to other organs, particularly the liver and lungs. At the time of writing, treatment usually included surgery, but often added radiation therapy. For advanced disease (also referred to as metastatic disease), systemic chemotherapy could also be employed. Without chemotherapy, median survival for people with metastatic CRC was about eight months. In general, treatment other than surgery was not curative, but might prolong life and improve its quality. Several drug regimens were in use, as either first-line (initial therapy) or second-line therapy. In Ontario, existing therapy was estimated to cost approximately $38,000 and the evidence suggested it could extend life by approximately 1.5 years. Questions now arose as to the potential role for a number of newer agents, including bevacizumab, known as Avastin.

## Avastin

In 1971, US scientist Dr. Judah Folkman published his observation that solid tumours required access to a constant supply of blood in order to receive oxygen and nutrients. He postulated that blocking angiogenesis (the growth of blood vessels) might be a valuable way to treat cancer. Although the particular agents he discovered proved disappointing in clinical trials, the overall concept appeared to remain valid. Researchers turned to one of the many growth factors involved in forming new blood vessels, vascular endothelial growth factor (VEGF). Bevacizumab (Avastin) is a monoclonal antibody that can selectively bind to and inhibit VEGF. By itself, it cannot kill the tumour cells, but in theory adding this compound to a treatment regimen can slow tumour growth by blocking the blood supply needed to feed the cancer. The usual form of administration is intravenously through the arm, every 14 days, until the underlying disease shows progression, which would suggest that Avastin is no longer being effective in blocking tumour growth. Avastin is manufactured by California-based Genentech, one of the pioneer biotechnology companies. (In March 2009, Genentech merged with the international pharmaceutical company Hoffmann-La Roche, and became a wholly owned member of the Roche Group.)

Most jurisdictions separate the decision about whether to allow a drug on the market (which is largely based on proving safety and effectiveness) from the decision about whether the drug will be paid for (which often incorporates questions of value for money). In the

United States, for example, the Food and Drug Administration (FDA) decides whether to approve drugs, but not whether to pay for them. In February 2004, the FDA approved the use of Avastin as a first-line treatment for patients with metastatic CRC, but only as part of a regimen in combination with either intravenous 5-FU/FA or with irinotecan plus intravenous 5-FU/FA (see Appendix A). This was the first angiogenesis inhibitor they had approved. The clinical trials suggested that adding Avastin did not cure the disease, but extended the lives of those responding to the drug by approximately five months. Soon after, Avastin was approved for use in CRC by the European Medicines Agency (EMEA) in January 2005, and by Health Canada in February 2005. Avastin has subsequently been licensed to be part of the treatment regimen for other solid tumours, including metastatic non–small cell lung cancer; clinical trials were ongoing for other tumour types. At the time of writing, Roche had recommended Avastin for the following indications: metastatic CRC; locally recurrent or metastatic breast cancer; advanced, metastatic, recurrent, non-squamous, non–small cell lung cancer, and advanced and/or metastatic renal cell cancer. As is often the case for new medications, however, there was some variation in (and controversy about) the extent to which its use for particular conditions was supported by clinical evidence, and in when (and whether) it was approved in various jurisdictions.

However, approval by these agencies did not mean that it would be paid for. (See Appendix B for the drug approval process in selected jurisdictions.) Roche has applied in many countries to have Avastin added to the formulary of drugs that would be covered by insurers, whether public or private. Various stakeholders have expressed their views. (See Appendix C for a summary of the views of key stakeholders.)

This in turn led to a series of efforts in all of these jurisdictions to weigh the costs and benefits. Determining whether the health benefits of a new drug or technology merit the expenditure is a process fraught with ethical and political dilemmas for payers, clinicians, and patients. Much debate surrounds the issue of who should be responsible for determining the treatments that patients receive, and ethical issues surround cost-effectiveness studies that attempt to place a monetary value on human life (see Chapter 1, section 3.6, Ethical Frameworks).

One of the most elaborate procedures existed in the United Kingdom, where an arm's length body, the National Institute of Health and Clinical Excellence (NICE) was set up to review new technologies and drugs on behalf of the National Health Service (Steinbrook, 2008). Unlike the situation in Canada or the United States, NICE was explicitly asked to look at the "value for money" of new therapies. The NICE review of Avastin was negative (Tappenden et al., 2007a, 2007b); in November 2009 they denied funding for Avastin for CRC because they found costs were high relative to benefits. Similarly, in the United States, insurance companies have often refused to pay for all or part of the costs of Avastin.

### Assessing the Costs and Benefits of Avastin

Technology assessment requires clarifying both costs and benefits. (Appendix D provides additional information on how a cost-effectiveness analysis might be performed.)

Several randomized controlled trials have attempted to evaluate the benefits of adding Avastin to chemotherapy regimens. Interpreting these studies is not always simple. Different studies have compared Avastin to different chemotherapy combinations, and used a variety of end points to measure outcomes, including: median time to disease progression in months, tumour response rate, median duration of survival in months, and one-year survival rate. All showed modest improvements over the short term. The drug also had side effects, largely related to increased blood pressure (which occurred in over 10% of those receiving Avastin), and to bleeding. Genentech reported that the risk of certain adverse events (transient ischemic attack, stroke, myocardial infarction, angina) approximately doubled among those receiving the drug.

One industry-sponsored study of 813 patients who had received no previous therapy for their metastatic CRC compared those who received one chemotherapy regimen (IFL) to those who received IFL plus Avastin (Hurwitz et al., 2004). The study found that in the group also receiving Avastin, median overall survival had increased from 15.6 months to 20.3 months, median progression-free survival had increased from 6.2 months to 10.6 months, and the proportion responding to therapy had increased from 34.8% to 44.8%. Another way of analysing this data would observe that this meant that over half of the patients received no benefit from chemotherapy (with or without Avastin), while still facing its often substantial side effects. Subsequent studies have suggested that even these modest gains may not persist over time; certainly these therapies do not cure the disease, and recent publications suggest that they do not appear to have prolonged disease-free survival when measured after three years (Van Cutsem et al., 2011). On the other hand, many patients and their doctors say the drug can improve the quality of life, particularly by enhancing a sense of well-being and the ability to carry out daily tasks without exhaustion or pain; such effects can be hard to measure or to place a value on. One problem with evaluating the impact is that the findings are often considered proprietary, and the manufacturer has been reluctant to publicly release data, particularly data relating to quality of life. Indeed, the publications posted on the NICE website concerning its analysis of Avastin included tables whose entries were largely blacked out because the company did not give permission for the data to be released.

In terms of costs, Avastin is an expensive drug; indeed, it is one of the most expensive drugs widely marketed. Prices vary, in part because dose is based on the patient's weight. Costs also depend on how many cycles of the drug are administered (as noted above, the dosing schedule is one intravenous injection every 14 days). When introduced in the United States, the average wholesale price was $4,400 per month; at the time of writing, the US FDA website estimated the cost as $7,500 per month. Costs per patient vary, but have been estimated at $100,000 per year in the United States, and $30,000–$40,000 per year in Canada. (Such estimates are difficult, because of variation in who pays what price, what discounts are negotiated, etc.) In 2008, sales of Avastin were nearly $2.7 billion. An editorial accompanying the report of the industry-funded study cited above focused on the median overall survival, and noted that the cost of extending life by an average of 4.7 months (from 15.6 months to 20.3 months) would add from $42,800 to $55,000 to the cost of noncurative care (Mayer, 2004). Another study estimated that the cost in Canada if all patients with early CRC received Avastin would be about $4 billion per year (Wright, 2009). Measured in terms of cost per quality adjusted life year (QALY), Avastin was computed as being in the range of $230,000 per QALY, considerably above commonly used threshold values of £20,000–£30,000 per QALY in the United Kingdom, and $100,000 per QALY in the United States (Brock, 2006).

Avastin has accordingly been controversial. It does not cure cancer, but in some cases it may prolong life, albeit for a relatively short time. It has thus highlighted issues about what benefits are worth purchasing, and what to do when the evidence is incomplete.

One ongoing dispute in financing health care is the extent to which patient choices should be influenced by (or insulated from) fiscal matters. A number of factors influence the ability of price signals to balance supply and demand in the way economic theory might predict (see Chapter 1, section 5.9, Insurance, Elasticity, and Moral Hazard). Traditionally, pharmaceutical companies have justified high prices on the defensible grounds that they needed to recover their costs for research and development. Genentech went beyond this, to justify the high price based on "the value of innovation and the value of new therapies." Given patent protection, however, companies would not face competitive pressures to lower prices on "necessary" products for many years. (Various payers have attempted, with varying success, to negotiate prices, but to be credible this would require that the payer refuse to purchase the product unless the price was lowered.) Either payers (public or private) would pay whatever price was asked, or people would be denied the treatment. From the standpoint of demand, economists often argue that good insurance coverage may create "moral hazard" and cause people to purchase goods and services they might otherwise not consider to be worth the money. Some also point to moral hazard for providers; there is an ongoing dispute as to whether insurance coverage (by government or by private insurers) has provided financial incentives for overtreatment of patients, rapid adoption of new brand name products over generic versions of therapies, and overuse of imaging services in the management of patients (Meropol & Schulman, 2007). Another view, however, is that access to potentially lifesaving care should not be limited to the rich (see Chapter 1, section 3.6, Ethical Frameworks). Some have suggested that very high prices for these drugs resemble extortion of desperate people and are not ethically justifiable (Brock, 2006).

### Coverage in Canada

The *Canada Health Act* (*CHA*) requires that medically required pharmaceuticals be paid for only if they are delivered within hospitals (see Chapter 1, section 7.2). Decisions about what will be covered by the hospital budget largely rest with hospital-based decision makers, primarily physicians. Should they decide that a particular drug is medically necessary for particular inpatients, it is expected to be covered from the hospital budget. (Many hospitals have attempted to manage this process by establishing their own formulary.) Historically, each Ontario hospital paid for its own intravenous cancer drugs, which resulted in considerable variation in what drugs were available. To help meet the costs of cancer drugs, Ontario set up the New Drug Funding

Program (NDFP), administered by Cancer Care Ontario on behalf of the Ministry of Health and Long-Term Care. The NDFP funds new and approved intravenous cancer drugs administered in hospitals; older drugs approved before the NDFP was created are covered through the hospitals' global budgets. The government estimates that the NDFP provides about 75% of the overall funding for intravenous cancer drugs in Ontario. However, the *CHA* is a floor, not a ceiling. If non-physician services, including pharmaceuticals, can be delivered on an outpatient basis, there is no requirement under the *CHA* that they be publicly paid for, although provinces/territories are able to pay for them should they wish to do so.

There are accordingly ambiguities as to how to deal with drugs that a province decides are not publicly covered, whether from hospital budgets or under provincial drug plans. Strict interpretation of the *CHA* would imply that hospitals could not allow private payment for insured services to insured persons; since all medically necessary pharmaceuticals for inpatients would count as insured services that are expected to be paid through the hospital budget, it might be deemed a violation of the *CHA* if hospitals allowed privately financed drugs to be administered within their facilities. Avastin is delivered intravenously and therefore requires professional supervision. If this drug could be administered in a non-hospital setting (e.g., a private clinic), however, private payment might be allowable. Such clinics soon appeared (Chafe et al., 2009). In downtown Toronto, a private clinic (Provis Infusion Clinic) opened in 2005, and would infuse drugs (particularly but not exclusively for cancer) as long as these were not publicly funded (Canadian Cancer Society & Turner and Associates, 2009). Another company, the Bayshore, has set up a similar network of 20 community care clinics in various cities, which can also perform infusions.

As noted, another option would be for drugs to be covered through public or private drug insurance plans. Provincial/territorial governments have varied in their decisions about what they cover and for whom, although most do have some form of provincial drug plan to cover some outpatient drug expenses. (At the time of writing, New Brunswick was the only province with no such public plan.) At the time of the case, Canada had 19 public drug plans, in addition to the myriad private plans, and each made its own coverage decisions. The Canadian Cancer Society estimated that 43% of Canadians had some coverage from a public drug plan, and 56% were covered primarily by private insurance. Public coverage for the cost of cancer drugs was higher than for other drugs (with the proportion with some public coverage estimated at 68%), because Saskatchewan, Alberta, and British Columbia fully covered cancer treatments regardless of the setting in which they were administered. However, caps and limitations on coverage, coupled with the very high cost of many new drugs (on average, $65,000 per year for a course of treatment with the newer cancer drugs), meant that a sizeable proportion of those with catastrophic expenditures faced very high out-of-pocket payments. The same report estimated that "one in twelve Canadian families still face catastrophic drug costs (defined here as greater than three per cent of net household income), even in provinces where universal coverage exists" (Canadian Cancer Society & Turner and Associates, 2009).

In Ontario, people older than age 65, those living in long-term care or receiving professional services through the home care programs, and people on social assistance were eligible for public coverage for all prescribed drugs on their formulary through the Ontario Drug Benefit Program (ODB). In addition, those with catastrophic expenditures exceeding a given proportion of their income were eligible through the Trillium Drug Program. Co-payments were required, but often were capped. In addition, Ontario introduced a process to allow compassionate access to approved drugs that were not yet on the provincial drug formulary for patients deemed to be in life-threatening situations (Canadian Cancer Society & Turner and Associates, 2009).

Nonetheless, people can be faced with substantial bills for pharmaceuticals, and patient groups have advocated strongly for improving access and coverage. This has been particularly pronounced for cancer, with a number of bodies (including the Cancer Advocacy Coalition of Canada, and a host of disease-related groups) advocating on behalf of patients. One of these groups, the Colorectal Cancer Association of Canada (CCAC), advocates for ensuring public payment for any systemic therapies which might prolong life. In April 2008, they publicly called on the Ontario government to fund Avastin. The Canadian Cancer Society has also advocated for better coverage for cancer drugs; they have subsequently noted that half of the newer cancer drugs were taken at home rather than in hospitals, and as such were not required to be publicly paid for. They noted the estimate that the average cost of treatment was $65,000; indeed, three quarters of the newer cancer drugs cost more than $20,000 per year. Even for those with private coverage, private insurers were reluctant to cover the full costs, and had required substantial co-payments (typically, 20%); some also capped coverage, on an annual and/or lifetime basis (Canadian Cancer Society & Turner and Associates, 2009). Media stories frequently appeared about particular individuals with high out-of-pocket bills for particular drugs; these stories often resulted in pressure for provincial ministries to pick up the costs (see Appendix C for some stakeholder views).

**The Ontario Process**

Most jurisdictions have established processes for determining what drugs should be approved, and what should be paid for. (See Appendix B for some information about these processes.) In Canada, although responsibility for approving drugs (based on safety and efficacy) rests at the national level, decisions about what should be paid for rests with payers (provincial governments for public plans; private insurers for private plans). This is often based on technology assessment, which attempts to compute potential benefits and weigh these against costs. As noted in Appendix B, a variety of processes have existed, including efforts to coordinate these activities rather than force each province to conduct its own technology assessments. Since such efforts are voluntary, their acceptance by provincial governments has varied considerably over time and across jurisdictions.

In Ontario, a number of different bodies existed which could make recommendations about funding pharmaceuticals. At the time of the case, the Committee to Evaluate Drugs (CED) (formerly known as the Drug Quality and Therapeutics Committee) had the mandate to review manufacturers' drug submissions to determine whether they should be listed on the Ontario Drug Formulary. In an effort to somewhat depoliticize the process, the executive director of the CED was given the power to make many decisions on behalf of the Ministry of Health. Other bodies existed with varying mandates, including some at the national level.

With respect to Avastin, the Ontario Ministry of Health and Long-Term Care was faced with various bodies making varying recommendations. Arguing for immediate public payment were patient groups and some oncologists. However, in January 2006, Ontario's Drug Quality and Therapeutic Committee (soon renamed the CED) had recommended that it should not be funded on the grounds of insufficient cost-effectiveness. This did not settle the matter; stakeholders continued to lobby for its approval. Pressure to reopen the decision not to fund was heightened because different provinces had reacted to this pressure by making different decisions. British Columbia, New-foundland and Labrador, Quebec, and Saskatchewan had all agreed to fund Avastin (for varying numbers of cycles) by 2008. Nova Scotia had rejected coverage. In April 2008, Cancer Care Ontario, the body coordinating and delivering cancer services in the province, had recommended that the province should fund Avastin for metastatic CRC patients. Documents suggested that adding Avastin to existing first-line chemotherapy regimens for CRC (which were already estimated to cost $30.6 million in 2008, rising to $37.8 million by 2010) would add between $16.7 million per year (if funding were capped at 16 cycles) and $25.4 million per year (for 22–23 cycles) to the province's bill. Resulting negotiations between the manufacturer and the CED led to an agreement; Roche would provide the drug at a discount, and the CED executive officer agreed that the province's New Drug Funding Program (NDFP) would pay for 12 treatment cycles (in combination with another chemotherapy drug, FOLFIRI) as a first-line treatment for patients with metastatic CRC, with the option of extending funding for another 4 cycles if these patients' condition remained stable. The additional cost for funding these 12 treatment cycles of Avastin over the next three years was estimated at $30 million.

This decision did not satisfy some stakeholders. In April 2008, the Colorectal Cancer Association of Canada issued a press release and started a write-in campaign to push for increased funding. Cancer Care Ontario also continued to recommend more funding. Several patients who were reaching the end of the 16 publicly funded cycles went public. One approached his provincial representative, who contacted the Office of the Ontario Ombudsman in May 2009. By September 2009, the Ombudsman released his report. Titled *A Vast Injustice*, it denounced the Ministry, arguing that there was a "paucity of medical evidence" to support the 16-cycle cap, adding "while a treatment cap may be an expedient way to control costs, it should not exist at the expense of compassion and consideration of individual circumstances. In the case of Avastin, it is impossible to justify the human price exacted by the current administration's inflexible and dispassionate application of the funding limit" (Marin, 2009). Others suggested that the cost of Avastin was excessive, given the expected benefits. Some pointed to the concept of "opportunity costs" and argued that alternative uses for the same funds might generate greater value for money. As noted, similar pressures were arising in all provinces/territories.

DECISION POINT

You are the Minister of Health of your province. What should you do?

SUGGESTED QUESTIONS FOR DISCUSSION

1. Who should make these decisions, and how? Discuss the potential roles of federal and provincial governments, cancer experts, and patients.
2. What are the views of key stakeholders, including patients, physicians, pharmaceutical companies, private insurers, and the various levels of government? How might these different views be considered in decision making?
3. Discuss the ethical implications of resource allocation for costly cancer drugs. How good does the evidence need to be? What should be done until the evidence is available?
4. Discuss the role of cost-effectiveness evaluations in the drug approval process.

APPENDIX A: COLORECTAL CANCER AND ITS TREATMENT

Cancer of the colon or rectum is commonly called colorectal cancer (CRC). It usually begins from polyps inside the colon or rectum. Polyps can take between 10 and 20 years to evolve into cancer. If they are detected and treated early, CRC can be often prevented, and the disease is highly curable (estimated at about 90%). However, there are few symptoms of early disease. Screening for colon cancer is thus considered extremely important.

CRC is more likely to occur in people over the age of 50, and the risk for developing CRC increases with age. Other risk factors include a diet high in fat and low in fibre; history of smoking; excessive alcohol consumption; physical inactivity; a family history (parent, child, or sibling) of CRC; and a history of Crohn's disease, ulcerative colitis, or having polyps.

The Canadian Cancer Society has estimated that about 8,900 people die from CRC in Canada each year. In Ontario, CRC was the second most common cancer diagnosed in men and the third most common cancer diagnosed in women. A 2010 estimate for the province was that 4,500 men and 3,800 women would be diagnosed with CRC, and 1,850 men and 1,550 women would die from that disease.

Two tests are commonly used to screen for CRC. The FOBT (fecal occult blood test) can detect small amounts of blood in the stool. Colonoscopy is a more invasive test; it involves inserting a small camera on a flexible tube passed through the anus to allow examination of the colon and part of the small bowel. Approximately 10% of people with a positive FOBT are found to have cancer during a follow-up colonoscopy. Currently, it is recommended that everyone 50 years and older be screened with FOBT every two years, with the recognition that a positive test requires a follow-up colonoscopy to determine if the person has CRC. In Ontario, screening with colonoscopy is recommended if the person has a positive FOBT or a family history of CRC. If a first-degree relative (parent, sibling, or child) had CRC it is recommended that such screening begin when the person at risk is 10 years younger than that relative was at the onset of disease.

**Treatment of CRC**

Cancers are commonly classified through the TNM Classification of Malignant Tumours system, which "stages" cancer according to the extent to which cancer has spread (metastasized) and whether nearby tissues or lymph nodes have been invaded. The mode of treatment, and the expected outcomes, vary by stage. Treatments for CRC include surgery, chemotherapy, radiation, or a combination.

The decision to *surgically* remove a tumour will depend on the size and location of the tumour. Invasive cancers that are confined within the wall of the colon (TNM stages I and II) are considered to be curable with surgery. If the tumours are small enough, it may be possible to remove them during a colonoscopy. Larger tumours may require removal of a part of the intestine. Depending on the size and location of the tumour, a permanent or temporary colostomy may be required. Improved preoperative imaging as well as improved surgical techniques have improved the ability to select appropriate patients, and have improved outcomes. CRCs that have spread to regional lymph nodes (stage III) still have a relatively good prognosis, with a cure rate of about 73% with surgery plus chemotherapy. However, once the cancer has spread to other organs (stage IV), outcomes are worse. For the most part, stage IV CRC is not considered to be curable, although surgery can still be deemed curative in 25% to 40% of those highly selected patients who develop resectable (surgically removable) metastases in the liver and lung. Chemotherapy can extend survival, and, rarely, surgery and chemotherapy together have resulted in a cure.

*Radiation therapy* uses a machine to direct radiation at the cancer and surrounding tissue. When used in high doses, radiation destroys cells in the area being treated. Radiation damages the cancer cell DNA, which prevents the cells from growing and dividing. When radiation therapy is done, both cancer and healthy cells are impacted, although most healthy cells can repair themselves. It can be used as the primary treatment approach, or combined with surgery and/or chemotherapy (often referred to as adjuvant radiotherapy). Combined modality therapy with chemotherapy and radiation therapy plays a significant role in the management of patients with rectal cancer. Adjuvant radiotherapy is sometimes used after surgery to reduce the risk of recurrence. The role of adjuvant radiation therapy for patients with colon cancer is not as precise. Currently, adjuvant radiation treatment does not play a standard role in the management of patients with colon cancer following surgery that is meant to be curative, but may play a role if patients have residual cancer.

*Systemic treatment/chemotherapy* may be given orally, by injection, or intravenously. Systemic treatment drugs interfere with the ability of cancer cells to grow and spread, but they also damage healthy cells. Chemotherapy is sometimes used after surgery to reduce the risk of the cancer coming back. Although there were a number of possibilities, the cost-effectiveness analyses reported by Roche in its submissions examined two regimens, each offered with vs. without Avastin. The first was IFL, which includes three drugs: ironotecan, 5-fluorouracil (5FU), and leucovorin. The second was 5-FU/FA (which includes 5-fluorouracil plus folinic acid). These alternatives are examined in the economic analysis in Appendix E.

## APPENDIX B: DRUG APPROVAL PROCESSES IN SELECTED JURISDICTIONS

Most jurisdictions separate the process by which drugs are approved for sale (usually based on safety and effectiveness) from the process used to determine whether they will be paid for (Wiktorowicz, 2003). Note that in all jurisdictions, the responsibility for testing drugs, including conducting the clinical trials and submitting evidence about their safety and effectiveness, rests with the pharmaceutical companies. There is accordingly some dispute as to whether such data are sufficiently reliable, given the potential incentives for drug companies to overstate benefits and/or understate costs. In general, decisions about whether to approve a drug consider only safety and effectiveness. In some but not all jurisdictions, decisions about whether third-party payers (both public and private insurers) will pay for drugs also include considerations of "value for money." In some jurisdictions, there may be additional processes to examine drug pricing, and/or negotiate lower prices. Note that "coverage" may still involve co-payments from patients, and that patients can still decide to pay for approved but uncovered drugs from their own pockets. Another dispute is the extent to which approved drugs can be used "off label" for conditions other than those for which approval was granted. There are also disputes as to the appropriate role for the public vs. experts in making these decisions (Abelson et al., 2007). Brief descriptions of the processes used in several jurisdictions at the time of writing follow, recognizing that the details are likely to change over time.

## Canada

In Canada, responsibility for approving drugs lies at the federal level, but coverage decisions rest with provincial/territorial governments and/or private insurers. At the time of writing, there were several independent processes at the national level, as well as different processes within each province/territory (Tierney et al., 2008). At the national level, Health Canada is responsible for regulatory review, to ensure that pharmaceuticals are sufficiently safe and effective and meet standards for the quality of manufacturing. (This also includes some responsibility for post-market surveillance to detect possible problems that become evident only after the product is in use.) Health Canada approval is required before a drug can be offered for sale in Canada. At the time of writing, these approvals were the responsibility of the Health Products and Food Branch (HPFB). Their decisions look at whether products work (compared to placebo), but usually do not consider their relative benefits, safety, or cost-effectiveness as compared to other pharmaceuticals that are approved for the same condition.

The Patented Medicine Prices Review Board is an independent, quasi-judicial body, at the national level, which examines the prices for patented medicines in Canada, and compares them to prices charged in other specified countries. This process is mandatory, but does not have the authority to consider value for money. Its procedures instead try to ensure that the costs of therapies are "not excessive." If a drug is classified as a "breakthrough drug" its prices are limited to the median of the prices for the same drugs charged in other specified industrialized countries that are set out in the Patented Medicines Regulations (France, Germany, Italy, Sweden, Switzerland, the United Kingdom, and the United States).

A third national process is voluntary, and arose from recognition of the duplication of effort associated with multiple provincial/territorial governments trying to review new medications. Under the auspices of the Canadian Agency for Drugs and Technologies in Health (CADTH), formerly known as the Canadian Coordinating Office for Health Technology Assessment, the federal, provincial, and territorial ministers of health established a Common Drug Review process in 2002 (Tierney et al., 2008). At the time of writing, all provincial/territorial publicly funded drug plans other than Quebec participated in this process, as did the federal payment plans run by Veterans Affairs Canada, Citizenship and Immigration (for refugees), and the Non-Insured Health Benefits for First Nations and Inuit. Under the Common Drug Review process, expert review teams would consider the information submitted by the pharmaceutical companies (including their pharmacaeconomic evaluations) and prepare a report for the Canadian Expert Drug Advisory Committee (currently called the Canadian Drug Expert Committee), whose members include two public representatives, plus health care professionals with expertise in clinical trial methodology, health technology assessment, drug policy, and health economics. This committee would then make positive or negative recommendations as to whether the medications they received were clinically effective and cost-effective. These recommendations were advisory only; each drug plan could still decide whether to list the drug on their formularies. On average, drug plans tended to follow these recommendations 90% of the time. The Common Drug Review process has been somewhat controversial, with many of the objections coming from the pharmaceutical industry (Tierney et al., 2008). Provinces/territories have also varied in the extent to which they wish to participate in the process and accept its recommendations.

The individual provinces/territories also have their own processes as to what should be paid for. As noted in the case, within Ontario, the CED has been given the mandate to review manufacturers' drug submissions to determine whether they should be listed on the Ontario Drug Formulary (which specifies which drugs will be publicly paid for under the Ontario Drug Benefit programs). The CED is expected to evaluate the quality and therapeutic value and costs of drug products, and to recommend to the Ontario Minister of Health and Long-Term Care both whether particular drug products should be considered for coverage under publicly funded drug programs and which (if any) conditions should be attached. The CED also makes recommendations as to which drug products should be deemed "interchangeable." Members of the CED are appointed for a renewable three-year term. To avoid conflict of interest, members cannot be employed by pharmaceutical companies. The terms of reference state that all members must have a professional degree in at least one of: medicine, pharmacy, pharmacology, or health economics. All must be in active practice or research, although two members must be "lay persons" and presumably might not have those professional credentials. To ensure communication with the Ministry, the Director of the Drug Programs Branch is designated as the Executive Secretary to the CED, and the Associate Director is designated as the Senior Consultant. The CED makes recommendations, but ultimate decisions were initially made by the Minister of Health and Long-Term Care. Subsequently, the policy was modified to have decisions made by the CED Executive Officer.

A new development is the emergence of cancer-specific review processes. In Ontario, the CED has a subcommittee (called CED/CCO) with the mandate to review new cancer drugs that have been submitted for consideration of public drug funding in Ontario via the Ontario Drug Benefits or the New Drug Funding Program (NDFP). The CED/CCO subcommittee uses the same evaluation criteria as the CED and incorporates Cancer Care Ontario's Program in Evidence-Based Care (PEBC) guidelines when making recommendations. The committee has recommended drugs for funding when they have found them to have clinically significant benefit when compared to the standard of care and they are convinced that the product is cost-effective. The mandate of the PEBC is to ensure that the best scientific evidence is applied in improving the quality of cancer care in Ontario.

Nationally, an interim cross-jurisdictional process to review all oncology drugs at the national level was implemented in March 2007, with the following provinces participating: Alberta, British Columbia, Manitoba, New Brunswick, Newfoundland, Nova Scotia, Prince Edward

Island, and Saskatchewan. The intention was that this interim committee, known as the Joint Oncology Drug Review (JODR), would be replaced eventually with a permanent process once recommendations had been made to the Deputy Ministers of Health based on an evaluation of the process. The JODR is based on Ontario's current cancer drug review process. Participating provinces have access to recommendations made by both Ontario's CED and the CED/CCO subcommittee; however, each jurisdiction is responsible for its own final funding decisions. In 2010, the provincial/territorial Ministries of Health (with the exception of Quebec) established the pan-Canadian Oncology Drug Review (pCODR) with a mandate "to assess the clinical evidence and cost-effectiveness of new cancer drugs and to use this information to make recommendations to the provinces and territories to guide their drug funding decisions." It began reviewing drugs in 2011, and its evaluative framework was developed in consultation with the patient advocacy community.

### United Kingdom

The National Institute for Health and Clinical Excellence (NICE), formerly called the National Institute for Clinical Excellence, is an independent, government-funded body that produces technology assessments. It uses the approach of estimating the cost per quality-adjusted life year (see Appendix D). As a rule of thumb, it considers treatments to be cost-effective if they cost less than £20,000, although it has on occasion accepted higher values of up to £49,000.

NICE was established in 1999, with the mandate of advising the British National Health Service (NHS). Since 2002, its recommendations have been binding on NHS organizations in England and Wales, who were required to provide any treatment recommended by NICE if prescribed by a clinician, although these organizations are allowed to provide treatments even if NICE has not recommended them. NICE's recommendations have been criticized, particularly by the pharmaceutical industry and patient groups (Steinbrook, 2008). Indeed, in 2011 the UK government announced that it planned to modify how NICE operates to make its views advisory, leaving decisions about which treatments should be paid for to the physician-led primary care trusts, although at the time of writing it had not implemented this proposal.

In the case of Avastin, NICE has continued to recommend against coverage, on the grounds that it (and several other expensive cancer drugs) "were not cost effective within their licensed indications." Its estimate was that the incremental costs per QALY of Avastin were over £170,000 (about US$300,000) (Steinbrook, 2008; Tappenden et al., 2007b).

## United States

The Food and Drug Administration (FDA) is responsible for approving drugs in the United States. Similar to the situation in Canada, FDA approval is based on evidence from clinical trials of safety and effectiveness only, without consideration of cost-effectiveness. FDA decisions thus do not determine whether these drugs are paid for. Those Americans without insurance coverage would have to pay out of pocket; for those with insurance, coverage decisions are made by third-party payers (public and private). However, even for those with coverage, co-payments and caps on total coverage are common, and a large and growing proportion of the costs for cancer drugs is born by individual patients (Meropol & Schulman, 2007).

Since 1992, the *Prescription Drug User Fee Act* has charged user fees to pharmaceutical companies to defray the costs of FDA review. These user fees accounted for over 40% of the budget of the FDA division that reviewed new drug applications; some have argued that this has led to a perception in the agency that they are accountable to the industry rather than to patients or payers (Avorn, 2007). However, the FDA has also taken the lead in mandating public disclosure of data from clinical trials, which in some cases (e.g., Vioxx) has led to reanalysis of the safety of those drugs and potentially their removal from the market.

## Australia

In Australia, the national government has responsibility for regulating medicines, as well as other "therapeutic goods" such as medical devices, blood, and blood products. This is handled by the Therapeutic Goods Administration (TGA), a division of the Australian Government Department of Health and Aging. The Advisory Committee on Prescription Medicines (ACPM) advises and makes recommendations to the TGA on prescription medicines; this committee replaced the Australian Drug Evaluation Committee (ADEC) in January 2010.

The Pharmaceutical Benefits Scheme (PBS) is a program under the Australian government that makes a range of necessary prescription medicines available at affordable prices to all Australian residents. At the time of writing, Avastin has been approved for initial PBS-subsidized treatment, in combination with first-line chemotherapy, for patients with previously untreated metastatic CRC who are functioning well. The criterion they use is the ECOG Performance Status, which is also used by the World Health Organization. This widely used scale has the following values. Grade 0 is "fully active, able to carry on all pre-disease performance without restriction." Grade 1 is "restricted in physically strenuous activity but ambulatory and able to carry out work of a light or sedentary nature, *e.g.*, light housework, office work." Grade 2 is defined as "ambulatory and capable of all selfcare but unable to carry out any work activities. Up and about more than 50% of waking hours." Grade 3 is "capable of only limited selfcare, confined to bed or chair more than 50% of waking hours." Grade 4 is "completely disabled. Cannot carry on any selfcare. Totally confined to bed or chair" and grade 5 is "dead" (Oken et al., 1982). Australia approved Avastin only for those patients classified as grades 0 or 1. Continuing PBS-subsidized treatment of Avastin, in combination with first-line chemotherapy, was permitted if the patient with metastatic CRC had previously been allowed a prescription for it, did not have progression of disease, and remained on first-line chemotherapy. The cost to the consumer (co-payment) in Australian dollars was $33.30 per cycle.

**European Community**

In those countries belonging to the European Union, there is a centralized process for approval through the European Agency for the Evaluation of Medicinal Products. Again, these decisions are based only on safety and effectiveness. Each member country makes its own decisions as to what it will pay for, and the price it will pay. In most of these countries, most people have first-dollar coverage through third-party payers. There is variation in the extent to which cost-effectiveness data is used. Another cost control mechanism being used by many jurisdictions is "reference-based pricing"; this approach defines a family of drugs deemed to be interchangeable, and then sets a baseline (reference) price for what will be paid for publicly, with costs above that level to be absorbed by the patient. As one study of access to cancer drugs across 19 countries has confirmed, considerable price variation exists (Drummond & Mason, 2007).

APPENDIX C: STAKEHOLDER VIEWS

Different stakeholders have taken different views about whether Avastin should be used at all, and who should pay for it if it is prescribed. Developing new drugs is expensive. An ongoing debate, in many countries, is how best to cover these costs.

*Technology assessment bodies* tend to examine cost-effectiveness (see Appendix D). One common measure of cost-effectiveness is the quality-adjusted life year (QALY). In the United States, many argue that treatments with incremental QALYs above $50,000 are not considered good value for the money, although different groups may use different cut-off points. It is also noteworthy that many criticize this approach; indeed, the current US government program to analyze clinical effectiveness has been explicitly prohibited from incorporating cost-effectiveness into its analysis.

The *pharmaceutical industry* points to costs of development and production, weighed against potential market size. The perspective of pharmaceutical companies is tied to financial incentives, defined by the inelasticity of demand for health care and drugs (see Chapter 1, section 5.9, Insurance, Elasticity, and Moral Hazard). Usually, the elasticity of demand for a good or service restrains firms from charging too much of a premium over their production costs. However, the inelasticity of demand for cancer care and monopolies for cancer drugs allow drug makers to set the price for new cancer drugs well above their costs of producing those drugs. In an inelastic demand situation, modest increases in production costs have a magnifying impact on the price companies can charge. This has led to very high drug costs and the ethical dilemma of how to measure what the resulting benefits are worth. The pharmaceutical industry has another advantage; without several competing, clinically identical products, it is difficult for payers to refuse to purchase a particular drug. Such a drug does not face competition, and therefore the pharmaceutical industry can exert monopoly power in setting prices. Roche, the pharmaceutical company which produces Avastin, does offer a patient assistance program that patients can access for drug funding. The nature of this assistance varies. For qualifying patients with private insurance coverage, Roche will pay the balance not covered by the insurer. Patients who do not have insurance may sometimes still be eligible for coverage, but Roche will determine the amount of financial assistance, based on the patient's ability to pay.

*Oncologists* have mixed views. On the one hand, they wish to provide the best care they can to their patients. On the other, they are conscious of the importance of receiving value for money. A 2006 poll of Boston oncologists found that, while 78% felt that patients should receive effective therapy, regardless of cost, a majority did not feel that these drugs necessarily offered good value (Nadler et al., 2006). In contrast, as noted in the case, Cancer Care Ontario, the body with responsibility for Ontario's cancer care system, has recommended use of Avastin.

In many jurisdictions, particularly but not exclusively in the United States, the increasing cost of cancer therapy has been placing a serious financial burden on patients and their families. The American Society of Clinical Oncology has set up the Cost of Care Task Force; in 2009, it released its first Guidance Statement on the Cost of Cancer Care (Meropol et al., 2009). The statement stressed the need to advise providers about how best to communicate with their patients regarding costs, but also determine how best to define the value of new innovations, and incorporate these into treatment recommendations. The statement suggested that it is important to "help physicians balance their desire to deliver optimal health care to each individual with their commitment to use societal resources wisely" (p. 3873). One particular concern was the "impact of cost on disparities in access to cancer care" (p. 3873).

Cancer *patients* may weigh risks and benefits of treatment differently than do the healthy policymakers, physicians, and guideline panelists who define acceptable standards of care and treatment paradigms. Faced with a high probability of death, people may be willing to try any treatment that offers hope. Much of the push towards approving these expensive drugs has come from patients facing extremely high costs to purchase these products. In general, the media have been highly sympathetic.

Patient groups have also been very active, including general cancer groups and more disease-specific ones (e.g., Colorectal Cancer Association of Canada). It is extremely difficult to convince patients and physicians to forgo drug therapy they believe would be beneficial just to save money. Increasingly, patient groups are receiving funds from pharmaceutical companies; some are referred to as "*astroturf groups*," which purport to be grassroots organizations representing the general public, but which are often funded by corporations seeking to influence government policy (Lyon & Maxwell, 2004). These groups, often backed by the media, make emotional pleas to pay whatever price pharmaceutical companies demand for the newest drug, placing significant pressure on governments.

*Insurers* have a desire to minimize their costs while providing good service to those clients they wish to retain. Understandably, private insurers have been reluctant to pay high drug costs. In some jurisdictions, they may be able to impose deductibles and cap the amount they will pay.

There has also been an ongoing dispute as to the role of the various levels of *government*. They may be involved in approving drugs, setting prices, reviewing technology assessments, and/or paying for pharmaceuticals. A number of reports have suggested that the federal government should become more involved, with suggestions including a national pharmacare plan to provide more universal coverage and/or a national role in purchasing drugs to ensure lower prices. To date, the federal government has resisted this push, on the grounds that health care is a provincial responsibility. Provincial governments also have a role as payer (for pharmaceuticals delivered within hospitals, as well as for those covered by provincial drug plans).

Note that various *political parties* have also become involved in these issues, particularly at the provincial level. For example, provincial health critics have criticized government decisions not to fund particular drugs for particular patients.

APPENDIX D: COST-EFFECTIVENESS ANALYSIS

As noted in Chapter 1, section 8.1, economic analysis basically compares the net costs and the net consequences of two or more possible courses of action. Further information on these issues can be found in these key readings (Drummond et al., 2005; Gold et al., 1996; Kattan, 2009). To perform such analyses, the analyst must identify the flows of costs and consequences over time of these possible courses of action.

One way (not the only way) to approach this comparison is to perform what is commonly called a decision analysis. The simplest illustrations use a decision tree; more complex examples often use Markov models or other approaches, which allow consideration of changes over time. A decision tree involves the following steps:

**Step 1**: Structure the problem. This involves several elements:

    a. Decide what possible actions might be taken, in what sequence. (If decision trees are being used, these are often referred to as *choice nodes*, or *decision nodes*.) They represent the choices that a decision maker can make among potential actions. In decision trees, they are often represented by squares. Note that the possibilities selected can be visualized as moving along one branch of the decision tree.

  b. Determine the possible outcomes as a result of each pos-
     sible action. For example, if one has surgery, one may die
     as a result of the operation, or live. (On decision trees, these
     are often referred to as *chance nodes*, and are represented by
     circles.) These chance nodes represent fate – the individual
     cannot choose which of these possible outcomes will hap-
     pen. At each chance node, the possible outcomes must be
     both mutually exclusive and exhaustive. Depending on
     how complex the tree is, there may be additional chance
     nodes (e.g., if one survives the surgery, one may be cured,
     or the disease may recur). Each branch of the decision tree
     will eventually lead to final outcomes, often called *terminal
     nodes*, usually represented by rectangles.

Step 2: For each chance node, determine how likely each event is.
        Mathematically, this requires that you assign probabilities to
        each branch at each chance node. Note that the probabilities at
        each chance node must sum to 1.0 (since the possibilities were
        defined as being mutually exclusive and exhaustive). These
        probabilities can be based on data about previous experience
        and/or on expert judgments.

Step 3: Value the costs and the consequences of each outcome. One
        common method to measure consequences is to assign utility
        scores to each terminal node. As noted in Chapter 1, section 8.1
        (Economic Analysis: Cost-effectiveness), there are a number of
        approaches that can be used to determine these values.

Step 4: Using this data, compute an expected value of the costs
        and the consequences for each choice node. This is done by
        multiplying the probability of each terminal node (step 2)
        by the costs and by the consequences (step 3) and summing
        them. This process is often referred to as *folding back* the
        decision tree.

Step 5: Choose the best action. This may involve selecting the branch
        with the best value for money, but other decision rules can
        also be employed (see below).

Step 6: Perform a sensitivity analysis. This means systematically
        varying the values assigned to key variables (probabilities,
        costs, consequences) to see how changes in those values
        would change the decision.

Approaches to how best to perform such analysis can vary considerably. For example, some simple models look at outcomes at one point in time; others use methods (e.g., Markov models) to include the natural history of disease. In effect, Markov models involve repeating the chance nodes, simulating the probability of moving from one state to another at each point in time. Another issue is how to handle situations where the estimated values attached to probabilities and utilities are uncertain; one valuable approach is to use probabilistic *sensitivity analysis* and systematically vary the estimates being used. Another issue is how much to *discount* future costs and consequences.

Note that utility measurement is also controversial among ethicists. Some argue that it is inappropriate to value certain health states as less than ideal; others note that if one does not, no value is affixed to interventions which might improve quality of life as opposed to affecting only life expectancy (Deber & Goel, 1990).

Regardless of how costs and consequences are computed, it is important to recognize that this method speaks only of relative cost-effectiveness; therapies are, by definition, compared against something. Analysts thus may speak of cost-effectiveness / cost utility, or incremental cost-effectiveness ratios (ICER). ICERs use a common denominator (e.g., years of life gained, QALYs gained). In turn, this allows comparison across conditions. These are sometimes referred to as *league tables*, akin to the rankings given to athletic teams. Technology assessment bodies may use formal or informal thresholds, arguing that therapies with costs per QALY above that threshold should not be funded. The literature varies in what this threshold is, but values of $50,000 to $100,000 per QALY are common in the United States (Yabroff & Schrag, 2009). In the United Kingdom, the National Institute for Clinical Excellence (NICE) has tended to use thresholds of £20,000 to £30,000 per QALY (US$33,000–$49,000 per QALY). In Ontario, the CED considers a range of $40,000–$60,000 QALY acceptable.

Note that use of ICERs is also controversial. A number of issues can arise, including the total cost (higher costs per QALY might be easier to justify for small numbers of potential recipients, since the total budgetary impact would be smaller); the magnitude of the potential benefit; and the equity implications of allowing some people to purchase potentially lifesaving therapy while withholding it from those who cannot afford the cost. There are strong advocates for the argument that people should have access to effective treatment, regardless of the cost.

Table 12.1. Adoption Zones

| | | | Cost of A compared to B | | |
|---|---|---|---|---|---|
| | | | More | Same | Less |
| Benefit of A compared to B | | More | Tough choice | Adopt | Adopt |
| | | Same | Don't adopt | Toss up | Adopt |
| | | Less | Don't adopt | Don't adopt | Tough choice |

Source: Deber (1992).

Others suggest that resources are not infinite, and that choices will have to be made. Whichever viewpoint is taken, economic analysis can at least clarify what the costs and consequences are likely to be.

One approach we have suggested is the concept of adoption zones (Deber, 1992). As shown in Table 12.1, it compares two alternatives (A and B) by analysing their relative costs and consequences and classifying them as More, Same, and Less. There are three clear "zones" where A should be adopted: (1) when the benefit is more and the cost is less than current treatment; (2) when the benefit is the same but the cost is less than current treatment; and (3) when the benefit is more but the cost is the same. Conversely, there are three scenarios in which adoption should clearly not occur: (1) when the benefit is the same but the cost is more; (2) when the benefit is less but the cost is more; and (3) when the benefit is less but the cost is the same. The challenge for decision makers arises in the corners of the schematic, where they must decide how much more should be paid for how much increased benefit, or, conversely, how much benefit should be sacrificed for how great a cost saving. The concept of adoption zones does not answer this question, but it does allow the decision makers to clarify where the policy choice lies, and hence whether it is necessary to confront these difficult decisions and calculations, or whether the choice lies in one of the zones where the choice is more obvious.

APPENDIX E: MODELLING THE COST-EFFECTIVENESS
OF AVASTIN

Avastin is used in combination with existing chemotherapy treatments as a means to reduce the progression of metastatic CRC and extend life. Analysing its cost-effectiveness thus requires looking at both the incremental cost and the incremental consequences. Several published decision analyses involve relatively complex sequences of possibilities, which we have simplified for the purposes of learning how to do a cost-effectiveness analysis. We will be employing a somewhat simplified version of the decision trees used by NICE for its assessment. Model 1 compares IFL alone to IFL plus Avastin; model 2 compares 5-FU/FA alone to 5-FU/FA plus Avastin. It is important to recognize that published work has used a variety of treatment alternatives, on a variety of patient populations, and that results may change as new trial results become available.

The simplest approach is to compute costs and consequences for each option. Let us assume, for example, that the following estimates are correct for model 1:

Mean cost of IFL chemotherapy treatment: $65,225 per patient
Mean cost of Avastin + IFL chemotherapy treatment: $104,000 per patient
Mean outcome of IFL chemotherapy treatment: 15.6 months of overall survival
Mean outcome of Avastin + IFL chemotherapy treatment: 20.3 months of overall survival

We can then compute an incremental cost-effectiveness ratio (ICER) for adding Avastin to IFL as follows:

The numerator is the incremental cost of using Avastin: ($104,000 − $65,225) = $38,775;
The denominator is the incremental benefit of using Avastin: (20.3 − 15.6) = 4.7 months;
Performing the math yields ($38,775 /4.7 months) × 12 months = $99,000 per life year gained.

A more complex analysis would build in more potential consequences (e.g., the probability that the therapy will be effective, the chances of adverse events, etc.). It might also build in a time element (e.g., the probability that someone would still be responding to the drug in the next time period); a common way of doing this is to use Markov models. A cost utility analysis will also incorporate the utility of each health state, on a scale of 0 to 1; for example, it might place a higher utility on months lived when the disease is not progressing and the person can conduct normal activities than months when the person is very ill.

The analysis conducted for NICE estimated that Avastin was effective in 40%–50% of patients. Adverse events were reported in 8%–21% of patients; these included GI perforation, hemorrhage, blood clots, and hypertensive crisis. The clinical benefit was an increase in progression-free survival of 1.2 to 4.4 months compared to standard chemotherapy regimens, and an increase in overall survival of 2.3 to 4.7 months. They placed a higher value on quality of life during the progression-free survival period. They computed that cost depends on patient weight (but is usually between $1,500 and $2,000 per treatment) and on the number of treatments. Various models, with different comparisons, have accordingly computed the benefits as between $93,000/QALY and $168,000/ QALY, and between $99,000 and $145,000 per life year gained.

A sensitivity analysis could then be conducted. For example, one might see what the impact would be of changing such variables as the cost of the drug, the survival time, or the quality of life resulting from treatment, on cost-effectiveness. In one such study, the authors concluded that to be cost-effective (where they set the threshold at the relatively high level of $117,000 per QALY), the drug should cost no more than $830 per dose. If survival were longer, or quality of life higher, the cost of the drug might increase somewhat to a maximum of $2,180. Both were considerably less than was being charged for the drug.

The NICE technology appraisal noted that the manufacturer submitted two simple-stage transition models, each with three states: *pre-progression* (alive without disease progression), *post-progression* (alive following disease progression), and *dead* (Tappenden et al., 2007b). Because patients are rarely cured entirely by this intervention, performing a cost-effectiveness evaluation of Avastin is challenging. If patients were cured entirely, the clinical outcome is binary: life or death. The measure of effectiveness is then the cost per life year gained. However, patients often live for long periods with the disease and have varying qualities of life during this period. The data is also somewhat controversial, in that some of the studies being used were done with a younger population, and showed slightly longer survival than might be expected for other populations. It must also be recognized that these numbers are averages. Many tumours do not respond to treatment; one estimate was a 34.8% response rate with IFL, compared to 44.8% for IFL plus Avastin.

Table 12.2. Cost-effectiveness Models for Avastin

| | Model 1: IFL with or without Avastin | | |
|---|---|---|---|
| | IFL only | IFL + Avastin | Difference |
| Outcomes: time (in years) with: | | | |
| Stable disease | 0.97 | 1.27 | 0.30 |
| Progressive disease | 0.59 | 0.7 | 0.11 |
| Total life years gained | 1.57 | 1.98 | 0.41 |
| QALYs stable disease (0.8) | 0.776 | 1.016 | 0.24 |
| QALYs progressive disease (0.6) | 0.354 | 0.42 | 0.066 |
| Total QALYs gained | 1.13 | 1.436 | 0.306 |
| Cost (£) | 23,645.84 | 43,006.57 | 19,360.73 |
| Cost (£) per life year | 15,061 | 21,720 | 47,222 |
| Cost (£) per QALY | 20,926 | 29,949 | 63,270 |

| | Model 2: 5-FU/FA with or without Avastin | | |
|---|---|---|---|
| | 5-FU/FA only | 5-FU/FA + Avastin | Difference |
| Outcomes: time (in years) with: | | | |
| Stable disease | 0.83 | 1.16 | 0.33 |
| Progressive disease | 0.57 | 0.43 | −0.14 |
| Total life years gained | 1.41 | 1.59 | 0.18 |
| QALYs stable disease (0.8) | 0.664 | 0.928 | 0.264 |
| QALYs progressive disease (0.6) | 0.342 | 0.258 | −0.084 |
| Total QALYs gained | 1.006 | 1.186 | 0.18 |
| Cost (£) | 21,459.35 | 37,113.45 | 15,654.1 |
| Cost (£) per life year | 15,219 | 23,342 | 86,967 |
| Cost (£) per QALY | 21,331 | 31,293 | 86,967 |

Using the data provided by the NICE assessment, one can perform a somewhat more complex (albeit still slightly oversimplified) analysis. Note that the NICE analysis included both a cost-effectiveness (cost per life year gained) and a cost utility (cost per QALY gained) component. Their models assigned the following utility scores to each state, on a scale of 0 to 1: Pre-progression = 0.8; Post-progression = 0.5 in one study and 0.6 in another; and Death = 0. Note that this model deliberately favours treatment, in that it does not reduce utility even if adverse events occur during treatment (Tappenden et al., 2007a). In Table 12.2, Model 1 compares IFL alone to IFL plus Avastin. Model 2 compares 5-FU/FA alone to 5-FU/FA plus Avastin. Note that the total life years gained has mild rounding error, and hence is not precisely equal to the sum of the first two rows. Costs are given in pounds rather than dollars. Also, the reported cost-effectiveness ratios in the published work differ very slightly from those that are derived using this spreadsheet.

Table 12.2 shows that, for Model 1, IFL alone would be expected to yield 1.57 life years (of which 0.59 would be spent with progressive disease). Adding Avastin would increase this by 0.41 life years, to 1.98 life years. (Other studies have estimated about 4.7 additional months.) Avastin would also increase the cost of treatment by about £19,361. Dividing the cost of IFL (£23,646) by the gains, one can compute the cost per life year gained, and per QALY. Similar computations can be performed for the cost per life year and per QALY of using IFL + Avastin. Note, however, that economic analysis requires us to compare alternatives. One would thus divide the increase in life years gained (0.41) by the increased cost, to determine that adding Avastin to IFL would cost over £47,000 per life year gained. Adjusting this figure for quality of life would reduce the gain to 0.31 QALYS, and hence increase the cost to over £63,000 per QALY gained. Because the gains in the 5-FU/FA comparisons are even smaller (0.18 life years, and also 0.18 QALYs), the cost-effectiveness is even weaker. Note that these estimates are quite sensitive to the assumptions made. However, all of these estimates are well above the rule of thumb NICE has traditionally employed, which says that treatments costing more than £30,000 per QALY are not cost-effective. For that reason, NICE has been reluctant to approve Avastin for CRC.

## APPENDIX F: REFERENCES CITED AND FURTHER READING

Abelson, J., Giacomini, M., Lehoux, P., & Gauvin, F.-P. (2007). Bringing "the public" into health technology assessment and coverage policy decisions: From principles to practice. *Health Policy (Amsterdam)*, *82*(1), 37–50. http://dx.doi.org/10.1016/j.healthpol.2006.07.009

Avorn, J. (2007). Paying for drug approvals: Who's using whom? *New England Journal of Medicine*, *356*(17), 1697–700. http://dx.doi.org/10.1056/NEJMp 078041

Brock, D. (2006). How much is more life worth? *Hastings Center Report*, *36*(3), 17–19. http://dx.doi.org/10.1353/hcr.2006.0036

Canadian Cancer Society & Turner and Associates. (2009, September). *Cancer drug access for Canadians.* http://www.colorectal-cancer.ca/IMG/pdf/cancer_drug_access_report_en.pdf.

Chafe, R., Dhalla, I.A., Dobrow, M., & Sullivan, T. (2009). Accessing unfunded cancer drugs in publicly funded hospitals. *Lancet, 10*(4), 306–7. http://dx.doi .org/10.1016/S1470-2045(09)70039-7

Canadian Cancer Society's Steering Committee on Cancer Statistics. (2011). *Canadian cancer statistics 2011, featuring colorectal cancer.* Canadian Cancer Society, Public Health Agency of Canada and Statistics Canada. http://pub lications.gc.ca/collections/collection_2011/statcan/CS2-37-2011-eng.pdf

Cookson, R., McCabe, C., & Tsuchiya, A. (2008). Public healthcare resource allocation and the rule of rescue. *Journal of Medical Ethics, 34*(7), 540–4. http://dx.doi.org/10.1136/jme.2007.021790

Deber, R. (1992). Translating technology assessment into policy: Conceptual issues and tough choices. *International Journal of Technology Assessment in Health Care, 8*(1), 131–7. http://dx.doi.org/10.1017/S0266462300007996

Deber, R., & Goel, V. (1990). Using explicit decision rules to manage issues of justice, risk, and ethics in decision analysis: When is it not rational to maximize expected utility? *Medical Decision Making, 10*(3), 181–94. http://dx.doi .org/10.1177/0272989X9001000305

Drummond, M.F., & Mason, A.R. (2007). European perspective on the costs and cost-effectiveness of cancer therapies. *Journal of Clinical Oncology, 25*(2), 191–5. http://dx.doi.org/10.1200/JCO.2006.07.8956

Drummond, M.F., Sculpher, M.J., Torrance, G.W., O'Brien, B.J., & Stoddart, G.L. (2005). *Methods for the economic evaluation of health care programmes* (3rd ed.). Toronto: Oxford University Press.

Gold, M.R., Siegel, J.E., Russell, L.B., & Weinstein, M.C. (1996). *Cost-effectiveness in health and medicine.* New York: Oxford University Press.

Hurwitz, H., Fehrenbacher, L., Novotny, W., Cartwright, T., Hainsworth, J., Heim, W., et al. (2004). Bevacizumab plus irinotecan, fluorouracil, and leucovorin for metastatic colorectal cancer. *New England Journal of Medicine, 350*(23), 2335–42. http://dx.doi.org/10.1056/NEJMoa032691

Kattan, M.W. (2009). *Encyclopedia of medical decision making* (Vols. 1–2). London: SAGE.

Lyon, T.P., & Maxwell, J.W. (2004). Astroturf: Interest group lobbying and corporate strategy. *Journal of Economics & Management Strategy, 13*(4), 561–97. http://dx.doi.org/10.1111/j.1430-9134.2004.00023.x

Marin, A. (2009). *A vast injustice: Investigation into the Ministry of Health and Long-Term Care's decision-making concerning the funding of Avastin for colorectal cancer patients.* Obudsman Ontario. http://www.ombudsman.on.ca/ Resources/Reports/A-Vast-Injustice.aspx

Mayer, R.J. (2004). Two steps forward in the treatment of colorectal cancer. *New England Journal of Medicine, 350*(23), 2406–8. http://dx.doi.org/10.1056/NEJMe 048098

Meropol, N.J., Schrag, D., Smith, T.J., Mulvey, T.M., Langdon, R.M., Jr., Blum, D., et al. (2009). American Society of Clinical Oncology guidance statement: The cost of cancer care. *Journal of Clinical Oncology, 27*(23), 3868–74. http://dx.doi.org/10.1200/JCO.2009.23.1183

Meropol, N.J., & Schulman, K.A. (2007). Cost of cancer care: Issues and implications. *Journal of Clinical Oncology, 25*(2), 180–6. http://dx.doi.org/10.1200/JCO.2006.09.6081

Nadler, E., Eckert, B., & Neumann, P.J. (2006). Do oncologists believe new cancer drugs offer good value? *Oncologist, 11*(2), 90–5. http://dx.doi.org/10.1634/theoncologist.11-2-90

Oken, M.M., Creech, R.H., Tormey, D.C., Horton, J., Davis, T.E., McFadden, E.T., et al. (1982). Toxicity and response criteria of the Eastern Cooperative Oncology Group. *American Journal of Clinical Oncology, 5*(6), 649–55. http://dx.doi.org/10.1097/00000421-198212000-00014

Steinbrook, R. (2008). Saying no isn't NICE – The travails of Britain's National Institute for Health and Clinical Excellence. *New England Journal of Medicine, 359*(19), 1977–81. http://dx.doi.org/10.1056/NEJMp0806862

Tappenden, P., Jones, R., Paisley, S., & Carroll, C. (2007a). The cost-effectiveness of bevacizumab in the first-line treatment of metastatic colorectal cancer in England and Wales. *European Journal of Cancer, 43*(17), 2487–94. http://dx.doi.org/10.1016/j.ejca.2007.08.017

Tappenden, P., Jones, R., Paisley, S., & Carroll, C. (2007b). Systematic review and economic evaluation of bevacizumab and cetuximab for the treatment of metastatic colorectal cancer. *Health Technology Assessment, 11*(12). http://www.hta.ac.uk/fullmono/mon1112.pdf

Tierney, M., Manns, B., & Members of the Canadian Drug Expert Committee. (2008). Optimizing the use of prescription drugs in Canada through the Common Drug Review. *Canadian Medical Association Journal, 178*(4), 432–5. http://dx.doi.org/10.1503/cmaj.070713

Van Cutsem, E., Lambrechts, D., Prenen, H., Jain, R.K., & Carmeliet, P. (2011). Lessons from the adjuvant Bevacizumab trial on colon cancer: What next? *Journal of Clinical Oncology, 29*(1), 1–4. http://dx.doi.org/10.1200/JCO.2010.32.2701

Wiktorowicz, M.E. (2003). Emergent patterns in the regulation of pharmaceuticals: Institutions and interests in the United States, Canada, Britain and France. *Journal of Health Politics, Policy and Law, 28*(4), 615–58. http://dx.doi.org/10.1215/03616878-28-4-615

Wright, C.J. (2009). *Too much health care: We can't afford life's creeping medicalization.* Literary Review of Canada. http://reviewcanada.ca/magazine/2009/11/too-much-health-care/

Yabroff, K.R., & Schrag, D. (2009). Challenges and opportunities for use of cost-effectiveness analysis. *Journal of the National Cancer Institute, 101*(17), 1161–3. http://dx.doi.org/10.1093/jnci/djp258

The following websites may also be helpful:

Canadian Cancer Society, http://www.cancer.ca/
International Society for Pharmacoeconomics and Outcomes Research, Canada Pharmaceuticals, http://www.ispor.org/HTARoadMaps/CanadaPharm.asp#4
pan-Canadian Oncology Drug Review (pCODR), http://www.pcodr.ca/wcpc/portal/Home?_afrLoop=273089772505000&_afrWindowMode=0&_adf.ctrl-state=gs8g5689w_91
Patented Medicine Prices Review Board, http://www.pmprb-cepmb.gc.ca/english/home.asp?x=1
US FDA, http://www.cancer.gov/cancertopics/druginfo/fda-bevacizumab

# 13 What to Do with the Queue?

## Reducing Wait Times for Cancer Care

*JOHN BLAKE, DANIEL BOLLAND, IAN DAWE, BRENDA GAMBLE,*
*GUNITA MITERA, NATALIE (WAJS) RASHKOVAN, SOMAYEH SADAT,*
*KENNETH VAN WYK, AND RAISA B. DEBER*

People with cancer may be treated with various combinations of surgery, radiation therapy, and chemotherapy. Radiotherapy cannot be administered in every hospital; it requires equipment and skilled technical staff. One such specialized hospital, the Princess Margaret Hospital (PMH) in Toronto, found itself faced with a growing wait list problem in its radiotherapy department. What should it do?

This case addresses several policy issues, including: queuing theory, wait lists and how to manage them, human resources planning, payment mechanisms and incentives, and the ethics of rationing.

**Appendices**

Appendix A: Treating Cancer: Radiotherapy
Appendix B: RT Training and Retention in Ontario
Appendix C: Characteristics of the Ontario Cancer System
Appendix D: Wait Lists
Appendix E: Queuing Theory
Appendix F: References Cited and Further Reading

**The Case**

Since cancer is in part a disease of aging, its incidence is rising in most industrialized countries. The province of Ontario, Canada, is no exception. Coupled with changes in treatment protocols, including greater use of radiotherapy, and increased survival time (which may often mean more treatments per patient), the demand for cancer treatment services had grown rapidly.

Since its founding in 1958, Toronto's Princess Margaret Hospital (PMH) had established a reputation as one of the premier teaching and cancer research facilities in Canada. In 1988, PMH saw 6,649 new cases and performed 78,399 radiotherapy treatments, which accounted for 27% of the cancer services delivered through the province's formal cancer care structure. However, the number of new cases continued to grow, increasing by over 46% between 1980 and 1990. Projections were that this growth would continue. By the spring of 1989, PMH began to develop a queue for radiotherapy.

**Cancer Care in Ontario**

Cancer can be treated in a number of ways, including various combinations of surgery, radiotherapy, and chemotherapy, alone or in combination. (See Appendix A for a brief description of radiotherapy.) Cancer care accordingly requires specialized expertise. Among the skilled personnel required are physicians (radiation oncologists), nurses (radiation oncology nurses), social workers, dieticians, medical radiation physicists, and radiation therapists (RTs), who administer the radiation treatment. RTs are a regulated health profession in Ontario. (See Appendix B for more information on RT training.)

At the time of the case, cancer services in the province of Ontario were delivered through both specialized cancer treatment facilities (including PMH) and/or through an informal network of internists, surgeons, and haematologists working in other hospitals and clinics. About half of cancer patients in Ontario were treated in formally structured cancer programs within regional cancer centres (RCCs); these tended to be located in teaching hospitals (usually affiliated with one of Ontario's medical schools), and to be under the auspices of the Ontario Cancer Treatment & Research Foundation (OCTRF). However, because of high capital and operating costs, all radiotherapy services in the province were concentrated in eight of the regional cancer centres. (See Appendix C for a brief summary of the organization of cancer treatment in Ontario.)

Reimbursement mechanisms also varied. At the time of the case, Ontario hospitals were largely funded on the basis of global budgets, while most physicians were paid on the basis of fee-for-service (FFS). Hospital staff other than physicians tended to be salaried. However, many of the specialist physicians in the RCCs were also salaried, and worked within group practices. (See Chapter 1, section 6.2, Payment Mechanisms and Incentives, for the incentive structures inherent in different ways of paying for care.)

In 1983, a cancer treatment role study commissioned by the cancer programs had documented reductions in staffing levels and noted the relationship between low staff levels and compromises in standards of practice. To alleviate quality of care issues, the study had recommended that provincial cancer treatment centres be refurbished, facilities at PMH be expanded, and that all the cancer centres be organized and managed by a single agency (at that time, the Ontario Cancer Agency). Plans were also made to move PMH from its existing site to a new building that would be closer to the University of Toronto's Faculty of Medicine and some of its other teaching hospitals (including the Toronto General Hospital and Mount Sinai Hospital).

**The "Mini-Crisis"**

Two of the 1983 cancer treatment role study's recommendations were acted upon immediately by the province; the Ministry of Health decided that PMH should be rebuilt and the RCCs should be updated over the next decade. In the meantime, the Ministry approved a program to update and/or replace PMH's existing equipment, and further supplemented capacity by providing four new radiation machines at Mount Sinai Hospital, which was located near the future site of PMH. (The study's recommendation for a provincial cancer agency was not implemented until 1997, with the creation of Cancer Care Ontario.)

Because it takes an average of one year to replace a radiotherapy machine, PMH's refurbishing program created a waiting list "mini-crisis" (backlog of patients) in 1987. PMH responded to this waiting list by decreasing the number of the resource-intense therapeutic care patients it treated. Reductions were achieved by moving some patients to another Toronto area RCC (the Bayview Regional Centre, which has subsequently been renamed the Sunnybrook Odette Cancer Centre) for treatment and by placing temporary caps on the number of new patients each radiation oncologist could accept. These measures were largely successful in allowing the hospital to maintain its waiting lists at an acceptable level during the machine retrofit. (See Appendix D for more information on wait lists.)

## The "Crisis"

Following the resolution of the 1987 "mini-crisis," a number of changes affected the ability to retain RTs at PMH. An economic boom had resulted in rapid growth in the Metropolitan Toronto area, which meant more potential patients. However, the boom also drove up the cost of living; this had a particular impact on RTs, whose wages had remained constant. Many PMH therapists opted to move from Toronto to RCCs located in less expensive communities, particularly since there was an unusual number of open positions at other facilities and a shortage of qualified personnel. Annual attrition at the hospital had been 8%–10%, but in the spring of 1989, with staffing already tight, PMH had lost 20% (approximately 12) of its RTs within a 3–4 month period. One consequence was that the director never had enough staff to comfortably schedule vacations or sick time. Staff, already feeling overworked, were frustrated.

Staff shortages created several repercussions. Beginning in February 1989, the hospital increased the RT workday from 8 to 10 hours. Staff morale declined as working overtime became routine. In addition, absenteeism increased and documented treatment deviations (errors in treatment not due to neglect) doubled. In April 1989, therapists collectively decided to limit overtime, to work 8-hour rather than 10-hour days, and not to staff 2 of the hospital's 10 radiotherapy machines. This action, which was presented as a quality of care issue, was supported by the hospital's medical staff. However, as a result of the therapists' decision, the hospital's treatment capacity was severely restricted; a full-fledged radiotherapy crisis ensued.

At full capacity, PMH's radiotherapy department was capable of providing about 400 treatment fractions per day. The therapists' action reduced the hospital's capacity to about 256 fractions per day. On an average day PMH received 28 new patient referrals, of whom 45% were prescribed radiation therapy. In total there was a daily demand for 302 radiotherapy fractions. With the decreased capacity brought about by the therapists' action, PMH now faced a daily deficit of 46 fractions. Every two days the number of patients waiting to receive radiotherapy increased by five.

PMH took immediate action to respond to the problem. In an effort to halt the exodus of RTs, the hospital's board approved an immediate 10% increase in RT salaries on April 1, 1989. The board also authorized a program to aggressively recruit RTs from overseas, primarily from the United Kingdom and Hong Kong (see Chapter 1, section 8.4,

Health Human Resources). These actions, while halting RT attrition, did little to augment the number of treatments that could be delivered, and the backlog continued to increase. In the period between April 1 and July 15, 1989, the number of patients waiting for radiotherapy grew from 140 to 300, while the number of backlogged machine hours (hours of treatment) increased from 1,130 to 2,400; patient waits for therapy rose from two to seven weeks. By the middle of July, it was obvious to all involved that the situation was no longer simply an administrative inconvenience; a serious problem existed. Drawing on its previous experience, the hospital, in conjunction with its staff oncologists, summarily reduced the number of new patients it would accept by 50%.

The hospital's cap on new patient referrals was only a partial success. The waiting list stopped growing, but the anticipated decrease in wait time did not materialize. Throughout August, the number of patients waiting to receive treatment remained constant; new patients entering the system continued to face a six- to seven-week wait for treatment.

The backlog of radiotherapy patients severely taxed PMH's ability to provide service. To compensate for changes in patient condition occurring between diagnosis and initiation of treatment, therapists were forced to revise the treatment protocols they had completed weeks earlier, further reducing the number of patients that they could treat. The extended waiting list also led to patients requiring specialized care (as inpatients or through home care) while waiting for radiotherapy. Neither PMH nor the local community agencies that provided some palliative care were able to cope with the extra demand. Since patients waiting for therapy must be examined every week, the PMH oncology clinics quickly became overbooked, forcing new patients to wait even longer before being given an appointment for assessment. Long patient wait times also caused the hospital's medical education program to suffer. Because of the six-week lag between the development and implementation of a therapy plan, medical residents were unable to follow patients through an entire treatment regimen. Staff instructors at the University of Toronto's Faculty of Medicine became increasingly frustrated with the quality of the educational experience being provided by PMH. In addition, the extensive waiting list hampered efforts to conduct randomized clinical trials. Oncologists, concerned that the backlog prevented patients from receiving necessary medical treatment within an adequate period of time, began to express the belief that patient safety could not be assured as long as a six-week wait for radiotherapy existed.

In early August, the hospital's president, Dr. Donald Carlow, sent a letter to doctors in eastern Ontario, asking that their cancer patients be referred to centres in Kingston (about 250 km from Toronto) and Ottawa (about 450 km from Toronto) rather than to PMH. These centres were associated with local medical schools, and in some cases might actually be closer than PMH to where the patient lived. On September 7, the hospital's Medical Advisory Committee (MAC) voted to temporarily stop accepting new patient referrals starting September 30 and lasting until such time as the number of patients waiting for radiotherapy reached more manageable levels. The MAC's recommendation was approved by the hospital's Board of Governors on September 12, with the proviso that assurances be obtained that patients who were refused care at PMH could be adequately accommodated elsewhere. All three Toronto daily newspapers attended a press conference called by Dr. Simon Sutcliffe, the vice-president of oncology, to announce the hospital's decision to stop accepting new patient referrals for a six-week period. At the press conference Sutcliffe stated that every effort would be made to ensure that patients affected by the service cuts would receive treatment at other cancer centres in Ontario and Canada. Sutcliffe also announced that a committee including representatives from PMH, the OCTRF, and the Ministry of Health had been set up to coordinate patient placement. Ministry officials promised that patients would not be forced to pay "for transportation, lodging, or medical expenses while being treated at centres outside of Metropolitan Toronto"; instead, extraordinary expenses would be covered by the Ministry of Health and/or by charitable organizations.

Front-page newspaper coverage of the hospital's decision was relatively sensationalistic (including such language as "malaise" and "crisis"), and reaction from patient and physician groups was unenthusiastic. On September 13, 1989 (the day the announcement was made public) an article in Toronto's *Globe and Mail* stated that "patients must wait for radiation treatment in every region of Canada," but also noted that the "length of wait varies substantially from region to region." The *Toronto Star* article quoted a Ministry official who described the situation as positive, arguing that under the proposed plan no patient would wait more than two weeks for therapy. Both newspapers published interviews with prominent ex-patients of PMH (one an ex-MPP serving on the hospital's fundraising committee, the other a senator), who decried the situation and called on the province to increase funding for cancer research and treatment. Both articles described PMH's physical plant as dirty, old, and tired, but praised the quality of care offered by the hospital's staff. The *Globe* article, which was supplemented with pictures of cancer patients receiving care at PMH along with a highly unflattering picture of the current Minister of Health, assigned responsibility for the problem to the provincial government. The Ontario Medical Association (OMA) was also highly critical of the government. Spokespersons for the OMA argued that by approving PMH's decision to limit service, the Minister of Health was institutionalizing substandard care.

In the two weeks between the provisional acceptance of the planned service cut and the Board of Governors' final review of the proposal, a number of events transpired. Six treatment centres in Ontario, as well as six in other provinces, indicated a willingness to take on additional patients (about 80 a week in total). In addition, several American sites were identified as potential providers in the event that all patients could not be accommodated at Canadian facilities. The province, in cooperation with PMH and the OCTRF, agreed to set up a hotline service to direct physician inquiries and coordinate new patient referrals during the crisis. The Canadian Cancer Society accepted responsibility for coordinating travel and accommodation for patients forced to travel to receive treatment. Funding for patient travel was obtained from the province through a special, one-time grant of $567,000, which was given to the OCTRF to administer.

In spite of the detailed planning and remarkable degree of cooperation between the Ministry, the Canadian Cancer Society, and the cancer centres (including OCTRF and PMH), the PMH Board of Governors, under pressure from patient advocate groups, balked at the proposal to stop accepting new patients. At its September 26 meeting, the board, arguing that there were no guarantees all patients could be treated elsewhere or that costs would be reimbursed equally under the proposed plan, overruled the recommendations of the MAC and reversed its decision to stop accepting new patients. The hospital's chairman, Mr. Kenneth Clarke, interpreting this as a vote of non-confidence, tendered his resignation on the spot. The board refused to accept it.

You are surprised to receive a call from an industrial engineer at the local university. She has read the newspaper stories, and suggests that queuing theory might help clarify how best to proceed (see Appendix E).

DECISION POINT

You are the hospital's president. The board's policy reversal places you in an awkward position with respect to the MAC; both cannot apparently be satisfied simultaneously. You have two days to develop an alternative to address the radiotherapy wait list. Your proposed solution, whatever it might be, must also be acceptable to the board, the Ministry of Health, and the hospital's Medical Advisory Committee.

SUGGESTED QUESTIONS FOR DISCUSSION

1. Suggest options for dealing with this issue. What are their advantages and disadvantages?
2. Discuss the potential options in terms of queuing theory. Which variables are they addressing?
3. Discuss the implications of various ways of paying providers, and how they affect the incentives to see/not see patients.
4. Discuss health human resources planning as it affects the ability to meet demands for radiotherapy, with particular emphasis on RTs.
5. Discuss the ethical issues involved in dealing with this issue.

APPENDIX A: TREATING CANCER: RADIOTHERAPY

Radiotherapy (also called radiation therapy), surgery, and chemotherapy are treatment modalities that can be used to treat cancer; they can be administered alone or in combination with one another.

A variety of specialized professionals are required to deliver cancer care. The Human Resources Policy Advisory Committee, a coordinating body set up in 1999 by the Canadian Association of Provincial Cancer Agencies, monitored four categories of providers: medical oncology, radiation oncology, medical physics, and radiation therapy (RT) (Padmos, 2008). Medical oncologists and radiation oncologists are physicians who have completed specialty programs. Medical physicists are scientists with graduate training in physics (MSc or PhD) and membership in the Canadian College of Physicists in Medicine (CCPM). The training programs for Ontario RTs at the time of the case are described in Appendix B.

The objective of radiotherapy is to deliver a measured dose of radiation to a defined tumour volume while minimizing damage to surrounding healthy tissue. Radiation may be delivered internally by implanting a radioactive source in the tumour region for a predetermined period of time, or externally by directing an external beam of ionizing radiation towards the tumour region in a series of treatments. Each treatment (fraction) is usually delivered daily over the predefined period of time, and thus requires a separate visit by the patient to the cancer centre. Each fraction lasts, on average, 15 minutes. Radiotherapy can be subdivided into radical and palliative therapy. *Radical* therapy represents an active attempt to reduce the tumour and possibly cure the patient. It is often combined with one or more other forms of treatment (e.g., surgery, chemotherapy). *Palliative* therapy is intended to aid in pain management, often through reducing pressure on vital organs created by a tumour; it consists of large doses of radiation delivered in a small number of treatments over a brief period of time.

A typical treatment course for someone requiring radiotherapy begins with referral to a treatment centre by a family physician or specialist. Once the diagnostic workup is completed, the next step is an initial evaluation by the radiation oncologist (specialist physician responsible for prescribing, interpreting, and coordinating radiation delivery in the management of cancer); this evaluation includes assessment of the biological and pathological characteristics of the tumour, its location and clinical manifestations, and the general health of the patient. A team, which includes the radiation oncologists, medical physicists, and radiation therapists, plans a course of treatment for the patient (also called the treatment protocol). After reviewing the findings of the initial evaluation, a therapeutic decision is made about the goal of therapy (cure or palliation) and the choice of therapeutic modality.

The radiation therapy treatment course begins with mapping out the area to be treated, calculating the individualized radiation dose to be delivered to the patient, performing quality assurance checks, and then delivering the radiation treatment. For radical therapy, patients will on average receive 25–35 treatments, delivered daily over 5–7 weeks, usually excluding weekends and holidays. Palliative treatment would usually be 1–10 treatments, delivered daily over 1–2 weeks. After the treatment course is complete, radical therapy patients are scheduled for follow-up in one of the regular clinics held by the attending radiation oncologist. The frequency with which patients are required to return to the clinic for monitoring and evaluation is based on their general health, the condition of their tumour, and the attending oncologist's estimate of prognosis.

Treatment planning has a number of steps. Typically, it starts with a computer tomography (CT) simulation; the patient receives a treatment-specific scan to allow the clinicians to map out the anatomic location where the radiation will be targeted while minimizing the dose to the surrounding normal tissues. This is followed by a set of therapeutic calculations called dosimetry, whereby the radiation therapists and physicists calculate the optimal radiation beam arrangement; this is individualized for each patient. The final radiation treatment plan computes the total radiation dose as well as the per treatment radiation dose; this too is optimized for each patient, as prescribed by the radiation oncologist.

During the course of treatment, the tumour response and general condition of the patient are monitored. In addition, the radiation oncologist works with the referring physician to coordinate the overall care of the patient and to integrate radiotherapy with other therapeutic modalities. Follow-up visits are scheduled after therapy to evaluate the general condition of the patient, assess the tumour response and the response of the surrounding tissues, and detect any recurrence.

At the time of the case, the annual new patient volume at PMH was 7,000 patients, of whom approximately 45% would undergo radiotherapy treatment in their first year of treatment. About half would receive radical therapy and would receive an average of 30 fractions per course of treatment; those prescribed palliative therapy would undergo an average of 10 fractions. Approximately 20% of all patients who receive radical therapy suffer a relapse and must be treated again. In total, there would be a demand for about 302 fractions per day. If each radiotherapy treatment, or dose fraction, required 15 minutes of machine time, recognizing the need for some downtime for maintenance, if each machine operated for 10 hours per day, it could deliver 40 fractions per day; if it operated for 8 hours per day it could deliver 32 fractions per day. If the PMH had 10 machines, and all were working for 10 hours per day, the hospital could deliver 400 treatments per day; running them 8 hours per day would deliver 320. At the other extreme, if 2 of the machines were out of service and the PMH was short-staffed, then running 8 machines for 8 hours per day would deliver only 256 treatments.

APPENDIX B: RT TRAINING AND RETENTION IN ONTARIO

A factor influencing the availability of radiotherapy in Ontario (and Canada) throughout much of the 1980s was a shortage of radiation therapists (RTs). An RT's professional duties include radiation treatment planning in collaboration with radiation oncologists, providing information to the patient on the procedure, properly positioning the patient for treatment, administering the radiation treatment, and monitoring patients during treatment.

Training of RTs has evolved over time. In the early years, this work was done by nurses under physician supervision. The first Ontario training program for RTs began in 1956 in a large general hospital and had three students.

At the time of the case, training was still embedded within hospitals. The only RT education program in Ontario, the Ontario School of Radiation Therapy, operated a program of approximately three years' duration that included an 8-month instructional component at PMH and a 19-month work term at one of the regional cancer centres. Up until 1988, the school accepted 25 students annually; the province then agreed to double this to 50. Subsequent to the time of the case, another small training program was established in connection with the OCTRF clinic at Sunnybrook Hospital.

One key issue was the ongoing problem of recruiting and retaining RTs. A number of reasons were suggested, including relatively low wage rates leading to RTs leaving the province (D'Souza et al., 2001), the perception of a low professional profile, constricted career paths (at the time of the case, RT credentials were not recognized as being equivalent to formal post-secondary credits), and the stresses involved in dealing with ill and frightened patients. An additional complexity was that many RTs working in Ontario had been trained overseas (often in the United Kingdom), and many of these recruits did not intend to remain in Canada over the long term. Completion rates for students entering Ontario radiotherapy schools averaged between 85% and 90%.

Subsequently, training has moved to academic centres. At the time of writing, there was a three-year full-time Radiation Therapy Degree/ Diploma program, offered jointly by the Michener Institute for Applied Health Sciences with the University of Toronto or Laurentian University (for students in northern Ontario). Entrants must have at least one year of university education, although the majority have already completed an undergraduate degree. A four-year full-time Ontario College Advanced Diploma in Health Sciences/Bachelor of Medical Radiation Sciences program is offered jointly by McMaster University with Mohawk College. All of these programs are accredited by the Canadian Medical Association.

For additional information, see the Canadian Association of Medical Radiation Technologists website (given in Appendix F).

## APPENDIX C: CHARACTERISTICS OF THE ONTARIO CANCER SYSTEM

Cancer care requires a variety of specialized services. Initially, these were provided within individual hospitals. Over time, most jurisdictions have set up coordinating bodies; some of these provide services directly, while others work with hospitals or clinics.

In Ontario, at the time of the case, there was a mixture of delivery modes. A 2004 history of the governance of cancer control in Ontario describes the evolution of several organizations with responsibility for planning and delivering cancer care (Cowan, 2004). The Princess Margaret Hospital (PMH), incorporated in 1952 and opened in 1958, was a stand-alone specialty hospital, with a strong research arm (the Ontario Cancer Institute). It provided a complete range of inpatient, outpatient, and remote community outreach services, plus strong education and research programs (including basic and clinical research, the University of Toronto's oncology training program, and Canada's largest school for radiation therapists). The Ontario Cancer Treatment & Research Foundation (OCTRF), established in 1943, was responsible for establishing, maintaining, and operating regional cancer centres (with mandates for research, diagnosis, and treatment); these were located in general hospitals across the province, usually associated with teaching hospitals affiliated with one of the province's medical schools. Some other hospitals not part of OCTRF nonetheless treated cancer patients (e.g., the Toronto General Hospital, a teaching hospital, had done so since the early 19th century). Note that at the time of writing, although not at the time of the case, both PMH and the Toronto General Hospital were part of the same hospital corporation (University Health Network).

A number of studies had been conducted in an effort to clarify future system requirements. A 1973 study by PMH and the OCTRF had recommended the expansion of PMH; although planning for the new facility was initiated, these redevelopment plans were aborted by the recession of 1981–2. One hope was that the opening in 1981 of Bayview Regional Cancer Centre (BRCC), a new regional cancer centre at a site in the north end of Toronto, would take on the additional cases. (This centre is now known as the Sunnybrook Odette Cancer Centre.) How-ever, delays meant that the new facility could not immediately absorb the anticipated volume during its first years of operation. In 1988, provincial cancer treatment capacity was further expanded through the creation of an eighth regional cancer centre in the city of Sudbury. While PMH once provided the bulk of cancer treatment in the prov-ince, by1992 OCTRF facilities were the predominant service providers. OCTRF had established clinics in Sudbury, Windsor, Thunder Bay, Lon-don, Hamilton, Ottawa, and Kingston, as well as the north Toronto site; together these clinics provided approximately 80% of the province's formal cancer treatment services.

In 1997, the OCTRF evolved into a new provincial government agency, Cancer Care Ontario (CCO), which currently has responsibil-ity for cancer care in Ontario. Rather than deliver this care directly, it works with hospitals. In 2004, the regional cancer clinics were renamed Integrated Cancer Programs, and were integrated with and managed by their 11 host hospitals, with their cancer services monitored, funded, and coordinated by CCO. At the time of writing, there were 14 such programs, including PMH. For additional information, see the CCO website (given in Appendix F).

APPENDIX D: WAIT LISTS

Considerable attention has been paid to the issue of wait lists and how to manage them. Indeed, in 2004, the federal government created a $5.5 billion Wait Times Reduction Fund (which is set to expire in 2014) to allow provincial/territorial governments to reduce wait times in five priority areas: cancer, cardiac care, hip and knee surgery, cataract sur-gery, and diagnostic imaging (CT and MRI). This has been accompa-nied by efforts to monitor success in reaching benchmark targets set by clinical experts.

There are a number of complexities involved in determining what an appropriate wait is. Even defining when someone is placed on a wait list is not always clear; should the clock start when the physician and patient agree to a treatment, when the facility is notified, when the treat-ment is booked, when the specialist is consulted, or when the patient visits the GP? In the case of radiation oncology, waiting time usually starts with the point of treatment decision; in contrast, wait times for an

MRI were measured from when the clinic was notified. Waits could be measured cross-sectionally, retrospectively, or prospectively. They can be reported in terms of the mean waiting time, the median waiting time, and/or the proportion of patients waiting for a given period. They may be based on questionnaires to random samples of physicians, random samples of patients, and/or registry data about what happens to actual patients. There may or may not be appropriateness criteria to ascertain who should receive that treatment in the first place. Another key issue is ensuring that the lists are accurate. One wrinkle is that when wait lists are managed by individual clinicians, patients may be on multiple lists; Sanmartin et al. (2000) noted that many of those purportedly on surgical wait lists were indeed duplicates, and that many had already had their surgery. Indeed, Canada's wait time strategy has led to considerable improvement in the accuracy of wait time data in addition to improving access.

Another complexity is determining what constitutes an appropriate wait, particularly when patients are put on lists well ahead of time. As one CIHI report noted,

> While in an ideal world all patients would receive treatment within these prescribed time frames, expecting 100% of patients to receive treatment within benchmarks is not practical for a number of reasons. For example, some patients may experience other illnesses or complications while waiting, making it temporarily inappropriate for them to receive surgery and extending the reported wait. Registry systems may not be sophisticated enough to adjust for this temporary delay. The same situation may occur when patients postpone surgery for personal reasons, such as waiting for a family member to assist with post-surgical convalescence or teachers waiting to have a procedure during their summer hiatus. As well, wait time registries require continuous management to ensure that only appropriate patients are waiting. There may be a time lag in removing patients who are palliative or have died, resulting in reported waits that are longer than the benchmark. On the other hand, unavoidable delays from the system side, such as cancelled elective procedures due to a lack of available beds or physician illness, can increase waits for some patients. (Canadian Institute for Health Information, 2011)

Several studies have pointed to the importance of using operations research approaches, including queuing theory, in improving the management of wait lists. Appendix E describes queuing theory.

APPENDIX E: QUEUING THEORY

A queue is defined as a line or sequence of persons, vehicles, etc., awaiting their turn to be served. Queuing theory is a branch of applied mathematics that describes waiting line situations. In queuing models, *customers* requiring service arrive at a system, over time, from an *input source*. Customers enter the queuing system and join a *queue*. At certain times, a member of the queue is selected for service by a rule known as the *queue discipline*. The required service is then performed for the customer by the *service mechanism*, after which the customer leaves the system.

Queuing systems are defined by specifying the following four factors:

1. the rate at which customers arrive to the system (inter-arrival rate, designated as $\lambda$),
2. the rate at which customers are served (service time, designated as $\mu$),
3. the number of servers in the system (designated as s), and
4. the manner in which customers are selected from the queue for service (queue discipline).

The equation $\rho = \lambda/(s^*\mu)$ describes the utilization factor of a queuing system, where $\rho$ refers to the proportion of the available resources which are being used. For a system to function well, $\rho$ should be less than 1.0. As $\rho$ approaches 1.0 (the average arrival rate begins to equal the exit rate) customers experience increasingly long waits for service. It can be shown that if the utilization factor of a queuing system equals or exceeds 1.0, the system will become unstable and the queue will grow without bound. In such a system, the number of customers waiting for service increases without limit.

In any queuing system, there are five mechanisms that can be manipulated to change the nature of the waiting line process. These are as follows:

1. Decrease the arrival rate. Slow the rate at which customers enter the system by erecting barriers to entry through price, geography, or eligibility constraints.
2. Increase the service rate. Speed up the process by which customers are served by reducing the amount of work that servers must expend on each customer, decreasing server idle time, or increasing system efficiency. Even simple mechanisms that distribute

workload evenly among servers, such as employing a single queue in a system with multiple servers, can reduce idle time and improve efficiency.

3. Increase the number of servers in the system. Since system utilization is defined as $\lambda/(s*\mu)$, that means that increasing s, the number of servers in the system, is functionally equivalent to decreasing $\mu$, the service time.

4. Modify the queue discipline. The criteria used to prioritize patients in a queuing system can have a significant effect on wait time parameters. A number of possibilities exist. First come/first served queuing disciplines are commonly perceived as equitable, but depending on the objective, might not be the most efficient way to select customers for service. Ordering the line by giving priority to those needing the lowest processing time might be more efficient in making the average patient wait less (although wait times for more complex patients needing longer processing times might grow); one common example is the "eight items or less" line in many supermarkets. Other possibilities are to "triage" and take the most severe cases first, or to select cases according to ability to meet some predefined wait target. All of these approaches can be modelled.

5. Place limits on the number of customers in the queue. Since $\lambda$, $\mu$, and s are unaffected by changes in queue capacity, placing limits on the number of customers who can wait in the system does not change any waiting line's structural characteristics. It does, however, force customers refused entry to seek alternatives.

The field of industrial engineering has been using queuing theory (and other related methods) to improve the operational efficiency of service delivery (Carter & Price, 2001).

APPENDIX F: REFERENCES CITED AND FURTHER READING

Canadian Institute for Health Information. (2011). *Wait times tables: A comparison by province, 2011.* https://secure.cihi.ca/estore/productFamily.htm?locale=en&pf=PFC1599

Carter, M.W., & Price, C.C. (2001). *Operations research: A practical introduction.* Boca Raton, FL: CRC Press.

Cowan, D.H. (2004). *Closing the circle: A history of the governance of cancer control in Ontario.* Cancer Care Ontario. https://www.cancercare.on.ca/common/pages/UserFile.aspx?fileId=13708

D'Souza, D.P., Martin, D.K., Purdy, L., Bezjak, A., & Singer, P.A. (2001). Waiting lists for radiation therapy: A case study. *BMC Health Services Research, 1*(3), 1–3.

Health Canada. (2006). *Final report of the Federal Advisor on Wait Times.* http://www.hc-sc.gc.ca/hcs-sss/pubs/system-regime/2006-wait-attente/index-eng.php

Health Council of Canada. (2007). *Wading through wait times: What do meaningful reductions and guarantees mean? An update on wait times for health care.* http://www.healthcouncilcanada.ca/rpt_det.php?id=127

Padmos, A. (2008, Winter). *Health human resources for cancer control in Canada* (Vol. 10). Report Card on Cancer in Canada. Cancer Advocacy Coalition of Canada. http://www.canceradvocacy.ca/reportcard/2007/Health%20Human%20Resources%20for%20Cancer%20Control%20in%20Canada.pdf

Priest, A., Rachlis, M., & Cohen, M. (2007). *Why wait? Public solutions to cure surgical waitlists.* Canadian Centre for Policy Alternatives and the BC Health Coalition. http://healthcoalition.ca/wp-content/uploads/2010/01/why_wait_surgical_waitlists.pdf

Sanmartin, C., Shortt, S.E.D., Barer, M.L., Sheps, S., Lewis, S., & McDonald, P.W. (2000). Waiting for medical services in Canada: Lots of heat, but little light. *Canadian Medical Association Journal, 162*(9), 1305–10.

Wait Time Alliance. (2011). *Time out! Report card on wait times in Canada.* http://www.waittimealliance.ca/media/2011reportcard/WTA2011-reportcard_e.pdf

The following websites may also be helpful:

The Canadian Association of Medical Radiation Technologists, http://www.camrt.ca/abouttheprofession/abouttheprofession/radiologicaltechnologists/

Cancer Care Ontario, Regional Cancer Program and Regional Cancer Centre Locations, https://www.cancercare.on.ca/cms/one.aspx?pageId=8226

# 14 Down the Tubes

## Should In Vitro Fertilization Be Insured in Ontario?

*TALAR BOYAJIAN, SUSAN BRONSKILL, SHERYL FARRAR, ERIN GILBART, SEIJA K. KROMM, LISE LABRECQUE, MINA MAWANI, WENDY MEDVED, PHYLLIS TANAKA, DAN TASSIE, JUDY VERBEETEN, AND RAISA B. DEBER*

Insurance cannot cover everything, and deciding what should (and should not) be included is not simple. In 1993, the government of Ontario had asked an arm's length panel to examine currently funded services that were deemed "unnecessary or of questionable medical benefit" so that they could be delisted from the provincial health insurance plan's schedule of benefits. Among the procedures deinsured was in vitro fertilization (IVF) for all infertility diagnoses other than women with bilateral fallopian tube blockage. The technology has since improved, leading to calls to revisit the decision.

This case addresses several policy issues, including: priority setting and rationing (including the ethical issues involved), interest groups, and the role of the media.

### Appendices

Appendix A: The Joint Review Panel Process
Appendix B: Treating Infertility
Appendix C: Funding IVF
Appendix D: References Cited and Further Reading

### Making Coverage Decisions

In any system of insurance, decisions must be made about what will be included in the "basket" of services and what won't be. In Canada, the

*Canada Health Act* (*CHA*) requires full public funding for all "insured services" to all "insured persons." As noted in Chapter 1 (section 7.2, *Canada Health Act*), the definition of insured services is based on where they are provided (all "medically necessary" hospital services) and by whom (all "medically required" physician services). Provinces are able to insure beyond these requirements, but are not obliged to.

However, the *CHA* does not define what services delivered by doctors or hospitals will be deemed "medically necessary" or "medically required." One policy question is who will make such determinations and on what grounds. In general, this is left to the judgment of the providers. There is some variation across provinces/territories, but also considerable agreement. Another issue is how the services are paid for (see Chapter 1, section 6.2, Payment Methods and Incentives). In general, providers have considerable autonomy in deciding not only which services to offer in hospitals but also to whom, particularly if they are funded through global budgets. Few payers attempt to micromanage which services are provided in hospitals when the hospital funding model does not involve billing for each service; for example, they do not attempt to dictate when, and how often, nurses will take vital signs of patients, although they do expect that the organizations, and the professionals who work in them, will do what is needed to ensure quality care. (To the extent this does not happen, regulators may find it necessary to set rules at various levels of detail.) For services paid on a fee-for-service (FFS) basis, however, it is necessary to determine what will be included within the fee schedule, and the amount (fee) that will be paid for each insured service. Although in theory the province (as the major funder of hospitals) is able to impose its decisions as long as it complies with the "reasonable compensation" condition of the *CHA*, in general, most provinces determine fee schedules with strong input from physicians through their provincial medical association.

In Ontario, the Ministry of Health and Long-Term Care (MOHLTC) has consulted and negotiated with the Ontario Medical Association (OMA), the exclusive bargaining agent for physicians, to determine the range of physician services that will be listed on the Ontario Health Insurance Plan (OHIP) Schedule of Benefits, and the price to be paid for each. In 1993, the OMA and the Ministry had agreed to work together towards improving the effectiveness and efficiency of the health care system. One result was a decision to experiment with a more systematic approach to determining what services should be insured.

## The 1993–4 Joint Review Panel (JRP)

The seven-member Joint Review Panel (JRP) was charged with reviewing a set of services and determining which might be removed from
the OHIP schedule of benefits ("delisted"). The goal was to reduce
physician billings by $20 million over three years. A list of 19 services
of "unnecessary or of questionable medical benefit" were targeted for
possible delisting, of which 8 had been proposed by the OMA and 11 by
the Ministry of Health (see Appendix A). The JRP was chaired by Dorothy Pringle, then the Dean of the Faculty of Nursing at the University of
Toronto. The other members of the panel included two representatives
from the Ministry, two physician representatives from the OMA, and
two public representatives.

One of the services that had been targeted for possible delisting by
the JRP was in vitro fertilization (IVF) (see Appendix B). Ontario had
been covering IVF for a maximum of three cycles for all women for
whom it had been prescribed, regardless of the specific infertility diagnosis. The JRP was informed that if all IVF services were delisted from
the provincial fee schedule, savings to the government would be in the
range of $4.4 million.

## The Royal Commission on New Reproductive
## Technology Reports

Coincidentally, on the day that the JRP was formed, the federal government's Royal Commission on New Reproductive Technologies released
its long-awaited report to the public (Canada Royal Commission on
New Reproductive Technologies, 1993). In its efforts to assess the clinical effectiveness of IVF and other related technologies, the Royal Commission had attempted to base its decisions on evidence. It accordingly
suggested that in order for a procedure to be categorized as effective
(i.e., as a treatment that would be of proven benefit for a specific infertility diagnosis) it would have to meet at least one of the following two
criteria: (1) It would have to be shown to be effective for a specific indication through "appropriately" designed randomized controlled trials;
this criterion further specified that there would have to be enough data
to allow a *meta-analysis* (combining data from all studies satisfying the
quality criteria) with, in total, at least 200 couples in each of the control
groups and the treatment groups; and/or (2) If a specific mechanism
was known to be causing the infertility, the procedure would have to be
shown to correct that problem in a way that was biologically convincing.

The commission suggested that procedures not meeting at least one of these criteria should be deemed to be of unproven value, and should be offered only in the context of research. "Effective" was defined as evidence that receiving the procedure was more likely to result in a live birth than receiving no treatment for a couple with a particular diagnosis.

Although the Royal Commission researchers had identified a total of 501 randomized control trials in the literature over the 24-year period they examined (1966–90), they had found relatively few studies that they judged to be of sufficient quality to perform a meta-analysis. In the end, their conclusions about IVF were drawn based on data from five studies. The pooled results led them to conclude that IVF could be shown to be effective only in cases of bilateral fallopian tube blockage resulting from tubal disease or damage, severe endometriosis, or previous surgical sterilization, and that IVF had not been proven effective for any of the other diagnoses for which it was being used. (This did not mean that it was proven to be ineffective, just that there was not enough data to allow them to reach a firm conclusion.) An additional barrier to determining the efficacy of IVF in the management of infertility was the lack of standardization in the definition of success rates across IVF clinics. Based on these findings, the Royal Commission had included among its recommendations two items regarding IVF: that IVF for bilateral fallopian tube blockage be an insured service under provincial medical programs within the regulatory framework recommended by the Royal Commission on New Reproductive Technologies (recommendation 128), but that Ontario discontinue coverage of IVF for indications other than bilateral fallopian tube blockage and that the resources be reallocated to fund clinical trials of unproven but promising techniques (recommendation 129) (Canada Royal Commission on New Reproductive Technologies, 1993).

### The JRP Process and Decisions

The JRP had solicited public input to help inform their decision making. In November–December 1993, they placed a bilingual advertisement in all Ontario daily and weekly newspapers, inviting voluntary written submissions and oral presentations from the public regarding their opinions on deinsurance of certain items on the OHIP Schedule of Benefits. The advertisements indicated that "the panel's deliberations will depend heavily on public input received during the review process" and assured Ontarians that "all medically necessary services will continue to be covered by OHIP." The deadline for written submissions was January 10, 1994, and the public hearing was to be held on January 19, 1994, in Toronto.

A total of 987 letters and briefs were received, 395 of which addressed deinsuring IVF (see Appendix A for a breakdown of the types of submissions received). Of the 395 written submissions, 140 supported delisting and 255 were against delisting IVF. At the public hearing, 32 presentations (each 15 minutes long) were made. Three of these (from the Ottawa and Toronto chapters of the Infertility Awareness Association of Canada, and from a consumer representative) addressed IVF; all three were against delisting it.

In their final report, the JRP recommended deinsuring IVF for all infertility diagnoses except for bilateral fallopian tube blockage. For those who met the criteria, only three cycles of treatment would be insured, excluding the cost of drugs. The panel justified its decision on the basis of the perceived low effectiveness of IVF for other indications. (See Appendix A for a list of other services that were proposed by the Ministry and the OMA for possible delisting, the potential savings, and the JRP recommendations.) The government of Ontario agreed with the recommendation; by June 1994, it had changed coverage rules for IVF and some other services.

## Subsequent Developments in Assisted Reproductive Technologies

Subsequently, technology has advanced. Appendix B describes approaches to treating infertility. Because it was common to implant multiple embryos in hopes that at least one would "take," infertility treatment had resulted in a multiple birth about 30% of the time. This rate was about 10 times greater compared to those who conceived naturally. Looked at another way, a high proportion of multiple births were the consequence of these approaches to assisted reproduction. Since multiple births are associated with elevated health risks for both mother and infants (related in part to a tendency for such children to be born prematurely with low birth weight) and higher health costs, increasingly experts are stressing the need to discourage implanting multiple embryos. Yet given the costs of one IVF treatment, those being treated for infertility had been resistant to such restrictions, particularly if this was seen as reducing the probability of a pregnancy during an IVF procedure. However, IVF now has a higher success rate than it had at the time of the JRP. Improved implantation rates allow for the transfer of single versus multiple embryos. Use of single embryo transfer (SET) procedures in turn reduces the incidence of multiple pregnancies from infertility treatment and the associated medical complications. The Infertility Awareness Association of Canada (IAAC) has continued to lobby the government for expansion of IVF coverage; one of their arguments was that using IVF can eliminate the risk of multiple pregnancies through restricting how many embryos could be transferred at one time. (They carefully did not note that such restrictions could still be imposed for procedures done in that jurisdiction even if the government does not pay for the procedure.) The IAAC argued that the strategy of funding IVF had already been proven to be successful in a number of other countries. (Appendix C summarizes coverage policies in selected jurisdictions.)

In response to this request, in 2006, the Ontario Minister of Health and Long-Term Care mandated the Medical Advisory Secretariat to conduct an updated health technology assessment to determine the clinical effectiveness and cost-effectiveness of IVF, and the role of IVF in reducing the rate of multiple pregnancies from infertility treatment. The Ontario Health Technology Advisory Committee (OHTAC) reviewed the evidence-based analysis and concluded, "Review of cost-effectiveness studies showed that due to its relatively high cost, IVF should not be recommended as the first line of treatment in the majority of cases. Two important exceptions, however, are bilateral tubal obstruction and severe male factor infertility, where IVF should be offered immediately" (Ontario Health Technology Advisory Committee, 2006).

In 2008, the Ontario Expert Panel on Infertility and Adoption was established to provide advice to the Minister of Children and Youth Services on how to improve Ontario's adoption system and how to improve access to fertility monitoring and assisted reproductive services. Its final report, *Raising Expectations*, was released in the summer of 2009 (Expert Panel on Infertility and Adoption, 2009). The panel recommended that the government of Ontario fund up to three cycles of IVF for women aged 42 and younger, and that the following ancillary services be covered when provided for a funded IVF cycle: (1) intracytoplasmic sperm injection (ICSI) when clinically indicated; (2) freezing and storage of embryos for women with any excess good quality embryos; and (3) up to two frozen embryo transfers per fresh egg retrieval when a patient has good quality frozen embryos. The panel insisted that public funding would reduce multiple births, and hence both reduce hospital and other health care costs and improve the health outcomes of mothers and babies across the province. In a relatively contentious analysis that was disputed by other experts, they estimated that by following their recommendations, Ontario could save between $400 and $550 million over the next 10 years from reducing the number of multiple births born from assisted reproduction, plus another $300 to $460 million in savings that would have been spent to support these children over their lifetimes. They suggest that the savings in health care costs could be used to offset the cost of providing access to assisted reproductive technologies. The Ministry of Children and Youth Services sent this report to the MOHLTC, since that ministry would be responsible for making the funding decisions.

Another report examining the impact of multiple pregnancies and assisted reproductive technologies on health resources in Alberta concluded that there would not be any net savings; it concluded that any cost savings associated with public funding of IVF and reduced multiple pregnancies/births would be offset by the additional IVF cycles (Chuck & Yan, 2009). If it was correct, this did not mean that the costs were not worth paying, but did mean that public funding of IVF would increase rather than decrease health care expenditures.

DECISION POINT

You are the chair of a committee that has been brought together to reconsider public funding of IVF and other related technologies. What do you recommend? Should IVF be publicly insured? If so, under what circumstances?

SUGGESTED QUESTIONS FOR DISCUSSION

1. What is infertility? Is it a disease or a social condition? Compare and contrast various alternatives that might be used by families wanting a child.
2. What, if any, aspects of IVF should be regulated, and by whom? What are the similarities and differences between: "natural" conception; assisted reproduction; and adoption? Which factors should/should not be taken into account in determining whether an individual or a couple should have a child? Prospective parents' history of violence? Single parenthood? Sexual orientation? Parental income? Age of prospective parent(s)?

3. Is IVF something the public should pay for? What factors or criteria should be considered in deciding whether to publicly fund health services, including infertility?
4. How do you define what is "medically necessary" or "medically required"? How would this relate to the services that were suggested for delisting by the JRP?
5. Who should be involved in making the decision about whether IVF should be funded? How should these decisions be made, and how should they be revisited?
6. Discuss the role of interest groups in this case.

APPENDIX A: THE JOINT REVIEW PANEL PROCESS

The following services were considered for delisting by the Joint Review Panel; the estimated annual physician billings at that time (in millions of Canadian dollars) are given in parentheses (Giacomini et al., 2000). They are listed by who proposed the potential cut (Ministry of Health, which is what the Ministry of Health and Long-Term Care was called at that time, or Ontario Medical Association), in decreasing order of the estimated annual physician billings at that time.

*Services Proposed by the Ministry of Health (MOH):*
  – Removal of certain benign skin lesions ($5.9)
  – In vitro fertilization for conditions other than complete fallopian tube blockage ($4.4)
  – Injection of simple varicose veins ($2.5)
  – Removal of acne pimples ($2.0)
  – General anaesthesia for uninsured dental procedures ($1.8)
  – Reversal of sterilization ($1.5)
  – Routine newborn, ritual, or cosmetic circumcision ($1.0)
  – Otoplasty to correct outstanding (protruding) ears ($0.5)
  – Removal of tattoos (except resulting from abuse) ($0.2)
  – Repair of torn earlobes (except from acute trauma) ($0.1)
  – Removal of port-wine stains on the face and neck ($0.3)
*Services Proposed by the Ontario Medical Association (OMA):*
  – Annual health examinations ($40)
  – Weight loss clinic referrals ($1.6)
  – Travel assessments/immunization clinics ($0.25)
  – Insertion of testicular prosthesis ($0.05)

- Insertion of penile prosthesis for impotence ($0.22)
- Intracorporeal injection for impotence (injection into the penis for problems with impotence) ($0.22)
- Uvulopalatopharyngoplasty (surgical resection of unnecessary palatal and oropharyngeal tissue in selected cases of snoring, with or without sleep apnea) ($0.22)
- Excision of calcaneal spur (surgical removal of spur on the heel bone) ($0.057)

A number of principles were established to guide the panel's process for reviewing the proposed services for delisting. They included: do not take costing into account in decision making; seek gender and age equity; and do not consider whether the OMA or Ministry had suggested that item.

**Members of the Joint Review Panel**

Chair
  *Dorothy Pringle*, Dean of the Faculty of Nursing, U. of Toronto
Government representatives
  *Dr. Ewen Mackenzie*, Senior Medical Consultant, Ministry of Health, Health Insurance Division
  *Mary Fleming*, Project Consultant, Ministry of Health, Alternative Funding Unit
Ontario Medical Association representatives
  *Dr. Kent Gerred*, General Practitioner, Toronto
  *Dr. William Redmond*, General Surgeon, Brockville
Public members
  *Angela Willson*, President, Consumers Association of Canada
  *Catherine Schuler*, Past Vice-Chair, Association of District Health Councils of Ontario

**Interest Group Submissions to Joint Review Panel**

The panel received 395 written submissions regarding the delisting of IVF. Of these, 140 submissions favoured delisting, of which 70 were from concerned groups or individuals, and 70 were Miraculous Medal (a church organization) questionnaires. Key issues raised in these submissions included: (1) IVF is too expensive, not proven to be sufficiently effective or medically necessary to be covered by OHIP; (2) "natural" parenthood is a privilege not a right; and (3) infertility is not a societal problem but a personal one.

The remaining 255 submissions opposed delisting IVF, of which 117 were from concerned groups or individuals, and 10 were Miraculous Medal questionnaires. There were also 52 petitions from an unknown source, and 76 form letters to the OMA. Key issues raised in these submissions included: (1) infertility is a disease, and hence treatment should be insured like other diseases; (2) Ontarians have the right to reproduce; (3) OHIP pays for abortions, and therefore it should also pay for IVF; (4) delisting will create a two-tiered system between those who can afford to pay for IVF and those who cannot; (5) infertile couples should be offered a fair choice of treatment options; and (6) it is important for families and infertile individuals to have this hope.

*Public Hearings*

A total of 32 presentations were made at the JRP Public Consultation hearings on January 19, 1994. Eight of these dealt with delisting in general; they were made by: Canadian Union of Public Employees, Ontario division; Employer Committee of Health Care Ontario; Dr. Michael Rachlis (a well-known policy analyst); Association of Ontario Health Centres; Medical Reform Group; City of Toronto, Board of Health; Advocacy Resource Centre of the Handicapped; and the Registered Nurses Association of Ontario. The remaining presentations dealt with specific items proposed for delisting. For example, eight dealt with the annual health examination, five spoke about anaesthesia for uninsured dental procedures, three about routine newborn circumcision, and three others about such items as removal of tattoos, removal of acne pimples, simple sclerotherapy, removal of benign skin lesions, removal of port-wine stains (adults), and intracorporeal injection for impotence. Two spoke about travel assessments / immunization clinics.

As noted in the case, the three presentations about IVF were made by the Ottawa and Toronto chapters of the Infertility Awareness Association of Canada (IAAC), and by one individual consumer. The IAAC was a national charitable organization dedicated to infertility, established in 1990 with a mandate to provide educational material, support, and assistance to Canadians who were experiencing difficulty conceiving or carrying a pregnancy. IAAC described itself as the "voice of the community for family building and fertility awareness." It noted that it was the only established patient advocacy group in Canada that had a nationwide network of support groups mandated to promote reproductive health. IAAC maintained that infertility was a reproductive health disease that deserved appropriate medical care like any other medical problem. They identified several reasons in favour of public funding of assisted reproductive technologies, including: (1) almost all other Western nations pay for IVF; (2) for some cases of infertility, IVF is the only treatment option; (3) IVF is used for only a limited time and has a high return in terms of improved quality of life; (4) many medical procedures are done to improve quality of life rather than to sustain life, and there is no other disease for which patients are expected to pay out-of-pocket for treatment; and (5) infertile Canadians pay for the abortion, maternity, and sterilization services used by the fertile, as well as for education and health care provided to their children.

### Results: Services Recommended for Delisting by the Joint Review Panel

Of the services listed above, the panel recommended deinsuring the following services, all of which had been suggested by the MOH: removal of certain benign skin lesions; in vitro fertilization for conditions other than complete fallopian tube blockage; injection of simple varicose veins; removal of acne pimples; reversal of sterilization; routine newborn, ritual, or cosmetic circumcision; removal of tattoos (except those resulting from abuse); and repair of torn earlobes (except from acute trauma).

They recommended not deinsuring the following services that had been suggested by the MOH: general anaesthesia for uninsured dental procedures; otoplasty to correct outstanding (protruding) ears; and removal of port-wine stains on the face and neck.

They also recommended not deinsuring the following services suggested by the OMA: annual health examinations; travel assessments / immunization clinics; insertion of testicular prosthesis; insertion of penile prosthesis for impotence; intracorporeal injection for impotence (injection into the penis for problems with impotence); uvulopalatopharyngoplasty (surgical resection of unnecessary palatal and oropharyngeal tissue in selected cases of snoring, with or without sleep apnea); and excision of calcaneal spur (surgical removal of spur on the heel bone).

No recommendation was made about weight loss clinic referrals, also an OMA suggestion.

APPENDIX B: TREATING INFERTILITY

Infertility is clinically defined as the inability to achieve pregnancy after one year of regular unprotected sexual intercourse. It is not uncommon; international estimates of the prevalence of infertility range from 4% to 14%, with a consensus estimate that it affects about 10% of married or cohabiting couples of reproductive age. There appears to be a growing prevalence of infertility; reasons include the continued trend towards delayed childbearing, as well as problems resulting from sexually transmitted infections.

Infertility affects both women and men at about the same rates; about 40% of infertility cases can be traced to a problem in the female, and another 40% to a problem in the male. The rest are caused by a combination of male and female factors or are idiopathic (cause is unknown). Major causes of female infertility include ovulatory disorders, blocked or damaged fallopian tubes, and endometriosis. Male factor infertility is attributable to sperm abnormalities, such as failure to produce sperm or low sperm motility.

There are a number of treatments available to address the problem of infertility. These range from relatively simple hormonal treatment to the assortment of complex and potentially invasive procedures collectively referred to as assisted reproductive technologies (ART). ARTs are procedures that involve the manipulation of eggs and/or sperm outside of the body for the purposes of establishing a pregnancy. Treatment options include (but are not limited to) the following:

*Controlled ovarian stimulation (COS):*
Pharmaceuticals are given to stimulate a woman's ovaries to promote the growth and development of multiple eggs in a single menstrual cycle. COS increases the chances of pregnancy by creating a greater number of eggs available for fertilization. It may also increase the incidence of multiple pregnancy if more than one egg is fertilized.

*Intrauterine insemination (IUI):*
Also referred to as artificial insemination (AI), this is a procedure in which washed and filtered sperm are injected directly into a woman's uterus around the time of ovulation. IUI improves the chances of pregnancy by increasing the number of sperm entering the uterus. IUI may be used in a natural cycle or with COS.

*In vitro fertilization (IVF):*
An ART procedure in which eggs are removed from a woman's ovaries and fertilized by sperm in a petri dish (in vitro). After fertilization, eggs are cultured in a laboratory for three to five days, after which time one or more of the resulting embryos are transferred to the woman's uterus in the hopes that implantation will occur. Embryos that are not transferred can be cryo-preserved for use in a future frozen embryo transfer (ET) cycle. IVF is most often performed using COS, but it can be done in a natural cycle.

*Single embryo transfer (SET):*
IVF where only one embryo is implanted; this reduces the incidence of multiple pregnancies from infertility treatment.

*Frozen embryo transfer:*
An ART procedure in which cycle monitoring is carried out with the intention of transferring frozen-thawed embryos.

*Intracytoplasmic sperm injection (ICSI):*
A technique used in combination with IVF in which a single sperm cell is injected directly into an egg to fertilize it; ICSI is mainly indicated for severe male factor infertility.

*Assisted hatching:*
This technique is sometimes used during an IVF cycle. A small opening is made in the outer layer surrounding the egg, which is thought to help increase the chances of implantation or attachment of the embryo to the endometrium.

*Gamete intrafallopian transfer (GIFT):*
An ART procedure in which one or more mature eggs and sperm are placed directly into the woman's fallopian tubes, and fertilization may then occur inside the body.

*Direct oocyte sperm transfer (DOST):*
An ART procedure in which one or more eggs are collected from the ovary and placed immediately in the uterus; sperm is then added, and if fertilization occurs, it occurs in the uterus instead of in the fallopian tube.

*Zygote intrafallopian transfer (ZIFT):*
An ART procedure in which eggs are fertilized outside of the body and the resulting zygotes are placed in the fallopian tubes.

Several commissions have studied how best to treat infertility, including Canada's Royal Commission on New Reproductive Technologies (1993). As noted in the case, in its 1993 report, the commission had determined that there was enough evidence to conclude that IVF was effective when infertility resulted from tubal defects, and ineffective if infertility resulted from defects in sperm, but that there was not enough evidence to categorize it as either effective or ineffective for other causes of infertility. They had concluded that there was not yet enough evidence to assess the other therapies they examined (GIFT, DOST, and ZIFT). In 2006, the Ontario Health Technology Advisory Committee had examined IVF; it recommended IVF with sperm injection (ICSI) for patients with severe male factor infertility and IVF-SET in infertile women with serious medical contraindications to multiple pregnancy. It added that couples who wished to avoid the risk of multiple pregnancy could consider IVF-SET as an alternative to IUI (which is usually done in conjunction with COS) (Canadian Agency for Drugs and Technologies in Health, 2010). The Ontario Expert Panel on Infertility and Adoption (2009) noted that rates of multiple births were indeed lower in those countries enforcing rules about how many embryos could be transferred.

APPENDIX C: FUNDING IVF

**IVF in Ontario Compared to Other Jurisdictions**

In 1985, Ontario had been the first Canadian province to fund IVF; it was covered for all clinical indications up to a maximum of three cycles. In 1994, following the JRP recommendations, the OHIP fee schedule had been amended to cover IVF only for women with bilateral fallopian tube blockage that was not due to voluntary sterilization.

No other Canadian province had moved to cover IVF until 2010, when the Quebec government announced that it would cover up to three IVF cycles and the associated medical services. Funding was dependent on regulations limiting the number of embryos that could be transferred for implementation; the province was quoted as saying that this initiative would save $30 million per year in treatments for premature babies that would otherwise have resulted from multiple births with unregulated IVF. Within the year, the rate of multiple pregnancies from infertility treatments was said to have dropped from 27.2% to 5.2%. In 2010, the province of Manitoba announced a 40% refundable tax credit for IVF (to a ceiling of $8,000 a year) if treatment was received in a Manitoba clinic.

In 2009, Nisker (2009) estimated that only 15% of Canadian women with clinical indications for IVF were accessing this therapy. Some other countries, including Australia, Belgium, Denmark, Finland, the Netherlands, and Sweden, were more generous in covering IVF, although various restrictions often applied, relating to such factors as age, number of cycles, and/or number of embryos to be implanted (Hughes & Giacomini, 2001). In Ontario, the costs of diagnostic and surgical management of infertility remained covered under the provincial health insurance plan. In addition, funding was provided for an unlimited number of intrauterine insemination (IUI) cycles.

## Cost of Assisted Reproductive Technologies

One barrier to accessing assisted reproductive technologies was the significant financial burden associated with each procedure; this limited access to those individuals/couples who could afford to pay for these treatments or lived in a jurisdiction where the costs were covered. In Ontario, the average cost of IUI was $350 for a natural cycle or $720 for a stimulated cycle (excluding fertility drugs). A 2009 consultant's report estimated the following costs for various procedures in each province, excluding the costs of fertility drugs, which could vary from $2,500 to $7,000 per cycle; the numbers for Ontario and the Canadian average are shown in Table 14.1 (Ovo Consulting, 2009).

Table 14.1. Cost of Selected Assisted Reproductive Technologies in Ontario and Canada

| Procedure | Ontario | Average Canadian price |
| --- | --- | --- |
| IVF (natural cycle) | $4,200 | $4,471 |
| IVF (with ovarian stimulation)* | $5,700 | $5,660 |
| IVF-ICSI (with ovarian stimulation)* | $6,914 | $6,996 |
| Assisted hatching | $313 | $406 |
| Frozen embryo transfer | $1,179 | $1,067 |

Source: Ovo Consulting (2009)

## APPENDIX D: REFERENCES CITED AND FURTHER READING

Canada Royal Commission on New Reproductive Technologies. (1993). *Proceed with care: Final report of the Royal Commission on New Reproductive Technologies* (Vols. 1–2). Ottawa, ON: Minister of Government Services Canada. http://epe.lac-bac.gc.ca/100/200/301/pco-bcp/commissions-ef/baird1993-eng/baird1993-eng.htm

Canadian Agency for Drugs and Technologies in Health. (2010). *Status of public funding for in vitro fertilization in Canada and internationally* (Issue 14). http://www.cadth.ca/products/environmental-scanning/environmental-scans/issue-14

Chuck, A., & Yan, C. (2009). *Assistive reproductive technologies: A literature review and database analysis.* Institute of Health Economics. http://www.ihe.ca/publications/library/2009/assistive-reproductive-technologies-a-literature-review-and-database-analysis/

Expert Panel on Infertility and Adoption. (2009). *Raising expectations: Recommendations of the expert panel on infertility and adoption.* Ontario Ministry of Children and Youth Services. http://www.children.gov.on.ca/htdocs/English/infertility/index.aspx

Giacomini, M., Hurley, J., & Stoddart, G. (2000). The many meanings of deinsuring a health service: The case of in vitro fertilization in Ontario. *Social Science & Medicine, 50*(10), 1485–500. http://dx.doi.org/10.1016/S0277-9536(99)00394-9

Hughes, E.G., & Giacomini, M. (2001). Funding in vitro fertilization treatment for persistent subfertility: The pain and the politics. *Fertility and Sterility, 76*(3), 431–42. http://dx.doi.org/10.1016/S0015-0282(01)01928-8

Mladovsky, P., & Sorenson, C. (2010). Public financing of IVF: A review of policy rationales. *Health Care Analysis, 18*(2), 113–28. http://dx.doi.org/10.1007/s10728-009-0114-3

Nisker, J. (2009). Socially based discrimination against clinically appropriate care. *Canadian Medical Association Journal, 181*(10), 764. http://dx.doi.org/10.1503/cmaj.091620

Ontario Health Technology Advisory Committee. (2006). *OHTAC recommendations.* http://www.health.gov.on.ca/english/providers/program/ohtac/tech/recommend/rec_ivf_101906.pdf

Ontario Ministry of Health and Long-Term Care. (2006, October). *In vitro fertilization and multiple pregnancies: Health technology policy assessment.* http://www.ontla.on.ca/library/repository/mon/16000/269307.pdf

Ovo Consulting. (2009). *In-vitro fertilisation in Canada: Cost structure analysis.* Canadian Fertility and Andrology Society. http://www.cfas.ca/images/stories/pdf/ivf_cost_structure_analysis.pdf

Shanner, L., & Nisker, J. (2001). Bioethics for clinicians: 26. Assisted reproductive technologies. *Canadian Medical Association Journal, 164*(11), 1589–94.

Steinbrook, R. (2008). Saying no isn't NICE – The travails of Britain's National Institute for Health and Clinical Excellence. *New England Journal of Medicine, 359*(19), 1977–81. http://dx.doi.org/10.1056/NEJMp0806862

# 15 Prescription for Conflict

*BEV LEVER, LAURA ESMAIL, LINDA GAIL YOUNG, AND*
*RAISA B. DEBER*

In 1992, Canada passed Bill C-91, which amended the Patent Act to extend the period of patent exclusivity for new pharmaceuticals in Canada from 17 to 20 years and eliminate compulsory licensing. Bill C-91 pitted social goals (and the interests of those using and paying for drugs) against economic goals (and the interests of those developing and selling these products). Under continued international pressure to liberalize trade markets, standardize intellectual property protection, and encourage a knowledge-based economy, some now question whether these provisions should be revisited. This case addresses several policy issues, including: policy goals, framing of issues, scope of conflict, pressure groups, and globalization. This case can also be taught as a role play exercise.

**Appendix**

Appendix A: References Cited and Further Reading

**The Case**

Canada's patent regime for pharmaceuticals has historically been passionately debated. Different stakeholders had a number of often contradictory policy goals, including: ensuring affordable drug prices; providing fair intellectual property protection for the innovative pharmaceutical industry; supporting the domestic generic drug industry; and ensuring that Canada met the requirements of its international trade agreements.

The pharmaceutical industry is global, high-tech, fiercely competitive, and often highly profitable; it is frequently viewed as being a part of the emerging knowledge base industries that will drive the global economic engines of the future. In 1992, when Bill C-91 was introduced to amend the *Patent Act*, approximately 24,000 Canadians were employed by the pharmaceutical industry. Many of those employed by this industry held well-paid research or marketing positions. At the time, Canada represented only approximately 2% of the world market, yet the pharmaceutical industry potentially provided significant research dollars to Canada.

Intellectual property (IP) refers to a variety of intangible creations and inventions. Intellectual property can be protected by giving its creators an exclusive right over its use for a stipulated period of time, using such legal approaches as patents, copyrights, and trademarks. However, the rights conferred are specific to particular jurisdictions, and hence are enforceable only to the extent that each jurisdiction agrees to respect them. Internationally, a number of efforts have been made to harmonize IP rules, including the World Trade Organization (WTO)'s Agreement on Trade-Related Aspects of Intellectual Property Rights (TRIPS), negotiated in the 1986–94 Uruguay Round. Nonetheless, each country retains considerable flexibility.

Within the trade policy arena, a number of issues relating to pharmaceuticals remained highly contentious. One was the question of patent protection. Patents give exclusive rights to the patent holder for a fixed time period. Canada had extended the term for pharmaceuticals to 17 years in 1987; Bill C-91 had called for increasing it to 20 years. Another question related to compulsory licensure. Canada had provisions which would allow its Commissioner of Patents to grant licenses to other companies to allow them to import, make, use, or sell a patented invention, in exchange for paying a royalty (at a level to be determined by the Commissioner of Patents) to the patent holder. Patent holders objected to this provision, which they felt undermined their intellectual property rights. Another issue was the powers given to the Patented Medicine Prices Review Board (PMPRB). This independent federal board was created in 1987, and had limited powers to regulate the prices of new patented medicines sold in Canada.

As noted in Chapter 1, section 7.2 (*Canada Health Act*), there is no requirement for provincial/territorial insurance plans to cover drug costs unless those drugs are administered in a hospital. However, most provincial governments have voluntarily implemented drug programs for certain populations. Those eligible for such programs vary; criteria may be based on various combinations of age (e.g., seniors), disease (e.g., cancer), and/or income (e.g., recipients of social welfare programs). There is also extensive private insurance coverage for pharmaceutical costs, much of this paid by employers, albeit with varying co-payments and deductibles. The affordability of pharmaceutical products remains a critical policy concern for many stakeholders.

## History of Federal Legislation on Pharmaceutical Patent Protection

In 1923, the Canadian *Patent Act* allowed compulsory licensing of pharmaceutical products. This provision permitted generic firms to receive a license to manufacture and sell a drug before the patent expired, on the conditions that royalties were paid to the innovating company and that all manufacturing was done in Canada. However, the cost of manufacturing the active ingredients of pharmaceutical compounds was often seen as prohibitive, and only 22 compulsory licences were granted between 1923 and 1969.

This policy was altered in 1969 when generic drug companies were permitted to import pharmaceutical compounds as long as they paid a 4% royalty fee to the patent holder. With this change in policy, more than 290 compulsory licences were issued between 1969 and 1982. In 1983, University of Toronto economist Harry Eastman was asked by the federal Liberal government to head an inquiry into the issue of compulsory licensing. In 1985, the Commission of Inquiry on the Pharmaceutical Industry, called the Eastman Report, recommended that compulsory licensing provision should be maintained with only minor changes (increasing the royalty payment to 14%, and not granting compulsory licenses during the first four years after the patent had been granted). It calculated that the savings from this policy in 1983 alone would be at least $211 million, in a total market for pharmaceuticals of $1.6 billion. It concluded that pharmaceutical manufacturing remained extremely profitable, and that the industry's profit in Canada was still higher than in most other countries (with the notable exception of the United States). It also stated its belief that the fear of the multinationals that they would lose significant market share to the generic drug companies was unfounded, suggesting that the generic companies had only gained 3.1% of the market between 1969 and 1983 (Eastman, 1985).

In 1987, Canada's newly elected Progressive Conservative government was in the midst of negotiating the Canada-US Free Trade Agreement (FTA). Throughout the negotiations for the agreement, the federal government had maintained that there was no requirement by the FTA that Canada amend its patent laws to extend Canada's patent term for pharmaceuticals. However, the federal government argued that Canada did need to extend the patent term to bring Canada's patent laws into line with other countries, and that doing this would also benefit the Canadian economy through the investment commitments of the multinational drug companies. In December 1987, the Conservatives' Bill C-22 was passed into legislation; it amended the *Patent Act* to provide a 17-year period of patent protection.

Immediately after the agreement was signed, the American press quoted US government officials as saying that, had Canada not agreed to change its patent laws, there would have been no FTA. When asked why the "drug deal" was not mentioned in the final version of the FTA, Bill Merkin, the US deputy chief negotiator in the free trade talks, was quoted as saying, "Ottawa didn't want it [intellectual property] to be in the free trade negotiations. They didn't want to *appear* to be negotiating that away as part of the free trade agreement. Whatever changes they were going to make, they wanted them to be *viewed* as 'in Canada's interest'" (Clarkson, 2002, p. 247).

Subsequent to the 1987 changes, Canada became one of the 108 countries negotiating the General Agreement on Tariffs and Trade (GATT). The GATT, if signed, would determine the trading and tariff regulations to be adhered to among the 108 signatories, whose most influential members were referred to as the Group of Seven (G7); they included Canada, France, Germany, Italy, Japan, the United Kingdom, and the United States. Canada was the only G7 country that allowed compulsory licensing and was not home to any multinational drug company headquarters.

Intellectual property rights were discussed at the GATT negotiations. What was referred to as the Uruguay Round of Negotiations had three main objectives: to reduce impediments to international trade; to secure adequate protection of intellectual property rights; and to ensure that the mechanisms used to enforce intellectual property rights did not themselves create barriers to trade. When talks deadlocked, Arthur Dunkel, Director-General of the GATT, submitted a report on December 20, 1991, that was designed as a draft agreement on a wide range of trade issues. It included provisions for intellectual property rights.

Canada's initial reaction came even before the report was released; Canada's Minister for International Trade, Michael Wilson, noted that Canada would abide, albeit reluctantly, with the recommendation to abolish compulsory licensing should other GATT countries agree.

However, Dunkel's report provided considerable latitude to individual governments in changing existing laws, including allowing an eight-year period for doing so. Clauses were accordingly incorporated into the GATT which would require the signatory countries to: (1) rescind compulsory licensing within eight years of the date of signing retro-active to December 20, 1991, and (2) bring patent laws into line with the majority of the countries. As a signatory, Canada would have to adopt a period of 20 years for patent protection. Reportedly, the US drug industry had hoped for stronger language, and began a lobbying campaign. However, a dispute between France and the United States regarding French agricultural subsidies led to the GATT talks being halted in 1992; the GATT remained unsigned until 1994. In 1995, these agreements moved into the new World Trade Organization (WTO), which also administered the Agreement on Trade-Related Aspects of Intellectual Property Rights (TRIPS).

Simultaneously, Canada was also negotiating the North American Free Trade Agreement (NAFTA). During these negotiations Canada agreed to amend its *Patent Act* by eliminating compulsory licensing and extending the period of patent exclusivity. However, as of December 1992 NAFTA had not yet been signed. The new US President-elect, Bill Clinton, had included in his platform a promise to review health care, in particular the cost of drugs, and initiate some action by the end of his first 100 days. One key area of comparison was with Canada, where it was noted that prescription drugs were, on average, 36% cheaper than in the United States.

To assess the likely financial impact of Bill C-91, Canada's federal government had compiled information regarding the impact of the pre-vious patent extension passed in Bill C-22. Paul Blais, the Minister of Consumer and Corporate Affairs at the time, had announced that the analysis found that these patent changes had benefited Canada, result-ing in a cumulative total of $1.1 billion (since 1987) of research and development (R&D) investments, the creation of 2,400 highly skilled jobs, and only "minor" increases in drug costs; others disputed these figures. The government analysis had also computed that Bill C-91 would increase the costs to the provinces for the prescription drugs they paid for by $125 million over the next five years, and argued that this would be more than offset by the $400 million which the multina-tionals had committed in further R&D investment.

A series of hearings was held in the federal legislature in 1992 as Bill C-91 moved through the House of Commons process. Approximately 153 groups or individuals applied to testify to the special legislative committee. Among the issues being discussed were: whether patent protection should be extended from 17 to 20 years; whether this should be retroactive; whether compulsory licensure should be maintained or eliminated; and what powers should be given to the PMPRB. Additional detail about key stakeholders and their views is provided below.

## Positions of Key Stakeholders

The *Pharmaceutical Manufacturers Association of Canada* (PMAC) was the trade association of the companies who produced patented medicines (Since 1999, the association has been called Canada's Research-Based Pharmaceutical Companies, or Rx&D.) PMAC, like the pharmaceutical industry, was global in scope; companies developed, manufactured, and sold products worldwide. PMAC argued that Canada was the only country in the industrialized world that did not treat new pharmaceutical products the same as they treated other inventions. The brand name companies asserted that it cost over 475 million Canadian dollars and took in excess of 10 years between the submission of a patent application and the launch of a new drug product onto the market, in large part due to the extensive time and effort required for product testing and regulatory approval. Consequently, they argued that pharmaceutical products enjoyed less effective patent life (market exclusivity) than did other classes of products where such delays did not exist. The brand name companies claimed that they were looking for a fair return on investment. They also emphasized that, while other products received 20 years of patent protection, Canada allowed pharmaceutical products, on average, only 17 years.

PMAC also objected to the system of compulsory licensing introduced in 1969, which automatically granted licences to generic manufacturers to produce a copy of the patented drug prior to patent expiry, in return for a royalty on sales paid back to the innovating company. They noted that they had already lost approximately 10% of market share to generic manufacturers, and their fear was that the generic drug companies would capture 35% of the market within the decade. They strongly suggested that, should this situation remain unchanged, research and manufacturing currently conducted in Canada would be moved to a more favourable market, noting that investment decisions were primarily based on a country's intellectual property protection. If, however, a more "favourable climate" would be created in Canada, they committed to increase their investment in Canadian research and development.

The Canadian generic drug companies (GDCs) and their association, the Canadian Drug Manufacturers Association (since 2003, referred to as the Canadian Generic Pharmaceutical Association [CGPA]), disagreed. They noted that it was not uncommon for generics to take over up to 50% of the market for a drug from its inventors once the patents expired. The savings this might generate for the consumer/payer varied but could be considerable, although the generic companies tended to charge somewhat higher prices in Canada than in some other jurisdictions. The nature of the generic industry, based on the use of compulsory licensing to copy drugs, made it highly dependent on government legislation and provincial drug formularies for business opportunities. If the period of market exclusivity and patent protection were extended to 20 years, the GDCs argued that it would unfairly limit their ability to compete. They noted that doctors have a tendency to prescribe newer drugs even though those products might not be more effective than what was already on the market.

Since the changes to the legislation in 1987, GDCs had fought to prevent further restrictions being placed on their industry. Bill C-91 evoked extensive lobbying by the GDCs, with their targets including the federal and provincial governments, pharmacists, and the public. The GDCs also attempted to stop the progression of the bill by taking the issue to court. The court ruled that their petition was premature, in that Bill C-91 was not yet law, and that it would be "contemptuous of Parliament" to intervene at this point. In addition, the GDCs pressured the provinces with threats of halting future investments. Manitoba, which was scheduled for a $100-million expansion over 10 years by Apotex (the largest generic drug company at that time), was told that investment prospects were dependent on there being no changes to the *Patent Act* until at least 1996, and hence that the expansion might be aborted if the bill were passed.

As the positions of the players become more entrenched, the GDCs also took issue with the federal government's figures for the number of jobs created by Bill C-22. The GDCs argued that the net increase in the number of jobs was much less than the government had presented and that almost half of those would be in marketing and sales as opposed to in research and development.

PHYSICIANS

The Canadian Medical Association (CMA) favoured the bill, with the caveat that the federal government should take necessary steps to ensure that sufficient price control mechanisms were in place. In a

November 27, 1992, press release, it stated, "We are in favour of eliminating compulsory licensing but we are also in favour of accessible and affordable health care for patients. The government must try to balance these policy objectives as fairly as possible." Doctors, especially those involved in research, had multiple interests. Some were funded by PMAC companies; these companies also subsidized conferences and educational activities. Doctors were also the major prescribers of medicines; as such, they wanted to ensure that a supply of effective treatments was available, but also had to respond to patients, hospitals, and payers who often complained about the high cost of these drugs. The CMA agreed that it would be advisable to review drug prescribing patterns and ensure that utilization was appropriate.

PHARMACISTS

Pharmacists were somewhat split in their position. Pharmacies made much of their profits from prescription sales, although increasingly they also received revenues from selling other merchandise. However, in most jurisdictions, pharmacists could charge the cost of the drug plus a mark-up and a dispensing fee. All provinces have attempted to curtail the rising cost of drugs, with varying success. Provincial governments have attempted to regulate the mark-up and dispensing fees they were willing to pay for recipients of provincial pharmaceutical insurance programs (which, depending on the jurisdiction, include various combinations of seniors, social assistance recipients, home care service recipients, those in long-term care facilities, those with specified illnesses, and/or those with catastrophic drug expenditures, depending on the year and the province). Other payers may or may not pay the same price. Another potential price control mechanism was a provincial drug formulary; at the time of Bill C-91, all jurisdictions except British Columbia, Alberta, and the Yukon had them. These formularies are lists of drugs that the provincial plan will cover; they often specify which drugs are deemed to be interchangeable (which includes generic drugs). Formularies may also set the price they will pay. The pharmacists were thus arguing on several grounds, including as health care professionals with an expertise in drugs, as business people with economic interests, and as a group with frequent contact with the users of drugs (and with their complaints and concerns about drug costs).

The Canadian Pharmacists' Association was called as a government witness to the committee reviewing Bill C-91, and argued that "patent protection and drug costs are two different concepts ... that can perhaps be best handled as separate issues." In contrast, the Ontario Pharmacists' Association argued that "we could not support extended patent protection since, in our view, this would undermine the moderating influence on drug prices provided by generic competition ... the issues of patent protection, compulsory licensing and drug costs are inexorably linked."

PROVINCIAL GOVERNMENTS

The provincial governments paid for a significant portion of drug costs, both through their funding of hospitals and through provincial drug plans. The federal Minister of Trade, Mr. Wilson, informed the provinces that there would be no additional funding to provincial governments if Bill C-91 passed. He argued that any increase in pharmaceutical expenditures would be balanced by the increase in provincial revenues coming from brand name industry investment. The provinces were not convinced, with the notable exception of the province of Quebec (where most of the drug company research laboratories were located). Indeed, all provincial health ministers (with the exception of the Quebec minister) wrote the federal health minister, Benoit Bouchard, strongly requesting that the federal government not lengthen the patent protection term for brand name drugs. If the federal government did nonetheless extend the patent term, the provincial ministers indicated three key concerns: (1) that the legislation not be made retroactive; (2) that the federal government compensate the provinces for the increases in drug program costs; and (3) that price controls be strengthened. The provinces called for the development of a joint federal-provincial strategy to address drug costs. They indicated that their overriding concern was the cost impact and the potential need to cut other health programs if the overall cost of health care was to be controlled. Individual submissions, including projected cost impacts, were presented to the House of Commons and the Senate. As well, the provinces joined together in the form of a presentation by the BC Minister of Health, Elizabeth Cull. They attempted to persuade the federal government to drop Bill C-91 altogether or, at least, to achieve such changes such as the elimination of the retroactive date of implementation and the strengthening of price controls.

The provinces also argued that the PMPRB, which had been created by Bill C-22 in 1987 with the mandate to monitor and limit patented drug prices, was ineffective. It was not required to consult the provinces, it relied on voluntary compliance by the multinationals rather than using the legislative clout it potentially had at its disposal, and it covered only 3% of drugs (the remaining 97%, including all older drugs, being outside of its jurisdiction). Indeed, 40% of new drugs introduced in 1991 were charging in excess of PMPRB guidelines. A big concern of the provinces was whether the changes proposed through Bill C-91 would result in more effective functioning of the PMPRB. They suggested adding provincial representatives to PMPRB. They also asserted that the amount which Ottawa had paid them to cover any increases in drug costs as a result of Bill C-22 ($25 million per year over the previous four years) was grossly inadequate. The costs for patented medicines had risen from $1 billion in 1988 to $1.9 billion in 1992 at a time when the number of prescriptions had increased by only 6.1% per year.

The province of Quebec however, supported the bill. As noted, Quebec was the Canadian centre for the majority of the multinational drug companies. (Ontario also was the location for some brand name pharmaceuticals and home to the largest number of generic firms.) Of the dollars reinvested by the multinationals into Canada for 1990 and 1991, Quebec and Ontario had received 45% each. Quebec was offered "enormous investments" according to Judy Erola, former MP, and at that time president of PMAC, which might "pass (Quebec) by" if patent protection was not extended.

PRIVATE INSURERS

Private insurance companies offered extended health service plans to cover at least a portion of drug costs (as well as dental, eye care, rehabilitation, and other services not included in publicly funded health insurance in Canada). These insurance plans were generally employer-paid or cost-shared with employees. As insurers of drug plans, companies such as Green Shield, Great West Life, and Blue Cross indicated that they would prefer more generic substitutions on the market to reduce their costs. The average cost of drug claims had risen at a rate in excess of 11% compounded annually for the period 1987–91, well above the CPI rate. This could mean that, if Bill C-91 was passed by the Senate and the projected increases to drug costs materialized, they would have to increase the premiums for drug payment plans. The fear of these companies was that employers might choose to eliminate drug benefits if premiums became too costly. However, drug plans were a relatively small component of the insurance business and some believed that the pressure applied by the brand name companies on the private insurers ensured that the insurance companies did not speak out too loudly.

PATIENTS

Patient groups expressed their fear that Bill C-91 would increase the cost of prescription drugs, increases which for the most part they would have to pay. Within this group, seniors (who are the largest users of pre-scription drugs) felt particularly threatened. Although many provincial drug plans paid all or most of the costs of drugs being used by seniors, there were fears that this benefit might be cut or eliminated should costs increase. The result could be higher taxes if benefits remained unchanged, significant reductions in the scope of provincial drug care plans, and/or some form of user payment system. The seniors, as well as poverty groups and other citizens' groups, attempted to put pres-sure on Ottawa to have the bill overturned, including appearances at the House of Commons and Senate committees dealing with Bill C-91. They strongly voiced their belief that outpatient prescription drugs should be covered under the *Canada Health Act*. As well, they expressed concern about what they felt was misleading information regarding the potential benefits of Bill C-91 to Canada. Specifically, they attacked the investments which the multinationals proposed to make if the bill passed. According to their submission, the figures quoted to the public did not take into account the considerable tax breaks that the provinces (particularly Quebec, Alberta, and Ontario) provided to these com-panies. They argued that, of the $400 million that the multinationals said would be reinvested, between $220 and $280 million represented these tax breaks, and hence would come out of Canada's revenue in the form of lost taxes. At that time, the multinationals had agreed to reinvest a percentage of their profits (10% by 1996 under Bill C-22), where profits were, by definition, after-tax dollars. This group argued that this meant that the 8.8% that Ottawa had announced as already being invested actually amounted to less than half that amount. Hence, these stakeholders argued that the public were getting the short end of the stick in two ways: higher drug prices and minimal invest-ments. However, it should be noted that it was unclear to what extent these groups really represented patients, since most patients would qualify as "diffuse" interests (see Chapter 1, section 4.1, Concentrated/ Diffuse Interests) and as such did not take the time to participate in these consultations.

## HOSPITALS

The voice of the hospitals was presented by the Canadian Hospital Association and the Ontario Hospital Association, each of which prepared briefs to the Legislative Committee on Bill C-91. Their primary concern was the potential cost impact of this bill on hospital operating expenses. They noted that the previous years had already seen massive cuts and layoffs to the hospital sector, and argued that they could not absorb the estimated increase of 15%–20% in drug costs. They noted that the national data provided by the Canadian Institute for Health Information (CIHI) about health expenditures suggested that the percentage of total health care costs going to the drug sector had risen from 8.9% in the mid-1970s to 13.3% by 1990. (Note that these numbers are somewhat misleading, since CIHI included the costs of drugs administered within hospitals in the hospital category. The shift from hospital to community thus also meant that some of this increase in drug expenditures reflected a reclassification of these costs; see also Chapter 1, section 9.1, Canadian Data.) The hospitals also noted that total drug costs probably exceeded the costs for physician services.

## LABOUR

Labour organizations, concerned that their members might be facing massive layoffs, responded negatively to Bill C-91. The decline in the sale and manufacturing of generic pharmaceuticals which would result from the passage of Bill C-91 was interpreted as threatening the jobs of more than 2,000 Canadians employed by the Canadian owned (generic) pharmaceutical industry. Further, it was feared that the bill would make it unlikely that the generic companies would create the thousands of new jobs which allegedly would have resulted from continued growth in the generic drug industry.

Labour groups outside the pharmaceutical industry were also opposed to Bill C-91. Submissions were made to the House of Commons and the Senate for the bill to be withdrawn because of concern regarding the negative impact the projected increases to drug costs would have on union members. Although unions were frequently covered by drug plans, many of those plans were cost-shared. The costs of these plans were often governed by the costs of the drugs. As costs rose, so did the premiums paid by the employers and employees. An additional concern put forth by the unions was underestimating the power and influence of the multinational drug company lobby. The Canadian

Table 15.1. Views of Key Stakeholders

| Group | Extend patent protection from 17 to 20 years | Retroactivity | Compulsory licensure | PMPRB role and powers |
|---|---|---|---|---|
| PMAC | Yes | Yes | Eliminate | Limit to maintaining exclusivity period |
| GDCs | No | No | Maintain | No comment |
| CMA | Yes | No | Eliminate | More powers |
| Pharmacists | Split | No | Split | More powers |
| Quebec | Yes | Yes | Eliminate | No comment |
| Ontario | Formal review required | No | Formal review required | Add provincial reps |
| BC | Formal review required | No | Formal review required | Add provincial reps |
| Insurers | No | No | Maintain | No comment |
| Seniors | No | No | Maintain | Not effective |
| Hospitals | No | No | Maintain | More powers |
| Labour | No | No | Maintain | No comment |

Auto Workers union, in its testimony before the Senate committee, gave one example. In negotiations with Ford in 1982, after much pressure by Ford, the union had reluctantly agreed to have its drug plan cover only generic drugs whenever possible. This would have resulted in over $1 million savings for the company. After the contract was signed, the American drug companies were said to have put such pressure on the US parent company that Ford changed this deal.

Table 15.1 summarizes the views of the key stakeholders on four key issues.

MEDIA COVERAGE

The media have played an important role in influencing societal needs and expectations relative to health care. They have affected patients' demands through the promotion or denigration of procedures, therapies, and drugs. With increasing frequency, the public, influenced by the media, want input into the type and/or amount of drugs prescribed by physicians. In a country where universal health care was so valued, news that some aspect of this was being threatened was felt likely to attract media attention. Surrounding Bill C-91 were such headlines as: "New drug law will hike costs by $1 billion, Lankin says" (Lisa Priest, *Toronto Star*, October 29, 1992); "Report says drug patent law will cost Canadians billions" (Canadian Press, *Globe and Mail*, November 17, 1992); "New drug law both an upper and a downer" (Ann Gibbon, *Globe and Mail*, June 24, 1992); and "Drug costs set to soar as MPs approve patent bill" (Shawn McCarthy, *Toronto Star*, December 11, 1992).

### Subsequent Developments

Bill C-91 became law in 1993. Despite efforts by the Liberal opposition to stop the passage of the bill or to at least change some of the clauses attached to it, it was approved as presented. For the first time in Canadian history, closure had been used to limit debate at every stage of the passage of this bill through the House of Commons and the Senate. At the time of writing, the law remained in effect.

Subsequently, other national and provincial initiatives have affected the industry, including the Common Drug Review (a process where most of the provincial governments work together to determine whether drugs should be approved for use on formularies), and provincial initiatives to attempt to control pharmaceutical prices (Canada has among the highest generic drug prices in the world).

Since then, there have been major changes in the pharmaceutical industry. The growth rate of brand name pharmaceutical research investment has slowed down. Many of the promised research jobs did not materialize, and others have been eliminated. One trend has been for the major companies to merge. Merck, for example, acquired Schering-Plough in 2009. The next year, it announced plans to save up to $3.5 billion by closing numerous research sites and manufacturing plants, and eliminating roughly 10% of their workforce (15,000 jobs) by 2012. Among the sites closed was their Montreal, Quebec, office; all of the researchers working there were either dismissed or transferred out of Canada.

Provincial governments are seeking modifications to allow them to reduce their drug costs. At the same time, Canada's attempt to negotiate a trade deal with the European Union led to demands that Canada modify its drug patent laws to further protect the brand name companies against competition from generic manufacturers, and further extend the period of patent protection (including giving up to five years "credit" for the time it took to get regulatory approval).

DECISION POINT

You are the federal Minister of Trade. It is 2013. You are under pressure from provinces and employers to reduce drug prices. What should you do? Should you revisit drug patent legislation?

SUGGESTED QUESTIONS FOR DISCUSSION

1. What policy options should you consider? How would each address such issues as return on investment; international trade policy; and affordability of drug prices?
2. Discuss framing and how this affected the debate.
3. Discuss the positions of the key stakeholders.
4. Discuss scope of conflict. Where might these questions be dealt with? How might that affect which issues were raised, and the powers of different stakeholder groups?

APPENDIX A: REFERENCES CITED AND FURTHER READING

Bell, C., Griller, D., Lawson, J., & Lovren, S. (2010). *Generic drug pricing and access in Canada: What are the implications?* Health Council of Canada. http://healthcouncilcanada.ca/rpt_det.php?id=156

Clarkson, S. (2002). *Uncle Sam and us.* Toronto: University of Toronto Press.

Eastman, H.C. (1985). *The report of the Commission of Inquiry on the Pharmaceutical Industry.* Minister of Supply and Services Canada. http://www.archives canada.ca/english/search/ItemDisplay.asp?sessionKey=1143478259019_206_191_57_199&l=0&lvl=1&v=0&coll=1&itm=257716&rt=1&bill=1

Lexchin, J. (1993). Pharmaceuticals, patents, and politics: Canada and Bill C-22. *International Journal of Health Services, 23*(1), 147–60. http://dx.doi.org/10.2190/UCWG-YBR3-X3L0-NWYT

Lexchin, J. (2007). *Canadian drug prices and expenditures: Some statistical observations and policy implications.* Canadian Centre for Policy Alternatives. http://www.policyalternatives.ca/sites/default/files/uploads/publications/National_Office_Pubs/2007/Canadian_Drug_Prices.pdf

Sibbald, B. (2001). Drug patent protection: How long is long enough? *Canadian Medical Association Journal*, *164*(9), 1331.

Sood, N., de Vries, H., Gutierrez, I., Lakdawalla, D.N., & Goldman, D.P. (2009). The effect of regulation on pharmaceutical revenues: Experience in nineteen countries. *Health Affairs*, *28*(1), w125–37. http://dx.doi.org/10.1377/hlthaff.28.1.w125

# 16 Ask Your Doctor

## Direct-to-Consumer Advertising of Prescription Medicines

CHRIS BONNETT, CHRISTOPHER J. LONGO, YEESHA POON, AND RAISA B. DEBER

What limits should be placed on the ability to advertise prescription drugs? Canada restricts direct-to-consumer advertising (DTCA); media companies and pharmaceutical companies argue that these regulations are unnecessary infringements on their ability to inform the public, particularly in an era when information flows easily across national borders, while others suggest that DTCA may harm consumers and increase drug costs. What should the government do?

This case addresses several policy issues, including: regulation, the role of the state, scope of conflict, interests, globalization, and framing. This case can also be taught as a role play exercise.

**Appendices**

Appendix A: Regulatory Structures
Appendix B: References Cited and Further Reading

**The Case**

Canada's national *Food and Drugs Act* includes a provision, under the Food and Drug Regulations, which regulates how pharmaceuticals can be advertised in Canada. This provision severely limited direct-to-consumer advertising (DTCA), a term which refers to advertising prescription drugs to the public in a range of media. Current interpretation of these regulations permits prescription drug advertising to give information only about the name of the drug and how much it would cost for a given quantity. The rationale was that this information would allow consumers to compare prices for any drugs they had been prescribed, while still allowing the physician to decide which drugs to order. The *Act* also prohibits advertising treatments for a set of serious diseases listed as Schedule A (see Appendix A).

On December 23, 2005, CanWest MediaWorks Publications Inc. filed suit in the Ontario Superior Court of Justice, arguing that these prohibitions were inconsistent with the Canadian *Charter of Rights and Freedoms*, and hence should be nullified (see Chapter 1, section 2.2.2, *Charter of Rights and Freedoms*). Its statement of claim in the Ontario Superior Court named the Attorney General of Canada as the defendant. At the time, CanWest published 10 major daily newspapers, plus another 23 smaller newspapers; it also owned the Global Television Network plus other specialty cable television channels. CanWest also objected to the fact that US magazines and television stations, which could be seen in Canada but were governed by US regulations, could publish such advertisements. CanWest wished to access that potentially profitable revenue source.

Other stakeholders soon weighed in, although not all became involved in the court case. Physicians and pharmacists, provincial and public payers, and consumers expressed a variety of differing opinions. Academics presented evidence that DTCA encouraged overuse of prescription medicines. Payers (both public and private) were concerned that pharmaceutical costs were high and growing (see Chapter 1, section 9.1, Canadian Data). However, although they worried that DTCA would further drive up costs, they did not become formally involved in the case. Workers covered by private drug plans were also worried that the viability of these plans might be threatened; indeed, several large unions were granted official intervenor status in the case. A related argument was that women might be particularly vulnerable, since much of this advertising targeted women. On the other side, the industry association for brand name drug manufacturers, Canada's Research-Based Pharmaceutical Companies (Rx&D), agreed with CanWest that the rules should be changed. It argued that DTCA would help ensure that patients, in consultation with their physicians, would have access to important information they would need to manage their health.

Supporters of DTCA claimed that it could benefit public health by educating the public, leading to earlier diagnosis and needed care of important illnesses, by improving patient compliance in taking prescribed medication, and by giving patients more autonomy to manage their own health care. Critics of DTCA focused their arguments on cost increases, the accuracy and appropriateness of drug advertising, and the underlying mission of advertising to sell products and make a profit. They argued that most advertisements had little or no educational value, left out important warnings and precautions, and made marketing claims which were not always supported by adequate evidence; they also raised concerns that patient demand might increase inappropriate prescribing (Hollon, 1999; Silversides, 2009). A systematic review in 2005 had found no evidence that DTCA led to health benefits (Gilbody et al., 2005).

The debate was not a new one. The Canadian federal government had already responded to the DTCA question through a series of studies, including a 1996 "consultation workshop." In March 2000, and again in February 2002, the federal government had introduced minimal changes to the DTCA regulations. It is now 2007. With CanWest heavily promoting the idea of DTCA, will Health Canada need to review this issue once again?

**Regulating DTCA**

In almost every country, including Canada, pharmaceutical drugs are regulated by the government. One key distinction is between prescription drugs, which must be prescribed by a physician, and non-prescription drugs (also called over-the-counter, or OTC, drugs), which are considered safe enough to be used directly by patients for conditions that do not need to be diagnosed by a physician. Like most countries, Canada does not permit prescription drugs to be sold until they have been approved by the appropriate governmental agency.

In Canada, the approval process is a federal responsibility. At the time of writing, the process was specified under Part C, Division 8 of the *Food and Drug Regulations*, and required the manufacturer to demonstrate the safety, efficacy, and quality of the product. This usually required that the manufacturer conduct (and pay for) a series of (expensive) clinical trials to generate the necessary data. Once a manufacturer has met Health Canada's regulatory requirements, it receives a Notice of Compliance (NOC). These products can be further subdivided into new drugs (sometimes called innovator drugs), which still have patent protection, and bio-equivalent products (generic drugs); generic drugs are products whose period of market exclusivity has expired and can thus be produced by competing companies.

Most pharmaceutical drugs are complex products which can have powerful effects on the body, both intended and unintended. People can have more than one health problem, and it is not uncommon for people to take multiple drugs. Their safe use often depends on clear written and spoken instructions to patients; these are often provided by physicians and/or pharmacists. Some patients may take an active role in this process, while others may have difficulty.

The purpose of the prohibition on DTCA for prescription drugs was to protect the purchasing consumer. Accordingly, false and misleading advertising is not allowed, nor is the advertising of any narcotic, or any drug before receiving its NOC from Health Canada. However, Health Canada does not actively monitor or enforce DTCA; it allows the industry to self-regulate. If problems or complaints arise, then Health Canada may (or may not) act. There are also questions relating to the quality of the evidence provided to those purchasing the drug (Mintzes, 2012).

The law makes a distinction between advertising and "other activities," which it defines as including non-promotional activities (such as disease education), "help-seeking" announcements that describe specific symptoms and encourage persons so affected to consult their doctors, as well as press releases about new research under development. The rules about DTCA of pharmaceuticals in Canada accordingly allowed two categories of advertisement. *Reminder ads* allowed companies to advertise a prescription medicine as long as they were careful not to state what the drug would be used for. *Help-seeking ads* allowed them to advertise that treatments were available for particular conditions as long as they did not mention a specific drug; these often used the tag line "Ask your doctor" (Mintzes et al., 2009). Increasingly, companies were running such ads. By late 1999, there were domestic billboards for Zyban (smoking cessation) and full-page, colour newspaper advertisements and transit posters supporting Xenical (anti-obesity). Ads for such products as Cialis (erectile dysfunction), Alesse (birth control), and others followed.

Detailed drug advertising is allowed in Canada if directed to health professionals; DTCA is somewhat more ambiguous. Health Canada (2010) has stated that it "supports and encourages the use of a voluntary health product advertising preclearance system that supports adherence to federal legislative requirements." This preclearance is done by recognized APAs (Advertising Preclearance Agencies) that Health Canada works with but explicitly "does not endorse." For prescription drugs, the recognized APAs in Canada include two voluntary agencies. The Pharmaceutical Advertising Advisory Board (PAAB) examines ads directed towards health professionals and attempts to ensure that they are accurate and balanced, while it and Advertising Standards Canada (ASC) can vet informational ads directed towards consumers. These bodies can give such ads a stamp of approval, or can express concerns. Thus, although the process is voluntary, there is a strong incentive for manufacturers to comply. Any DTCA is expected to be reviewed by at least one of these APAs to ensure that such advertisements follow the Canadian guidelines. As noted, although Health Canada has emphasized that it does not recognize or endorse these agencies, it does provide information about these preclearance agencies on its website, and states that the preclearance of advertising material by these arm's length agencies is highly recommended. Both PAAB and ASC charge preclearance fees for reviewing DTCA.

Globalization has added an additional complication, to the extent that information can flow across jurisdictional boundaries. International websites now allow those surfing the Internet to access US consumer information on drugs. American television stations and magazines are seen daily by Canadian cable and print subscribers, while pharmaceutical companies often sponsor disease agency websites (one example being the website of the Arthritis Society of Canada).

Among the arguments made in the CanWest case by Canadian media companies was that it was unfair that they could not capture any of this advertising revenue, and that Canadians were entitled to get information about pharmaceutical products. Both those for and against DTCA also brought up ethical issues, particularly as they related to the principles of autonomy, non-maleficence, and justice (see Chapter 1, section 3.6, Ethical Frameworks).

An interesting advertising parallel concerned tobacco. In a 1995 Charter case, the Supreme Court of Canada turned down the federal government's changes to the *Food and Drug Act* that disallowed all tobacco product advertising. In a split 5–4 decision, the court upheld a right to freedom of commercial communication. However, although some pharmaceutical companies used this decision to argue that DTCA should be allowed, other observers noted that the analogy might not hold. They also noted that the membership of the Supreme Court had changed somewhat since that decision.

### International Views

The costs of prescription drugs were increasing in many countries. Inflation-adjusted prescription drug expenditures per capita had doubled in Canada from $250/capita in 1995 to $600/capita in 2005, but had increased even more rapidly in the United States, from $250/ capita in 1995 to $1,000/capita in 2005 (Morgan, 2007). Payers wondered whether some of this difference was related to the flourishing of DTCA in the United States.

In the United States, some drug companies had been using reminder ads on television to promote their products; these ads provided very little information to consumers. One example was a set of advertisements that stated the names of particular drugs, accompanied by images of bright sunny meadows and the statement "At last, a clear day is here." These ads resembled Canadian "reminder ads"; they did not provide information about when these drugs should be used, or about their possible side effects. Accordingly, in 1997, the US Food and Drug Administration (FDA) issued new guidelines. These allowed full product advertising, including brand name, health claims, and major statements about side effects. They also relaxed provisions as to what constituted adequate provision for labelling information for broadcast DTCA as long as specified sources for further information were available (including toll-free telephone lines, websites, and/or printed material). In addition, they required that the advertisement must contain a major statement about side effects. This decision to relax the conditions regulating DTCA had led to a jump in spending on consumer advertising by pharmaceutical companies, from about US$1 billion in 1996 to US$4.2 billion by 2005 (Donohue et al., 2007; Morgan, 2007). Sales of these products increased. So did DTCA as a share of the total spent on promoting these products (Gagnon & Lexchin, 2008). As noted above, much of this US advertising could also be seen in Canada and Mexico because satellite and cable TV providers were not required to replace US ads. Canadian media companies felt that they should be able to get a share of this revenue.

Advocates of DTCA suggested that advertising was helpful because it could increase awareness of undiagnosed and undertreated diseases and thus improve public health. One paper cited examples of the effect advertising had on patient visits (Holmer, 1999). The Pharmaceutical Research Manufacturers of America (PhRMA) also argued that prescription drugs are a legal product, and that drug manufacturers have a right and a responsibility to inform people about their products.

The World Health Organization did not agree; it said that it did not believe prescription drugs should be advertised to the general public. At the time of writing, among OECD countries, only the United States and New Zealand permitted DTCA. A 2002 proposal by the European Commission to relax the ban on DTCA for three disease states (AIDS, asthma, and diabetes) had been rejected by the European Parliament and by the European Council in 2003. In April 2003, the New Zealand Medical Association had asked the government to prohibit DTCA of prescription medicine, although at the time of writing the government had responded with a consultation but little action. However, both the volume of and consumer exposure to these ads were much lower than in the United States (Mintzes, 2012).

**The Task Force**

A Canadian government committee was struck to develop an orderly plan to review the rules surrounding DTCA, and present a new regulatory structure (if needed) to the Federal/Provincial/Territorial Task Force on Drug Utilization, which would pass these recommendations on to the federal and provincial Ministers of Health. If the class wishes to use this case as a role play exercise, where the different stakeholders will provide input to the task force about their views of the pros and cons and the related health outcomes of DTCA in Canada, they may wish to select roles chosen from among as many of the following groups as seem appropriate.

*Government Groups*
- Federal government (including Health Canada, Industry Canada, and the Patented Medicine Prices Review Board)
- Provincial government (Ministries of Health from various provinces/territories)

*Professional Associations*
- Canadian Medical Association (physicians)
- Canadian Pharmacy Association (pharmacists)

*Others*
- Academics (including health policy and/or drug utilization experts)
- Canada's Research-Based Pharmaceutical Companies (Rx&D), the brand name manufacturers' trade association
- Canadian Drug Manufacturers' Association (trade association for generic drug manufacturers)

- Canadian Life & Health Insurance Association (representing private insurance industry that administers drug benefit plans for employed Canadians)
- Conference Board of Canada (representing employers who fund private drug plans)
- Consumers' Association of Canada (consumer advocacy)
- Media companies
- Pharmaceutical Advertising Advisory Board (independent review of advertising standards)

There were common interests across various groups (e.g., both public and private payers were all concerned that consumer-driven demand would increase costs), as well as tensions (e.g., brand name vs. generic manufacturers). However, personal relationships were quite strong; that "policy community" was relatively small in Canada, and many of the key players knew one another (see Chapter 1, section 4.2, Policy Communities).

The views of key groups are briefly indicated below.

**Stakeholder Perspectives**

*Supporting Full DTCA*

PHARMACEUTICAL INDUSTRY

The pharmaceutical industry, their advertising firms, and some media companies were strong advocates for more relaxed rules on consumer advertising. Rx&D, the industry association for brand name drug manufacturers, argued that the federal laws governing medication advertisements were written more than 40 years ago. These groups argued that Canadians would benefit from DTCA through increased awareness of disease symptoms and new treatment options. Rx&D also noted that Canadians were already affected by the US policies because they could see US media and the ads they carried. The Rx&D position paper cited a 1998 survey reporting that 78% of Canadians supported drug advertising that was monitored, regulated, and controlled, as well as other polls suggesting that most Canadians wanted more information about their medications.

MEDIA

Media companies noted that they could gain significant new advertising revenues from pharmaceutical companies. The editor of a Canadian women's magazine, *Chatelaine*, was quoted as saying, "Banning ads only infantilizes consumers, treating them as if they need to be protected from information they would misuse."

## Opposing Full DTCA

The organizations opposing DTCA included professional associations for physicians and pharmacists, government health ministries, and the Consumers' Association of Canada.

### CANADIAN MEDICAL ASSOCIATION (CMA)

The CMA referred to a policy on DTCA passed by their board of directors in 2002 (Canadian Medical Association, 2002). In it, the CMA argued that it supported objective, evidence-based, reliable plain-language information for the public about prescription drugs but opposed DTCA in Canada. They added that, in their view, current DTCA did not provide good information, but rather was a marketing ploy and sent the message that a prescription drug was a "consumer good" rather than a health care benefit (see Chapter 1, section 5.9, Insurance, Elasticity, and Moral Hazard). They expressed concern about negative impacts on the doctor-patient relationship, particularly if physicians refused patient requests for the advertised drug or were unaware of the drug at all, and also about the potential for increasing health costs and promoting inappropriate use of drugs. Physicians also expressed concern that DTCA would generate visits from patients to physicians ("ask your doctor"), leading to more and longer appointments that might or might not be appropriate. Depending on the payment model, this might or might not be profitable for physicians (see Chapter 1, section 6.2, Payment Mechanisms and Incentives). The CMA was also concerned about the need for busy physicians to keep up with the accuracy of information posted on the Internet.

### CANADIAN PHARMACISTS ASSOCIATION (CPHA)

Pharmacists argued that they were the most logical source for information about pharmaceuticals. They noted that their fee guide was moving to incorporate "cognitive services" as a reimbursable service; they defined this in terms of more consistent and higher-quality patient counselling and disease management services. Such services were reimbursed by public drug plans in five provinces, but rarely by private payers. In preparing for the 1996 federal workshop, the CPhA stated "its strong opposition" to DTCA; it believed that consumers were generally uninformed about their medications, and the association accordingly had strong concerns about patient safety and the additional cost burden to the system. If DTCA were to be permitted, the CPhA wanted offences punished first by fines and then by product withdrawal. On the matter of educating patients, the CPhA proposed that patient groups, governments, pharmaceutical manufacturers, and health care providers should develop objective information about pharmaceuticals and disseminate this information broadly in plain language. They noted that, although some provinces would reimburse pharmacists for such cognitive services as patient counselling as well as for dispensing drugs, the criteria were stringent and the amounts often low. One example, which began in 2007, was Ontario's MedsCheck program. Initially, it applied only to patients who were taking at least three chronic medications; the pharmacist would be reimbursed $50, once per year, for reviewing the chronic medications, although the program has since expanded somewhat (Ministry of Health and Long-Term Care, 2011). CPhA declared that they had a strong interest in consumer education and improving communication between health providers and patients.

CONSUMERS' ASSOCIATION OF CANADA (CAC)
The CAC made a distinction between "persuasive advertising" (which it opposed) and "balanced information" (which it supported). It expressed concerns that advertising might encourage misuse and overuse of medications. However, the CAC also advocated for patient involvement in personal health decisions and health policy development, in collaboration with health professionals. It also suggested that consumers might have different interests in their role of patient (where gaining access to new medications might be desirable) and as taxpayers. In its 2001 submission to the Commission on the Future of Health Care in Canada (Romanow Commission), CAC had maintained its position that the existing prohibition on DTCA should be maintained.

OTHER CONSUMER GROUPS
A related movement was the move towards empowered consumers, particularly given the availability of information through the Internet. Report cards in the United States, patient satisfaction surveys in Europe, and hospital scorecards in Ontario were among the manifestations of this new emphasis on accountability. A wide variety of other consumer groups existed, some of which took positions on DTCA. Most such

groups were linked to particular diseases. The positions varied. Some of these groups were even funded in part by the pharmaceutical industry, while others were highly suspicious of prescription drugs.

## Policy Options

In terms of policy options, it was suggested that Health Canada might, depending on the product, either continue with the status quo of limited prohibition based on types of information (e.g., name, quantity, price) and/or select various combinations of: general prohibition; limited prohibition based on time (e.g., not allowing DTCA for the first two years a drug is on the market, to allow more time to assess the safety of the product); allowing the industry to self-regulate with criteria for balanced presentation of drug information; requiring regulatory preclearance (e.g., by Health Canada or PAAB or ASC or both); and/or allowing information dissemination and treating prescription drugs like any other consumer good.

DECISION POINT

You are the chair of the task force. What do you recommend?

SUGGESTED QUESTIONS FOR DISCUSSION

1. What are your options? Discuss the advantages and disadvantages of each. Discuss regulation as a policy instrument.
2. Discuss the various conflicting policy goals, and how these relate to individual autonomy and the role of the state. How would you balance such issues of freedom of speech, public safety, and costs?
3. Discuss the role of interests, and the views (and influence) of such stakeholder groups as: pharmaceutical manufacturers (new products, generics), physicians, pharmacists, federal government, provincial governments, private payers, consumers, Pharmaceutical Advertising Advisory Board (PAAB), Advertising Standards Canada (ASC), and media.
4. Discuss how these issues might be framed.
5. Discuss the role of jurisdictions, particularly given electronic new media. How does this relate to the scope of conflict?

APPENDIX A: REGULATORY STRUCTURES

**Advertising Preclearance Agencies**

The Pharmaceutical Advertising Advisory Board (PAAB) is an independent review agency founded in 1976 whose primary role is to ensure that advertising of prescription drugs is accurate, balanced, and evidence-based.

Advertising Standards Canada (ASC) is a non-profit, self-regulatory body founded in 1957 whose primary role is to foster community confidence in advertising and to ensure the integrity and viability of advertising in Canada. ASC facilitates regulatory compliance by providing a fee-based service to industry to help them pre-review their advertising copy.

For other advertisements that would not be classified as DTCA, both PAAB's and ASC's major roles are to: maintain a Code of Advertising Acceptance; preclear advertising prior to publication or broadcasting; and encourage code compliance by monitoring ads, adjudicating complaints, reporting infractions, and administering penalties.

There are three major differences in processes for DTCA as compared to advertisements for other products: (1) the term advertisement cannot be used, because advertising prescription drugs to Canadians is illegal; (2) manufacturers can, on a voluntary basis, provide "non-promotional information" submissions to PAAB requesting advice to determine whether they are in compliance with Health Canada guidelines; and (3) complaints are handled only by Health Canada, rather than by PAAB or ASC.

The PAAB code includes advertising of prescription and OTC products to health professionals in all media, including Internet advertising. PAAB also reviews veterinary medicine journal advertising and provides advisory comments on direct-to-consumer materials for prescription drugs. ASC reviews advertising of OTC, cosmetics, and alcoholic products to consumers in all media and print advertising. ASC is not responsible for reviewing veterinary medicine advertising to consumers.

The organizations that were members of PAAB and represented on its board included: Association of Faculties of Medicine of Canada; Association of Medical Advertising Agencies; Canadian Association of Medical Publishers; Canadian Generic Pharmaceutical Association; Canadian Medical Association; Canadian Pharmacists Association; Best Medicines Coalition; Consumer Health Products Canada; Canada's Research-Based Pharmaceutical Companies (Rx&D); CARP (an advocacy group for seniors); and Fédération des médecins spécialistes du Québec (FMSQ) (Pharmaceutical Advertising Advisory Board, 2010).

The members of ASC were listed on their website (Advertising Standards Canada, 2011); most were in industries other than those associated with health care. The Therapeutic Products Directorate (Health Protection Branch), Health Canada, was an ex officio observer to the board of directors.

### The PAAB and ASC Framework for DTCA

PAAB was viewed sometimes as not being independent from the pharmaceutical industry. Although preclearance can be helpful, if enforcement is weak and the punishment is not sufficient, many argue that self-regulation will not work. In 1999, the then–Interim Commissioner of the PAAB, Ray Chepesiuk, argued that the existing approach to drug advertising was unsustainable. He suggested that consumers wanted more pharmaceutical and treatment information in order to make informed decisions, and that individual nations would be limited in their ability to control the flow of information by globalization and the treaties and trade agreements accompanying it. Chepesiuk recommended that DTCA have: an effective regulatory and review agency (perhaps the PAAB); plain-language, comprehensive risk information; a six-month deferral of advertising to allow physicians to become conversant with new medications; a mandatory message about the physician's role, and enforceable standards, especially with respect to comparative claims. Rx&D further suggested that such ads should also include information on alternative, reputable information sources, but specifically disallow comparative advertising between like products.

### The PAAB Complaints Process (for non-DTCA)

Complaints may be lodged by: health professionals, health care organizations, pharmaceutical companies, federal and provincial regulatory bodies, and drug payer organizations. For non-DTCA advertisements, PAAB has three different levels of administrative response. In stage one, the complaint is sent directly to the advertiser by the complainant or to the advertiser via the PAAB commissioner. The advertiser responds in writing to the complainant. The complainant then has three options: continue discussion with the advertiser; accept the advertiser's response; or seek review by the PAAB commissioner in stage two. Either the complainant or advertiser has the right to appeal the commissioner's reassessment ruling to a stage three independent review panel made up of three qualified individuals selected by the commissioner from individuals named by national organizations.

### ASC Complaints Process (for non-DTCA)

ASC may also receive complaints from health care professionals, advertisers, pharmaceutical companies, and consumers. ASC will investigate the complaint and may sometimes act as the "middleman" between the complainant and the advertiser to resolve the complaint. If it is a consumer complaint, then the Consumer Response Councils (composed of volunteer representatives from the advertising industry and the public) adjudicate the complaints with the goal of ensuring an objective, balanced, and fair process.

### PAAB and ASC Complaints Process for DTCA

Both PAAB and ASC may receive complaints from difference sources, review and clear advertising material, and conduct complaints adjudication. Health Canada retains ultimate authority for compliance and enforcement in relation to drug advertising, and to provide advice and guidance relating to advertising activities to these bodies as required. The independent agencies are expected to obtain voluntary compliance in the case of some types of advertising violations; where this fails, the issue can be referred to Health Canada.

### Health Canada's Role

Health Canada is the national regulatory authority for health product advertisements. They provide policies to effectively regulate marketed health products, put in place guidelines for the interpretation of the regulations, and oversee regulated advertising activities. They are committed to ensuring that information in a health product advertisement is not false, misleading, or deceptive. They may intervene when an advertisement poses a significant safety concern, in the event that resolution is not achieved through the independent agencies' complaints mechanism, when a prescription drug is illegally advertised to the general public, and/or when an unauthorized health product is promoted. However, if complaints do end up with Health Canada, the response to complaints tends to be slow; some observers suggest that this may reflect Health Canada's undercapacity to regulate DTCA.

The Health Canada website includes an overview for physicians on regulation of health products advertising in Canada. It notes that advertising is defined broadly to include "any representation by any means whatever for the purpose of promoting directly or indirectly the sale or disposal of any food, drug, cosmetic or device." It attempts to distinguish between advertising and information. Advertising must "comply with the advertising provisions of the Food and Drugs Act and associated regulations." Section 9(1) of the *Food and Drugs Act* prohibits false, misleading, or deceptive advertising of drugs; section 20(1) similarly prohibits misleading advertising for medical devices. An additional provision, Section 3(1), prohibits consumer-directed ads for health products (including medical devices) which make claims to treat, prevent, or cure any of the serious diseases listed in Schedule A to the *Act*; however, prevention (although not treatment or cure) claims are permitted by regulation for over-the-counter drugs and natural health products. The conditions listed in Schedule A are: acute alcoholism; acute anxiety state; acute infectious respiratory syndromes; acute, inflammatory, and debilitating arthritis; acute psychotic conditions; addiction (except nicotine addiction); appendicitis; arteriosclerosis; asthma; cancer; congestive heart failure; convulsions; dementia; depression; diabetes; gangrene; glaucoma; haematologic bleeding disorders; hepatitis; hypertension; nausea and vomiting of pregnancy; obesity; rheumatic fever; septicaemia; sexually transmitted diseases; strangulated hernia; thrombotic and embolic disorders; thyroid disease; and ulcer of the gastro-intestinal tract (Department of Justice Canada, 1985).

Section C.01.044 of the *Food and Drug Regulations* prohibits consumer-directed prescription drug advertising beyond the drug's name, price, and quantity, which means that advertisements for prescription drugs directed towards consumers that mention the name of the drug cannot mention its therapeutic use and/or benefits. Section C.08.002(1) prohibits any advertising of new drugs before they are authorized for sale by Health Canada.

APPENDIX B: REFERENCES CITED AND FURTHER READING

Advertising Standards Canada. (2011). *Advertising Standards Canada: Home.* http://www.adstandards.com/en/

Canadian Medical Association. (2002). *Direct-to-consumer advertising (DTCA).* http://policybase.cma.ca/dbtw-wpd/PolicyPDF/PD03-01.pdf

Department of Justice Canada. (1985). *Food and Drugs Act*. R.S. c.F-27. http://laws-lois.justice.gc.ca/eng/acts/F%2D27/

Donohue, J.M., Cevasco, M., & Rosenthal, M.B. (2007). A decade of direct-to-consumer advertising of prescription drugs. *New England Journal of Medicine, 357*(7), 673–81. http://dx.doi.org/10.1056/NEJMsa070502

Gagnon, M.-A., & Lexchin, J. (2008). The cost of pushing pills: A new estimate of pharmaceutical promotion expenditures in the United States. *PLoS Medicine, 5*(1), 1–5. http://dx.doi.org/10.1371/journal.pmed.0050001

Gilbody, S., Wilson, P., & Watt, I. (2005). Benefits and harms of direct to consumer advertising: A systematic review. *Quality & Safety in Health Care, 14*(4), 246–50. http://dx.doi.org/10.1136/qshc.2004.012781

Health Canada. (2010). *Guidance document: Health Canada and advertising pre-clearance agencies' roles related to health product advertising*. http://www.hc-sc.gc.ca/dhp-mps/advert-publicit/pol/role_apa-pca-eng.php

Hollon, M.F. (1999). Direct-to-consumer marketing of prescription drugs: Creating consumer demand. *Journal of the American Medical Association, 281*(4), 382–4. http://dx.doi.org/10.1001/jama.281.4.382

Holmer, A.F. (1999). Direct-to-consumer prescription drug advertising builds bridges between patients and physicians. *Journal of the American Medical Association, 281*(4), 380–2. http://dx.doi.org/10.1001/jama.281.4.380

Ministry of Health and Long-Term Care. (2011). *MedsCheck: About MedsCheck*. http://www.health.gov.on.ca/en/public/programs/drugs/medscheck/medscheck_original.aspx

Mintzes, B. (2012). Advertising of prescription-only medicines to the public: Does evidence of benefit counterbalance harm? *Annual Review of Public Health, 33*(1), 259–77. http://dx.doi.org/10.1146/annurev-publhealth-031811-124540

Mintzes, B., Morgan, S., & Wright, J.M. (2009). Twelve years' experience with direct-to-consumer advertising of prescription drugs in Canada: A cautionary tale. *PLoS ONE, 4*(5), e5699. http://dx.doi.org/10.1371/journal.pone.0005699

Morgan, S.G. (2007). Direct-to-consumer advertising and expenditures on prescription drugs: A comparison of experiences in the United States and Canada. *Open Medicine, 1*(1), E37–45.

Pharmaceutical Advertising Advisory Board. (2010). *Members/Directors*. http://www.paab.ca/members.htm

Silversides, A. (2009). Charter challenge of ban on direct-to-consumer advertising to be heard by Ontario court in mid-June. *Canadian Medical Association Journal, 181*(1–2), e5–6. http://dx.doi.org/10.1503/cmaj.091050

# 17 Rehabilitating Auto Insurance

*PAUL HOLYOKE, MARIE BALITBIT, LEE TASKER,
AND RAISA B. DEBER*

Auto insurance is compulsory in Ontario, and there are many insurers who offer to sell it to the general public. The 2011 Auditor General's Report has noted that, compared to other provinces, Ontario drivers paid much higher premiums and had a higher average injury claim. Various stakeholders pointed to such issues as the likelihood of fraud, the extent to which those injured received benefits, and the rate of return paid to insurance companies. What should the government do?

This case addresses several policy issues, including: insurance and moral hazard, policy/governing instruments (including regulation), and coverage for services falling outside the *Canada Health Act* requirements.

## Appendices

Appendix A: Concepts and Principles of Insurance
Appendix B: The Automobile Insurance System in Ontario
Appendix C: References Cited and Further Reading

## The Case

Who should bear the financial consequences of loss, damage, or injury arising from motor vehicle accidents (MVAs)? Such costs may roughly be divided into the costs associated with property damage (i.e., repairing the damage to the vehicles and other property they hit) and the costs associated with bodily injury (medical care, rehabilitation, etc.). These losses may be monetary, or can also include non-economic costs (e.g., pain and suffering).

One potential answer relates to who was responsible for the damages. Were the costs incurred by the party at fault, or by an "innocent" third party? *No-fault* models require that damages be paid by the person incurring the loss (and/or his or her insurer), regardless of why the accident happened. In contrast, *fault*, or *tort-based*, models may require victims to go to court to prove that the other driver was at fault before they can be reimbursed for their costs. Various combinations are also possible. For example, models may require that the victim and/or his or her insurer pay costs up to a set limit, and/or may restrict use of the courts to *severe* cases (often defined in terms of meeting a definition of severe impairment or injury). Different insurance models may also cap damages, limit what expenses can be claimed, and/or require co-payments or deductibles.

To help protect victims (particularly those not at fault), most jurisdictions have made automobile insurance compulsory for anyone wishing to operate a vehicle on public roads. There is considerable debate about how much profit insurers should make for providing this service. By definition, profit-making bodies have an incentive to charge the highest rates that the market will bear. Some provinces, including British Columbia, Manitoba, Saskatchewan, and Quebec, have chosen to use a public auto insurance system. Others, including Ontario, rely on private insurers (see Chapter 1, section 6.1.1, Public and Private). Provinces also vary in how much coverage is required, leaving drivers the option to purchase additional coverage should they so desire.

However, the logic of insurance (see Appendix A, and Chapter 1, section 5.9, Insurance, Elasticity, and Moral Hazard) would imply that insurers would be reluctant to cover people likely to be high-cost. Actuarial considerations might accordingly imply that higher-risk groups (where risk might be defined in terms of their age and sex, where they live, how much they drive, and/or the vehicle they drive, as well as their driving record) would be charged higher rates. Some of these distinctions may be seen as valid by the public, while others may not be. Particularly when insurance is compulsory, most governments have set up regulatory bodies to control what insurers can and cannot do (see Chapter 1, section 5.2.1, Regulation).

### The Ontario Experience

In 2011, Ontario had about 9 million licensed drivers, and about 7.5 million passenger cars and trucks (Office of the Auditor General of

Ontario, 2011). Auto insurance has been compulsory for Ontario drivers since 1980. The auto insurance market is also heavily regulated; at the time of the case, responsibility rested with the Financial Services Commission of Ontario (FSCO), an agency of the provincial Ministry of Finance. More than 100 private-sector companies offered auto insurance, with about 20 holding about 75% of the market. See Appendix B for additional information about automobile insurance in Ontario.

What insurance people are obliged to buy and sell in Ontario has changed dramatically over time. Between 1989 and 1996, successive Ontario governments led by the Liberals (Premier David Peterson, 1985–90), NDP (Bob Rae, 1990–5), and Progressive Conservatives (Mike Harris, 1995–2002) had each imposed major changes on Ontario's auto insurance policyholders, auto insurance companies, and regulators. Each change was preceded by at least a year or two of double-digit percentage increases in average premium rates. Each time, the resulting reform induced modest decreases in premiums for a short time, followed by another jump in rates.

The insurance model has accordingly varied. Prior to 1990, Ontario had used a tort-based auto insurance system, which required victims of MVAs to go to court to recover damages if they could prove that another driver was at fault. The damages that the courts could award were subdivided into economic losses (e.g., lost wages, the cost of repairs to a vehicle) and non-economic losses, such as pain and suffering. In Canada, the *Canada Health Act* (see Chapter 1, section 7.2, *Canada Health Act*) requires that the provincial/territorial health insurance plans fully cover all medically necessary hospital and doctor costs for all legal residents, but does not require coverage of such services as outpatient rehabilitation or outpatient pharmaceuticals, although provinces/territories can choose to do so. This meant that basic hospital and doctor costs for residents would be covered by the provincial/territorial insurance plan regardless of whether a victim sued. Some provinces accordingly included a provision that, in the case of a successful lawsuit, the provincial insurance plan would have a right to receive a portion of the proceeds of the lawsuit to cover its costs (referred to as "subrogation"). Any additional goods or services a victim might need, including outpatient rehabilitation, were to be paid out of the settlement he or she received from the lawsuit. This litigation-based system sometimes led to large settlements, but also could result in delays in treatment until the lawsuits were decided. Year-over-year premium increases were often in the double digits, with much of this going to pay legal costs. Another approach (which Ontario employed at the time of writing) was to require the insurance industry to pay the province a set amount intended to reimburse the government for the publicly funded hospital and physician services used by MVA accident victims.

The 1987–9 price increases in auto insurance premiums led the provincial Liberal government to move to a "no-fault" Ontario Motorist Protection Plan (OMPP) in June 1990. The OMPP eliminated the right to sue in court and the need to prove "fault" except in cases where a victim could show his or her injuries exceeded a "threshold" of "permanent" and "serious" injury. Those whose damages fell below that threshold and could not sue had a right to claim against their own insurer for three categories of regulated benefits, referred to as Statutory Accident Benefits: (1) medical, rehabilitation, and care benefits; (2) funeral and death benefits; and (3) weekly loss-of-income benefits. Medically necessary hospital and doctor costs were still paid by the provincial health insurance plan, but the provincial plan no longer had the right to recover its costs if the victim sued. Removing these costs from insurers led to a decline in premiums in 1990 and 1991, but by 1993 premiums started to increase again. Since 1993, Ontario's regulators have also required automobile insurers to sell auto insurance to just about anyone who applies for it, as long as they have an Ontario driver's license; this has been called the Take All Comers rule.

In January 1994, the NDP provincial government modified the OMPP to include a number of provisions, including obliging insurers to start paying benefits sooner (within 10 days of receiving a claim) and to pay significantly higher medical and rehabilitation benefits. A multifaceted dispute resolution process was instituted. The first step was to set up Designated Assessment Centres (DACs) to act as neutral assessors of victims' health status and treatment plans; opponents suggested that they were an additional (and costly) layer of bureaucracy. Should insurers or victims disagree with the DAC decision, they would have access to optional conciliation and arbitration services provided by the Ontario Insurance Commission (now called the Financial Services Commission of Ontario, or FSCO). The courts were still available for lawsuits should the DACS and the arbitrators fail to reach agreement, but only for victims with "permanent" and "serious" injuries. Hospital and doctor costs were paid out by the provincial health insurance plan regardless of whether there was a lawsuit, but the province now had a right to recover its costs if the victim sued. These modifications were not fully successful. Instead, higher costs for rehabilitation and treatment, plus the costs of dispute resolution, and suspicions that fraudulent activities were occurring led to double-digit increases in premiums, particularly in 1994 and 1995.

In November 1996, the Progressive Conservative (PC) provincial government changed the insurance model again. Its legislation instituted a basic auto insurance policy that was fairly similar to the pre-1994 coverage, and allowed consumers to choose whether they wished to purchase additional coverage. There were also measures to reduce fraud and abuse and to ensure appropriate treatment. All victims once again had the right to sue for a broader range of economic damages as long as they met a "catastrophic injury" threshold. As before, hospital and doctor costs were paid by the provincial insurance plan. However, rather than use subrogation to recover payments awarded to victims with successful lawsuits, auto insurers as a collective group were now obliged to make a special payment of $80 million per year to the government; the payment was prorated among insurers by their share of auto insurance premiums. Insurance premiums did decline 12% between 1996 and 1999, but then started to rise again. By the end of the third quarter of 2003, the average cost of insurance was 19.43% higher than a year prior, and 27.67% higher than it had been in late 1996.

The reactions to this round of premium increases included one measure to reduce costs for insurers; in 2000, the PC provincial government announced that the 5% retail sales tax on auto insurance premiums would be gradually phased out. It would be cut by 1% per year, which meant that that tax would be totally eliminated by April 1, 2004. Another set of initiatives, introduced in 2001, were anti-fraud measures; these required benefit claimants to be examined under oath if there was reasonable concern about accident circumstances, and required victims and their health professionals to sign treatment plans.

Beginning in 2000, the Ontario Physiotherapy Association had taken the lead in initiating the formation of the Coalition of Regulated Health Professional Associations and Allied Organizations. The coalition argued that one reason for rising premiums was red tape; it was accordingly set up to negotiate collectively with the insurance industry and government, and to come to collective solutions about fees and costs. Those negotiations eventually led to an agreement that was announced by the PC government in July 2003, for implementation on October 1, 2003, to introduce "Pre-Approved Frameworks" for treatment for whiplash injuries (the most common auto accident injury); such a framework would allow victims to proceed directly to treatment within strict guidelines for these injuries without having to seek pre-approval from their insurers. Another indication of the efforts of providers and insurers to work together was a joint website developed by the Health Care Coalition and the Insurance Bureau of Canada (IBC), the insurance industry's trade association, to publicize the achievements they had made and to show the results of their joint work in containing costs.

The insurers, however, remained concerned. In May 2001, the heads of some of Ontario's biggest insurers had said that the main reason for the need for large premium rate increases was competition among insurers, leading to overly low prices being charged for policies, particularly given the high costs they faced to pay claims. George Cooke, CEO of Dominion of Canada General Insurance Company, had argued that companies had hidden this because they had enjoyed good returns in the stock and bond markets, but that "companies have been fighting for market share at the expense of sound underwriting." The industry suggested that the barriers to entry in the industry were too low. In 2001, the provincial Ministry of Finance had started a relatively low-key consultation designed to examine potential solutions to rising premium rates. In its brief to the government, the IBC had pointed out that cars were pervasive in Ontario society, and that more people paid car insurance premiums than paid taxes in the province. It added that car insurance, with an average annual premium of $913, constituted a major expenditure in almost every household, but that "consumers will find it difficult to understand why their car insurance premiums have been squandered on dubious medical and rehabilitation services over the years."

The IBC said that the highly competitive nature of the auto insurance business, with over 150 insurers licensed to do business in Ontario, "has kept premiums artificially low." The cost to drivers were said to be: huge increases in health care claims, which rose from about $300 million in 1991 to over $1 billion in 2000 (this included the cost of assessments at DACs and related expenses, estimated to be about $150 million in 2001 and $220 million in 2002), and the rising costs for auto repairs, which it attributed to increases in the costs of parts and labour, the increasing complexity of cars, and the cost of towing and storing damaged cars. Because the IBC did not think that insurers had the market power to be able to reduce costs through negotiations with the health providers, it had advocated: imposing maximum fees for health care providers; allowing insurers to dispute treatment more easily in the first weeks after an accident; prohibiting all people except nurses, occupational therapists, physiotherapists, and physicians from being "case managers" for those with injuries; making health professionals accountable for their treatment recommendations; giving the government regulation-making power over treatments because "health care cost issues require [giving] the government [such] authority to grapple with the emerging issues"; abandoning the existing DAC system that cost $150 million a year; allowing fast-track DACs; allowing increased access to the courts for certain victims; ensuring that other, nonauto insurers were paying their "fair share" as first payers; and streamlining the way FSCO approved new rates.

In 2003, the Association of Designated Assessment Centres (ADAC) commissioned a study by management consulting firm Deloitte & Touche to address complaints about the DAC system, particularly quality and cost issues, and to make recommendations for improvements. The study concluded that the costs of the DAC system were not as great as insurers had claimed, but agreed that improvements could be made to streamline paper flow and to develop closer collaboration with stakeholders, particularly insurers.

## Auto Insurance as an Election Issue

The cost of auto insurance was an issue not only in Ontario. New Brunswick had held a provincial election in the spring of 2003. Although the Premier and leader of the Progressive Conservatives (PCs), Bernard Lord, had not addressed the issue of high and rising auto insurance premiums at the beginning of the campaign because he did not see it as a big issue, the other parties and the public had a different view. Stories about people in remote areas of NB not being able to drive their cars any more, and about the size of some people's premium rate increases, had stirred major discussions, and the issue came to dominate the campaign. In reacting, Lord first said that he would cut benefits, but then announced he would freeze rates and seek policy options after the election. On Election Day, June 9, the PCs came one seat away from defeat, with some observers suggesting this may have been related to their neglect of the issue of the cost of car insurance.

Automobile insurance rates were also an issue in Ontario's October 2003 election. Premier Harris had resigned for personal reasons in 2002, and had been replaced as Premier by former Minister of Finance Ernie Eves. The government was also dealing with the aftermath of the Walkerton tragedy (see Chapter 5, Trouble on Tap).

In June 2003, Ontario's PC government called an election; voters would go to the polls on October 2, 2003. In an effort to pre-empt the issue of auto insurance prior to the campaign, it had issued a white paper in July, discussing various options it was considering for bringing rates into line, including reining in health care spending and fraud. The white paper outlined the following causes the authors believed were leading to premium increases: (1) the average cost of repairs to cars had increased by 34% from 1998 to 2002, reflecting more purchases of more expensive vehicles, including light trucks and sport utility vehicles (SUVs); (2) health care costs had risen from $200 million in 1990 to $540 million in 1996 (170% increase over 1990 costs), and then again to $1.5 billion in 2002 (177% increase over 1996 costs); (3) higher costs of fraud in the system, estimated to be approximately 15% of costs; and (4) lower returns from investments during the stock market slump of 2000–3. The government outlined the steps it had already taken to control premium rates, including: the introduction of the Pre-Approved Frameworks for whiplash; restricting the use of medical examinations by insurers; prohibiting cash settlements for accident benefits until one year had passed so that injured people continued to get treatment and income replacement benefits; establishing a code of conduct for paralegals who helped car accident victims get benefits; defining unfair or deceptive acts or practices to apply to health care providers and paralegals in the auto insurance system; and increasing deductibles for pain and suffering awards in lawsuits. The white paper also sought the public's views on various means for further reducing premiums.

The opposition Liberal Party had promised their own set of reforms, with a goal of reducing auto insurance premiums by 10%–20%. During the 2003 campaign, the Liberal Party had argued that the standardized auto insurance product was not flexible enough, and required individuals to pay for coverage that they did not need or want. They also said that some premium hikes had been made by insurers on spurious grounds; for example, when a not-at-fault driver was involved in an accident or was issued an NSF cheque, his or her insurer sometimes increased the premiums. Another complaint was that insurers sometimes overemphasized geographic boundaries in rate setting. More fundamentally, the Liberals believed that the Designated Assessment Centres only repeated an auto accident victim's primary health provider's assessment of health needs, and therefore the DACs constituted a complete redundancy of effort and cost. They therefore called for the abolition of DACs. Fraud and conflict of interest (health professionals' self-referrals and kickbacks for referrals) were also pointed out as significant issues. The New Democratic Party advocated setting up publicly operated, not-for-profit auto insurance.

Stakeholders also weighed in. The Ontario Brain Injury Association (OBIA) had made a presentation to the Liberal Party's Insurance Committee on July 31, 2003. It argued that the crisis in auto insurance was not because of the costs of health care, adding that it was important to support the DAC system to ensure consumers had somewhere to go to get unbiased opinions and to get the medical and rehabilitation benefits they needed when challenged by their insurers. It also recommended not moving forward with treatment guidelines (such as the Pre-Approved Frameworks for whiplash) because these guidelines could turn quickly from "recovery recommendations" to "treatment barriers."

In September 2003, the Consumers' Association of Canada had released a study that it had conducted on the cost of auto insurance across Canada. Among its key findings were the following: (1) public auto insurance systems offered the lowest rates for consumers; (2) Toronto consumers paid the highest rates in Canada; (3) Ontario's rates were much higher than the rates in western provinces who used public auto insurance models; (4) Quebec's rates were much lower than Ontario's rates; and (5) under private auto systems, good young male drivers paid more than bad older drivers with high-priced vehicles, which seemed unfair.

### Government Action and the Reaction

On September 18, 2003, FSCO had taken health care providers by surprise and issued a guideline specifying maximum fees that insurers could be obliged to pay for treatment by health professionals; these fees were 30% less than the previously allowed fees. The PCs, in mid-campaign, claimed responsibility for these fee cuts and for the lower auto insurance premium rates that they expected would result.

According to the Ontario Physiotherapy Association (OPA), the Liberal Party indicated that, if elected, they would not implement the fee schedule announced by FSCO on September 18 and would immediately engage the health care professions in fee negotiations. The OPA said, "If the fees announced on September 18th are implemented, many practitioners will simply be unable to treat MVA patients and MVA patients will have increasing difficulty obtaining timely and appropriate care.

Ironically, the situation will generate additional costs for insurers and the health-care system generally as acute problems become chronic."

The Progressive Conservative government was defeated on October 2, 2003, and the Liberals, led by Dalton McGuinty, formed the Ontario government. The new government made a number of changes, including eliminating the DAC system as of March 1, 2006, and instead relying on the assessment made by the claimant's own health care provider. When the insurer disagreed, the case would be referred to FSCO's dispute resolution system. Another element was to incorporate a no-fault component, whereby victims of a MVA would be reimbursed by their own insurance company up to a fixed level for health care costs and wage losses; if the costs exceeded that level, victims could still sue the at-fault driver to recover these (as well as non-economic awards for pain and suffering). As a result of these changes, premiums stabilized, but then increased again.

In September 2010, a new series of reforms reduced the mandatory minimum benefits, made some coverage optional, and capped the costs for assessments (at $2,000 per assessment) and the benefits for specified minor injuries (at $3,500).

**The Issue of Fraud**

An additional issue was the extent to which insurance rates were being increased by organized fraud. Disquieting stories began to emerge about organized fraud rings. In the most egregious cases, criminal organizations who controlled body shops, towing companies, and/or physiotherapy clinics recruited participants to stage collisions (often driving vehicles obtained from salvage yards that had been written off as scrap after another accident) and to file claims. Early on, concern had been expressed that Ontario's requirement to pay benefits within 14 days left little time to scrutinize dubious claims (Baer, 1997). The extent to which health professionals were involved in fraud was also unclear. Regulators were faced with a trade-off between denying or delaying legitimate claims, and allowing fraudulent ones.

Two trends were visible. The number of people being killed and injured in motor vehicle accidents had declined significantly (by about 25% over the 10-year period ending 2009). At the same time, claims were climbing, with the average injury claim in Ontario ($56,000) being five times the average claim in other provinces, with premiums accordingly being far higher. Two 2011 reports highlighted the concerns. The

Office of the Auditor General of Ontario (2011) issued a report on auto insurance regulatory oversight. A related report was issued by a task force set up by the Ministry of Finance (Ontario Auto Insurance Anti-Fraud Task Force, 2011). Both concluded that fraud was now a major concern. Another cost driver noted by the Auditor General was the "reasonable rate of return" set in 1996 by FSCO at 12%; this had not been adjusted down to reflect decreases in long-term bond rates.

DECISION POINT

What should the Ontario government do to make good on its promise to reduce automobile insurance premiums?

SUGGESTED QUESTIONS FOR DISCUSSION

1. Why is the government obliged to do anything at all? What interest generally should the state have in insurance? How does this relate to ideas about the role of the state?
2. Does the state's interest and role in insurance vary with different types of insurance (e.g., health care, property damage, income replacement)?
3. Discuss the consequences of competition in an insurance market. Are there natural monopolies? What is the role of community rating? What is the role of the Take All Comers rule? What would the likely consequences of a fully competitive free market in insurance be?
4. What policy instruments are available to a government that wants to do something about insurance? Give examples of how the various instruments could be applied in this case.
5. How have the various interest groups framed the issue in this case and what options do or might they support?

APPENDIX A: CONCEPTS AND PRINCIPLES OF INSURANCE

Insurance is a very important feature of all market economies. The fundamental principle of insurance is *pooling of risk*, whereby the financial consequences of loss or peril are spread by an insurer across the members of the pool, so that those who actually incur the risk can be reimbursed for all or part of their losses. *Underwriting* refers to the overall process of examining risks, deciding whether they can be insured, and, if they can, working out how much would need to be collected.

The definition of the pool by the insurer is called *risk selection*. Once the insurer makes a decision about the pool to be covered, the costs that result when a risk materializes may be equally distributed across all people in the pool or the insurer may decide to spread the costs unequally across the pool, according to the proportion of risk each member brings. The amount of money each person contributes to the pool is often called a *premium*. (In contrast, government-run plans may choose to finance these costs through taxation rather than through premiums.)

There are many ways of setting premiums. One possibility is often called *community rating* and means that everyone is charged the same premium for the same coverage. However, if there are differences in the costs of claims by subgroups, insurers may wish to differentiate and charge higher premiums to higher-risk subgroups, or even deny them coverage. One ongoing policy issue is when such differentiation is acceptable. For example, should all unmarried males under age 25 be charged higher rates because, on average, this group experiences a significantly increased risk of loss? Is this fair to young men who drive safely? If the insurer wants to set premiums on a group basis rather than at the community level, each group's risk level and expected claims costs are taken into account and a premium is set for each group. Selecting who should be included in a group is therefore very important.

*Moral hazard* refers to situations where one party is insulated from the consequences of his/her decisions (see Chapter 1, section 5.9, Insurance, Elasticity, and Moral Hazard). It is a major issue in insurance, since moral hazard introduces several disquieting possibilities for an insurer. These may include: (1) the risk has already materialized for a person who purchases a policy and the purchaser is finding someone to subsidize already-existing costs – for example, if one has already had an accident, one may wish to find someone to help pay for repairing the automobile; (2) the insured person will make the risk materialize to get the policy's benefits – for example, a person may burn down a money-losing business to collect the insurance; and/or (3) the insured person will increase his or her estimate of damages after the occurrence of the event to get more benefits under the insurance policy. Moral hazard may also affect providers, particularly if they are the ones who determine what services are required. For example, tow truck drivers and repair shops may exaggerate the level of service needed to repair a damaged car. Similarly, health professionals (including physicians and rehabilitation providers) are usually the ones who decide what care is needed, which could be influenced by what they will be able to bill for.

The way the insurer compensates the insured person for his or her loss varies with the nature of the risk insured. *Indemnity insurance* focuses on the extent of the insured's monetary loss, which can be paid for in the form of money or in services (such as health care). *Non-indemnity insurance* applies when the amount of the loss itself cannot be "made good" (e.g., loss of life cannot be "made good" to the deceased person) but when a set amount of money or service, usually predetermined, is paid or delivered to a beneficiary of the policy upon the occurrence of that event or condition.

Some types of insurance may be compulsory. Under Ontario's *Compulsory Automobile Insurance Act*, all people who operate motor vehicles must be insured under an automobile insurance policy. For other potential damages, insurance is optional and the decision to purchase insurance is based on individuals' choice of whether they wish to personally bear a particular risk, along with the financial consequences to them if the risk should materialize. In theory, people should be able to protect themselves against the financial consequences of almost any type of loss or peril if they could find an insurer willing to take on the risks and issue a policy.

## Premium Rate Setting: How the Price of an Insurance Policy Gets Set

To carry out insurance business, an insurance company must be *solvent* and have sufficient assets to pay every likely claim under the contracts of insurance it has sold. The insurer acquires these assets by collecting premiums and by investing a certain portion of premiums. Some of the insurer's assets are kept on hand as cash (or short-term investments easily convertible to cash) so that it can pay for the immediate claims submitted by those it has insured; other assets can be invested on a longer-term basis. When government is the insurer, it can exempt itself by law from the requirement to be solvent in relation to the insurance liabilities, since it can draw on government revenues if necessary. Instead of setting aside certain tax receipts to pay future liabilities, it can focus only on ensuring that it has enough money to pay any claims that arise in a given year; this is called a "pay-as-you-go" scheme. From an insurance perspective, this approach can be risky; if the liabilities vary unexpectedly over time due to characteristics of the insured population or to environmental factors, the government may still have to find the money, which may involve borrowing, cutting other programs, and/or increasing taxes.

Premium setting is a complicated process. To simplify, there are four key components to the price: (1) expected claims costs arising from already-issued insurance policies (taking into account expected frequency and expected cost of these claims); (2) the insurer's overhead costs (e.g., costs of marketing, sales, investor relations, claims processing, investment of assets, and regulation); (3) the amount required to maintain the insurer's solvency relating to previous claims and assets; and (4) profit for shareholders. The assets set aside by the insurer for the first and second components are often called the *reserves*.

The insurance company actuaries usually estimate the future claims and administration costs by analyzing historical payment trends for similar policies and projecting the effect of any relevant environmental factors (e.g., rising health costs, increases in benefit payments, inflation, changes in likely length of claims due to improvements in length of life of beneficiaries, changes in accident rates, etc.). To assess the value of the assets, the actuary analyzes the quantity and current market value of the stocks, bonds, cash, etc. that make up the asset pool, and estimates the future value of those assets based on the return on investment of the various types of assets in the past, and the likely trends in the investment market. Actuaries tend to be conservative in the assumptions they make about the probable value of future assets and future liabilities, because they can be held professionally and legally liable for improperly valuing them. For example, if current stock market returns were in the range of 15% per year, an actuary would look at the long-term historical trends and use a lower return figure when estimating the likely future value of an insurance company's investment portfolio. If it turns out that the actuary's valuation of the assets was too high or the valuation of the liabilities too low, future premiums would have to be higher to cover the shortfall. If the actuary's valuation of the assets was too low, or the valuation of the liabilities too high, future premiums could be reduced or the insurer could take the surplus as profit.

In setting premiums, insurers have to satisfy their shareholders' desire for predictable and reasonable profit and their customers' desire for predictable and reasonable prices. If one or more of the components of the price have changed in a way the insurer did not expect, the insurer may react by: raising premiums to cover any shortfall; changing the composition of the pool (e.g., not renewing certain policies, not accepting new customers with certain risk profiles); reassessing its expectations of the future and adjusting premiums to reflect those new expectations; reassessing why it did not expect the component of the price to change as it did, so that premium setting in the future can be accurate and predictable; and/or making changes to the insurance policies to improve the predictability of the losses.

To reduce some of the variation in the costs that may arise under their issued policies as a result of moral hazard and unknown environmental factors, insurance policies can have some or all of the following features: not covering intentional damage caused by a policyholder with a view to receiving insurance benefits (extreme examples would include refusing to cover damages from suicide, arson, and/or murder); not covering medical conditions or faults known prior to the issuing of the insurance policy (often called pre-existing conditions exclusions); capping an indemnity at a particular level (e.g., fee limits, maximum benefits per insured period); requiring a *co-payment* by the insured person (the insurer will pay only a portion of the costs); having a *deductible* (the insurer pays the amount of the loss less a specified amount, the deductible, which the insured must pay him/herself); requiring the insured person to mitigate the loss where mitigation is within the scope of his or her control (e.g., compulsory attendance at medical appointments or a requirement to search for a job if wage loss is a covered risk); giving the insurer a right not to renew the policy of a person whose risk profile changes or who has incurred "excessive" costs; specifying that any services to be provided under the insurance policy are to be provided only by accredited service providers (to ensure effectiveness and efficiency); specifying that services will be paid for only if provided by service providers under contract to or employed by the insurer (to ensure a specific price and the conditions of delivery); and/or specifying that services will be paid for only in accord with standard fees and protocols negotiated by the service providers and insurers in advance so that there are common expectations of extent and cost of service in at least the most common cases.

In addition, insurers may have some opportunities (depending on the nature of the insured risk) to control claim costs through their claims processing approaches. The insurer can aggressively manage costs by demanding proof of need and by controlling access to insured benefits, by such measures as requiring a medical certificate before approving access for certain benefits. Another strategy is to challenge certain types of claims by policyholders with the expectation that a certain number will abandon their claims or will not be able to sustain the costs of dispute resolution (or to sustain going without benefits before the dispute is resolved). This strategy can be highly risky, because if an insurer is doing more than merely discouraging illegitimate claims, it may get a reputation for providing poor customer service and its future policy sales may decline as a result. Furthermore, by delaying payment, the insured's losses may increase and the insurer may ultimately be liable to pay more out on the policy than if the claim had been paid more quickly. Yet another approach is for the insurer to attempt to have its policyholders, especially those who have previously made claims, avoid recurrences of their losses or liabilities through loss prevention efforts; this can be a "win-win" situation.

*Reinsurance* is insurance for insurers. Reinsurers are generally international organizations that spread their risks by supporting "primary" insurers in several countries and in many regions around the world. Insurance companies pay premiums to reinsurers in exchange for an agreement to have a proportion of their claims paid for them, particularly in the event of a major loss or catastrophe. Reinsurance is one of many tools available to insurers to guarantee that they will meet every obligation to pay legitimate claims.

If the insurer does not do a good job of setting premiums, collecting them, investing assets, and/or paying claims, it may go out of business. To avoid situations where legitimate claims would go unpaid, in many jurisdictions (including Ontario), "compensation corporations" are compulsory for many types of insurance. As one example, all property and casualty insurers (which include automobile insurers) operating in Ontario are members of and pay into the industry-funded, non-profit Property and Casualty Insurance Compensation Corporation (PACICC), which will then respond to such claims.

APPENDIX B: THE AUTOMOBILE INSURANCE
SYSTEM IN ONTARIO

In 2003, when the Liberal government took office, there were approximately 9.4 million registered vehicles, 8.3 million drivers, and 75,000 commercial carriers in Ontario. Ontario's fatality rate had been 1.02 per

10,000 licensed drivers in 2001, the lowest in all of North America. In 2001 92.5% of Ontario drivers wore seatbelts, more than ever before. Several approaches had been used to try to minimize accidents. For example, in addition to efforts to curb drinking and driving, on April 1, 1994, Ontario had become the first jurisdiction in Canada to implement a Graduated Licensing System for new drivers. The cost of collisions, fatalities, and injuries in Ontario in 2003 was estimated at $9 billion per year.

As noted in the case, under the *Compulsory Automobile Insurance Act*, all drivers and owners of automobiles were required to be insured under an automobile insurance policy. If they drove (or permitted someone else to drive) and were not insured, they were guilty of a provincial offence with a fine of up to $100,000 on first conviction and up to $200,000 for any subsequent convictions.

Since 1993, insurers were allowed to refuse to offer a policy or renew a policy if a person had been at fault in an accident but otherwise were largely prohibited from declining or refusing to issue an auto insurance contract to other high-risk drivers, including those who had been insured by the Facility Association (discussed below) or had been refused insurance by another auto insurer. As noted in the case, the auto insurers refer to this as the "Take All Comers Rule" (Revised Regulations of Ontario, Regulation 664, section 5). If an insurer could show that the Take All Comers Rule would threaten its solvency, it could apply and receive an exemption from that rule, but this has been an extremely high threshold to overcome.

The Facility Association was a non-profit organization whose members were all the auto insurers who sell insurance in Alberta, New Brunswick, Nova Scotia, Newfoundland and Labrador, Northwest Territories, Nunavut, Ontario, Prince Edward Island, and Yukon. The Facility Association took on all the highest-risk drivers and had strict rules for returning those drivers to regular insurance companies for coverage at the appropriate time. In 2002, the Facility Association had 0.86% of the Ontario market.

In 2003, the IBC argued that the Take All Comers Rule did not serve a public policy role since car drivers could have access to a specialized high-risk insurance market that had developed since the rule had been instituted in 1993. In any event, the IBC argued, the process for filing relevant underwriting rules was "highly bureaucratic for insurers" and the rule should at least be more flexible, if not eliminated entirely. This did not happen.

If an insurer had not been exempted from the Take All Comers Rule, it was eligible to pool the highest-risk situations with other insurers' high-risk customers in the Risk-Sharing Pool (RSP) of the Facility Association. The RSP was created as a voluntary mechanism to keep the highest-risk customers out of the regular lines of the auto insurers while continuing to comply with the Take All Comers Rule. The Risk Sharing Pool had 1.94% of the Ontario market, as measured by the proportion of all premiums charged and collected. In addition, if an insurer had an exemption from the Take All Comers Rule, the insurer's potential customers whose risks were too high or who belonged to specific groups (e.g., people who had been refused insurance because of their at-fault accidents, or owners of historic vehicles or motorcycles) could apply to be insured by the Facility Association.

No auto insurer (regardless of whether they were exempt from the Take All Comers Rule) could consider the following factors in deciding whether to issue, renew, or terminate a policy or to continue any coverage or endorsement under a policy: a person's physical or mental disability; the number of persons who would become insured under a policy; a person's health status or life expectancy; a person's occupation, profession, or employment; a person's income; a person's other health or income continuation insurance; a person's request for an optional benefit under the policy; and/or a person's past claim for auto insurance benefits if he or she was not at fault. However, these factors could be taken into account by an insurer in setting premiums, as long as they were included in the underwriting rules the insurer submitted to FSCO.

Three kinds of *coverage* could be purchased under an auto insurance policy: (1) personal injury or damage, (2) third party liability, and (3) property damage. In Ontario, the coverage for personal injury or damage was entirely determined by FSCO, which was the regulator of the entire insurance industry; FSCO's coverage rules were approved by the provincial cabinet and published in regulations under the *Insurance Act*. Note that the precise categories and levels of coverage have varied over time, as have what is mandatory/optional, what (if any) caps were placed on benefits, and how severe an impairment must be before being eligible for compensation (Ontario Auto Insurance Anti-Fraud Task Force, 2011).

(1) *Personal injury or damage* benefits (sometimes referred to as the *Statutory Accident Benefits Schedule*, or SABS) were paid on a no-fault basis

to anyone injured in an accident, regardless of who had caused it. This coverage was mandatory, and included the following subcategories:

*Medical and rehabilitation benefits* could include various combinations of medical, dental, nursing, chiropractic, physiotherapy, medications, counselling, vocational training, and home and vehicle modifications. Note that for this category of benefits, at the time of the case, other insurance, including the publicly funded Ontario Health Insurance Plan (OHIP), would pay first, with the automobile insurance plan stepping in only where other payers would not cover the cost. There were also ceilings, which have been modified (up and down) over time.

*Attendant care benefits* covered "reasonable and necessary expenses" of up to a monthly ceiling; this varied depending on how catastrophic the injury was. Benefits were capped, although clients could choose to increase this coverage. In 2009, these benefits were eliminated for all but catastrophic claims.

*Death and funeral benefits* were also capped, with clients able to purchase additional optional coverage (up to preset limits).

*Income replacement benefits* applied to earners who, as a result of the accident, would be substantially unable to perform the essential tasks of their employment; these were set at 80% of net weekly income, up to a capped amount. Again, optional coverage could be purchased (to preset limits), and some benefits were available even if the injured person was not a paid worker.

(2) *Third-party liability* protected the insured person if someone else was killed or injured and their property was damaged. It would cover the claims against the insured made in a lawsuit plus the third party's costs of settling the claim. This coverage was also mandatory for a minimum of $200,000; clients could optionally purchase coverage up to $2 million.

(3) *Property damage* in general did not specify a minimum limit. At the time of the case, coverage was mandatory for *direct compensation*, which covered damage to an insured vehicle to the extent someone else was at fault for the accident, and for *uninsured automobile coverage* to protect drivers from damage caused by an uninsured motorist. Optional coverage allowed clients who so wished to purchase coverage for *collision* damage even if they were at fault, and/or for *comprehensive* coverage of losses from theft, fire, and non-collision damage. *Optional enhancements* included coverage for *transportation replacement* (e.g., a rental car), *family protection* for the insured person's family on the same basis as third-party liability coverage, and/or *removing depreciation deduction*, which

would pay the replacement value of the car rather than the depreciated value (Ontario Auto Insurance Anti-Fraud Task Force, 2011).

As noted in the case, some of these benefits were offered on a no-fault basis (up to a given level), whereby victims would be reimbursed by their own insurance company. If damages exceeded the no-fault level, victims had the option of suing the at-fault driver. The Auditor General estimated that over 99% of Ontario drivers purchased more than the mandatory coverage. In the 2010 calendar year, 9 million Ontario drivers paid $9.8 billion for auto insurance coverage; in turn, there were about 584,000 claims totalling $8.7 billion. This had increased by 61% in just five years, with most of the increases coming from the SABS benefits (Office of the Auditor General of Ontario, 2011).

The law also included certain statutory exclusions, defined as conditions that reduce the amount of coverage that would otherwise be available under the auto insurance policy. These included: (1) mechanical failure unless caused by the insured peril; (2) driver unable to maintain control of the car because he or she was under the influence of intoxicating substances; (3) driver criminally convicted for: causing death or injury by criminal negligence; dangerous operation of the car; failure to stop at the scene of the accident; driving when impaired or with more than 80 mg of alcohol in the blood; refusal to provide the police with a breath sample; causing injury when driving a car while impaired or with or over 80 mg of alcohol in the blood; and/or driving the car while disqualified from doing so; (4) owner used or permitted the car to be used in a race or speed test, or for illegal activity; (5) driver drove the car without a valid driver's licence; (6) driver used the car to carry explosives or radioactive materials; and/or (7) driver used the car as a taxicab, bus, or sightseeing vehicle, or to carry paying passengers.

At the time of the case, over 140 insurance companies were licensed to sell automobile insurance products in Ontario (this was down from 170 a few years earlier). Many of the insurers were global giants with operations in Ontario; others were small Ontario insurers operating only in their locality. Their assets varied accordingly, from about $65 million to over $3.3 billion.

To insure automobile risks and perils, an insurance company was required to have a licence from FSCO. Since 1993, it has been difficult for companies to cease doing auto insurance business in Ontario; specific rules governing this were instituted in 1993 by the NDP government after the auto insurance industry threatened to leave Ontario because of their opposition to the government's policies. Commencing in 1993, if an auto insurer wanted to cease writing auto insurance policies, it had to give 180 days' notice to FSCO and to its policyholders, along with additional information that FSCO might require.

## APPENDIX C: REFERENCES CITED AND FURTHER READING

Baer, N. (1997). Fraud worries insurance companies but should concern physicians too, industry says. *Canadian Medical Association Journal, 156*(2), 251–6.

Office of the Auditor General of Ontario. (2011). *Auto insurance regulatory oversight. 2011 Annual report*. Toronto: Queen's Printer for Ontario. http://www.auditor.on.ca/en/reports_en/en11/301en11.pdf

Ontario Auto Insurance Anti-fraud Task Force. (2011). *Ontario auto insurance anti-fraud task force: Interim report*. Ministry of Finance. http://www.fin.gov.on.ca/en/autoinsurance/interim-report.pdf

The following websites may also be helpful:

Financial Services Commission of Ontario, Understanding Automobile Insurance, http://www.fsco.gov.on.ca/en/auto/brochures/Pages/brochure_autoins.aspx#six

Insurance Bureau of Canada: Car Insurance, http://www.ibc.ca/en/Car_Insurance/index.asp

IBC's Ontario page, http://www.ibc.ca/en/Car_Insurance/ON/

Ontario Automobile Insurance Anti-Fraud Task Force: Final Report of the Steering Committee, http://www.fin.gov.on.ca/en/autoinsurance/final-report.pdf

# 18 Everybody Out of the Pool

## Financing Health Expenditures through Medical Savings Accounts

*KENNETH CHEAK KWAN LAM, MARK ROVERE,*
*AND RAISA B. DEBER*

What is the best way to pay for health care? As health costs increase, governments are increasingly seeking ways of controlling costs while ensuring adequate levels of coverage. Economists have suggested that greater use of market mechanisms, including encouraging patients to choose among competing providers, could improve quality and curb costs. One proposal is for greater use of personal medical savings accounts.

This case addresses several policy issues, including: financing, insurance and moral hazard, policy goals, and justice.

### Appendices

Appendix A: Public and Private Health Care Financing in Canada
Appendix B: The Distribution of Health Expenditures
Appendix C: References Cited and Further Reading

### The Case

There are various models used to finance health care. At one extreme, people can pay their own bills. At the other, they may be assured that all of their costs will be covered by the government. Other alternatives include various forms of private health insurance. As noted in Chapter 1, sections 6.1.1 (Public and Private), 6.1.2 (Financing and Delivery), and 6.1.3 (Models of Health Systems), different countries use different models to cover different services for different people.

Considerable attention has been paid in Canada, and in most industrialized countries, to the rising costs of health care. Increasingly, some ask whether the publicly funded system is sustainable. At the same time, there has been considerable attention to ensuring access, and making sure that people do not have to wait too long to receive care. An additional complication is that the *Canada Health Act* (see Chapter 1, section 7.2) requires public financing only for medically required services delivered in hospitals or by physicians. As care shifts from hospitals to home and community, an increasing share of care is moving outside these guarantees. Depending on the jurisdiction, population, group, and service, some of the costs for these services may still be covered by public insurance, some by private insurance, and some only by out-of-pocket payments.

To what extent should people expect others to help pay for the costs they incur? One proposal has been to empower consumers to make "wise purchasing decisions" by limiting their insurance coverage and ensuring that they have a financial stake in the choices they make. In turn, this rests heavily upon views about insurance, and how having it might affect people's behaviour (see Chapter 1, section 5.9, Insurance, Elasticity, and Moral Hazard).

One possible way to manage this is to use the tax system. For example, government might allow individuals to set up tax-sheltered medical savings accounts (MSAs). MSAs represent a shift from models of collective payment to more individualized models where the individual consumer decides what care to purchase, from whom, and at what price. However, to the extent that the individual was already paying these bills, MSAs could be viewed as public subsidy of these costs by allowing them to be paid with pre-tax rather than after-tax dollars, evoking questions about which purchases warrant such subsidy.

Variants of MSA models have been used in such countries as Singapore and the United States (Deber & Lam, 2011a, 2011b). In 2001, Alberta's Mazankowski Report recommended that the province use MSAs to replace the existing way of paying for health care, arguing that the opportunity to invest in MSAs would enable Albertans to take control of their personal medical needs through increased patient choice.

Although MSAs were not implemented at that time, Alberta's Wildrose Alliance Party had stated in 2010 that, if elected in the 2012 provincial election, they would introduce the opportunity for Albertans to set up tax-free MSAs. The precise details concerning how MSAs would be organized have varied; the Wildrose proposal emphasized that, initially, they could be used to purchase preventative and alternative health services (including naturopathy) that were not fully covered by the province's public insurance plan. (In that sense, they are similar to an existing Canadian model, called Health Spending Accounts, that has existed since 1986, initially only for large employers; it was expanded in 1998 to include small businesses and the self-employed. See Appendix A for more details.)

The case addresses several issues regarding MSAs, including: financing health care services in Canada, the fundamental concepts of insurance, the arguments for and against MSAs as a viable financing scheme, stakeholder positions, and ideological perspectives that could influence support or opposition to MSAs.

### Health Care Financing in Canada

In Canada, about 70% of health care costs are paid publicly, largely through the public insurance plans that are administered by each province. Although the provinces have some flexibility in determining what services will be covered publicly, the *Canada Health Act* (*CHA*) sets out the rules and principles that the provinces must abide by in order to receive the full federal health transfer to which they are entitled (see Chapter 1, section 7.2, *Canada Health Act*). The universality condition of the *CHA* requires that all "insured persons" (defined as including those legally residing in Canada) be fully covered for all "insured services"; the comprehensiveness condition of the *CHA* defines insured services as all medically necessary care delivered in hospitals or by physicians. In turn, this means that a number of services do not have to be covered publicly and must be paid for out-of-pocket or through private insurance. For instance, unless delivered in hospital, the following services are typically not covered under provincially funded public insurance plans: dental care, rehabilitation, vision care, drugs (delivered out of hospital), long-term care, and home care. Diagnostic imaging (e.g., MRI and CT scanners) is another potentially contentious area; it is typically delivered in hospitals, but private clinics offering these services have become widespread in a number of provinces.

The approximately 30% of health care financed privately represents a variety of services (see Appendix A for some data on public and private health care financing in Canada). Although individuals or households can purchase private insurance to cover some of this care, private insurance in Canada, like such coverage in the United States, is typically employer-based. Under this structure, premiums are either partially or fully paid by the employer. Depending on the jurisdiction, there may be regulations affecting coverage for those at higher risk (e.g., under Canadian law, large organizations, defined as those employing more than 25 workers, are not allowed to deny coverage or charge higher premiums to higher-risk employees, should they decide to offer private insurance). However, there are no requirements that employers provide private health insurance, and fewer are doing so.

In the absence of private insurance coverage, individuals are responsible for either purchasing insurance themselves in the private market, or paying for services out-of-pocket. It has been suggested that prepaid personal accounts such as MSAs would provide economic incentives for individuals to use medical care more responsibly, while upholding individual freedom. (Another potential feature is to allow individuals to use their funds to access new and often untested therapies, including complementary/alternative medicine, that are not funded by public or private insurers.) However, opponents of this type of financing contend that risk pooling through a properly structured insurance scheme is the optimal way of financing medical care. Both types of financing models have benefits and drawbacks.

**Insurance**

The fundamental principle of insurance is to hedge oneself (or one's organization) against the risk of uncertain losses (see also Chapter 1, section 5.9, and Chapter 17, Rehabilitating Auto Insurance). Insurance can be purchased against a wide range of eventualities (e.g., life insurance, home insurance, automobile insurance, health insurance). In general, insurance is used to hedge against the risk of a substantial loss that would otherwise be difficult to manage. For example, if a house is destroyed in a fire, it is very unlikely that most people would easily be able to afford to rebuild it. However, given a properly built house, such disasters should be relatively uncommon. It is thus common for people to pool the risk by purchasing insurance, each paying premiums to an insurer, who can in turn use these pooled premiums (and the money obtained through investing them) to cover losses when they occur. Risk pooling relies on what is often termed "the law of large numbers." For example, let us assume that, in a group of 1,000 people, each has a 1% risk of incurring a loss of $50,000 in a given year. The expected losses for that group would thus total 10 (1% of 1,000 people) times $50,000, or $500,000. If each person pays $1,000 in annual premiums to insure against that loss, the insurance company will have $1 million, an amount easily enough to cover those anticipated losses and to make a substantial profit. The model also recognizes that there is likely to be some variability in the exact number of people incurring that loss, with the amount collected providing some flexibility to cover years where the losses are particularly high. The basic principle behind "risk pooling" is that enough people must be included in the pool (law of large numbers) and that everyone in that pool should face a relatively low probability of loss. To avoid paperwork to pay for small losses, insurers may also require an annual *deductible* (where the insurance does not pay until losses cross a predetermined threshold), and/or *co-payments* (where the insurer pays for some but not all of the losses); they may also *cap* total coverage. In contrast, *first-dollar coverage* refers to situations where all losses are covered by the insurer.

To the extent that the logic of insurance applies to health care, it has several implications. One is that the risk of loss should be relatively similar among the members of the pool, and that those at higher risk should be charged higher premiums and/or be excluded from coverage (a practice sometimes referred to as "adverse selection"). In order to maximize profit, an insurance company has a disincentive to insure people who are likely to become sick or who have a "pre-existing" medical condition (Arrow, 1963). The extent to which these implications are seen as ethically appropriate clearly varies. In situations where it is agreed that everyone should be covered, one might then argue that health insurance represents a "market failure" that might warrant some form of government intervention (see Chapter 1, section 5.2, Policy/Governing Instruments).

Another issue relates to the concept of "moral hazard" (see Chapter 1, section 5.9), which implies that those insulated from risk may have an incentive to behave in a riskier fashion, and hence that first-dollar coverage should be avoided. The concept of moral hazard is based on the premise that individuals may change their behaviour if they have insurance because they are no longer responsible for the "full costs" if something goes wrong (Pauly, 1968, 2002). Moral hazard would thus suggest that well-insured people will "overutilize" health care services because they are not responsible for the full costs of those services. The theory thus implies that if individuals were responsible for paying the full costs of the medical services that they use, then they would be less inclined to demand "unnecessary" care.

One way to account for moral hazard when structuring an insurance scheme is to have a high-deductible insurance plan, under which individuals are responsible for paying a significant amount out-of-pocket until the predetermined threshold is reached. If people are price-sensitive, they will be reluctant to pay for services not covered by the deductible, and will be less likely to demand care that they might not need. On the other hand, if they are not sufficiently knowledgeable about what care is necessary, they may also be less likely to demand care that they did need, and hence may incur higher costs by avoiding early detection and treatment. The precise balance clearly depends on the patients and the potential treatments.

## Medical Savings Accounts (MSAs)

As noted above, medical savings accounts (MSAs) refer to a family of financing approaches that use a personal health spending account, often combined with a high-deductible insurance plan, to pay for specified health care services (Hurley & Guindon, 2008). MSA plans divide expenditures into three zones: (1) the *allowance*, paid (by someone) to each individual, and available to be used (for some things); (2) the *threshold*; all costs above this level are considered "catastrophic" and (in most versions) insured (to varying extents); and (3) the *corridor* between the allowance and the threshold, where all costs must be paid out of pocket (Deber & Lam, 2011b). Different countries use different nomenclature for these plans; they may also differ in such details as: whether enrolment is voluntary or compulsory; who makes the contributions (individuals, employers, and/or government); size of contributions (including maximums and/or minimums); size of "corridor" between the account and the level where catastrophic insurance coverage would begin; who owns the account (the individual or the employer); provisions for rolling over unused contributions to subsequent years (whether "use it or lose it" applies); the extent to which MSAs are sheltered from taxation; and what the contributions can be used for. Nomenclature also varies; such plans may also be called flexible savings accounts (FSAs), health savings accounts (HSAs), consumer-driven health insurance, consumer-directed health plans, defined contribution health plans, consumer allowances, and/or consumer-centric health plans (Baker et al., 2007; Gabel et al., 2002; Gauthier & Clancy, 2004; Hurley & Guindon, 2008; Shearer, 2004). This case will use the term MSA, recognizing that such variation exists.

The fundamental premise of MSAs derives from economic theory; it assumes that people will be more responsible when consuming/

purchasing medical services if they have to pay for them than they would be if someone else meets those costs. Advocates accordingly suggest that a number of potential benefits will arise, including: enhanced patient choice and empowerment; reduced government expenditures; improved system efficiency/effectiveness (including reduction of wait lists and enhancing innovation); reduced costs for processing small insurance claims; more cost consciousness; reduced utilization; and broadening the array of people and services covered. Opponents suggest that many of these benefits are unlikely to emerge, in large part because of how skewed health expenditures are in the population (see Appendix B). They suggest that adopting MSAs has a number of potential risks, including: undermining insurance arrangements, transferring resources from the sick to the healthy, increasing total costs, subsidizing services of questionable value, and producing worse health outcomes (particularly if people do not receive preventive services).

As mentioned above, MSAs can be structured in a number of ways. One possibility is to replace current public insurance plans with MSAs. Under this scenario, provincial governments would replace much of their public funding going to hospitals and physicians with money flowing directly to individuals so that they could set up MSAs. These public funds might be adjusted to patient characteristics (often, only age and sex, although in theory adjustments could also be made for other factors, including health status). Funds could also be placed in MSAs by employers and/or individuals. Recipients would use these funds to purchase whatever services are allowed by that model until the threshold (deductible) amount is reached, at which stage catastrophic coverage might step in. Depending on the model, MSA funds could be used for various combinations of medically necessary services delivered in hospitals and by physicians, medically necessary care not currently paid for publicly (e.g., in Canada, this could include, depending on the province, various combinations of outpatient pharmaceuticals, dental care, vision care, and long-term care), and/or other services (e.g., homeopathy). In most models, unused funds could then be rolled over to subsequent years; under some models, unused funds could be transferred into tax-free savings accounts that could be used for other purposes at the individual's discretion. Again, the fundamental argument for MSAs is the notion that people will be more responsible when using health care services (regardless of whether they are medically necessary) because they will have an incentive to use "fewer" services if they are able to keep unused funds.

One of the most commonly cited discussions in Canada advocating for the use of MSAs was included in Alberta's Mazankowski Report (2001).

## Mazankowski Report

The Mazankowski Report, also known as the Premier's Advisory Council on Health Report, was co-written by Donald Mazankowski, a former Deputy Prime Minister of Canada. It focused on the sustainability of health care financing in the province of Alberta, and provided a number of recommendations and potential strategies for ways in which to restructure health care financing in the province. One prominent recommendation in the report was that MSAs would create the necessary economic incentives for people to use the health care system more responsibly, save for future needs, increase accountability, and provide the flexibility and freedom for people to use their "savings" on a wide range of health promotion and medical services of their choice (Mazankowski, 2001). The report emphasized the notion that MSAs would provide an opportunity for individuals to "take control" of their medical needs.

The report accordingly proposed that individuals have a set amount of funding allocated to their account each year (through premiums), which could be partially funded publicly. It recommended that children be exempt and people with low incomes receive subsidies that would be deposited in their personal accounts. Under the proposal, individuals could use their account to pay for medical services, with the assumption that they would shop around in order to obtain the best price. If individuals did not use all of the money in their account by year's end, they would have the ability to keep it, which could be rolled over into another type of savings account. Depending on exactly how the MSAs were structured, unused money could be used for additional services that were not publicly insured or could be saved for future use (e.g., to pay for long-term care or home care). The report suggested that individuals would be responsible for replenishing their account on an annual basis. The report also recommended that MSAs be linked to patient cost sharing; for example, they argued that all adults should be required to use their personal account to pay a "co-payment" for a fixed portion (e.g., 20%) of the health services that they used, including for all publicly insured services (Mazankowski, 2001).

The report did recognize some potential concerns with implementing MSAs, and called for further study. It suggested that MSAs might increase government expenditures through increased administrative costs. In addition, the report recognized that if individuals had the ability to purchase a wide range of medical services with their account, including services not currently covered, then health care costs could significantly increase. The report's authors also identified the possibility that the ability to "roll over" unused savings might not be enough of an incentive for people to reduce their health care utilization. Finally, if people were obligated to pay for a portion of medically necessary services out-of-pocket once their account had been exhausted, the authors recognized that it could violate the conditions of the *Canada Health Act* (prohibition on user fees and extra charges) (Mazankowski, 2001).

### Stakeholders

There are many powerful stakeholders involved in the delivery and financing of health care services that could influence a government's decision to allow MSAs. However, the political, financial, and policy implications differ depending on how the MSA plan is designed. For instance, if employers are not responsible for contributing to the MSA, then from a payer's perspective, MSAs transfer risk from the insurer (employer/payer) to the patient (employee). Under this scenario, employers are less likely to be concerned about the breadth of coverage. In contrast, if employers are responsible for contributing to an employee's personal account, they are more likely to be concerned about what is covered and how it is structured (i.e., premiums and deductibles).

From a provider perspective, what is covered under MSAs can become quite political, especially if the breadth of coverage is mandated by government. Providers have a clear economic incentive to ensure that their services are included, particularly for price-sensitive care.

### Ideology

Support for MSAs is also related to views about the role of the state. Libertarians or individuals who advocate for personal choice and freedom tend to support MSAs, arguing that they enhance patient choice. As believers in personal responsibility, they support the notion that patients should have the freedom to take control of their personal medical needs. They commonly argue that health care should be treated like any other consumer good and should thus be based on an individual's willingness to pay. In contrast, individuals who take a solidarity orientation may argue that sick people should be helped. Views may also vary concerning the distribution of wealth, the extent to which accessing medical care should be dependent on an individual's ability to pay, and the extent to which health care should be treated as a regular consumer good (e.g., the distinction between demand and need).

Another issue relates to sustainability, and what can be afforded. Again, the extent to which care should be universal, or those with more resources should be able to buy more, may depend on views about the roles of individuals and of the state.

DECISION POINT

You are the newly elected health minister of Alberta. Should you implement MSAs?

POSSIBLE QUESTIONS FOR DISCUSSION

1. What sort of good is health care? Discuss the differences among utilization, demand, and need.
2. Who should pay for what? Does this vary by type of service? How does this relate to views of the role of the state? About resource allocation ethics?
3. Discuss how financing approaches relate to such policy goals as: equity, security, liberty, and efficiency.
4. What are the advantages and disadvantages of MSAs? If you decide to implement MSAs, how will you deal with the following issues: What medical services can they be used to purchase? Where does the money for the allowance come from (government? employers? individuals?) Should the allowance be uniform, or vary (and, if so, on what basis)? What should be done with unused funds?

APPENDIX A: PUBLIC AND PRIVATE HEALTH CARE
FINANCING IN CANADA

The Canadian Institute for Health Information (CIHI) (2013) classifies health spending by "source of funds" and "use of funds."

The source of funds classification is divided into public and private shares. Public share includes the following: *provincial/territorial governments* (which include federal health transfers to the provinces/territories); *federal direct spending* (e.g., for veterans and Aboriginal peoples, as well as for health research, and health promotion and protection); *municipal governments*; and *social security funds* (including workers' compensation boards). Private share includes private *out-of-pocket* (OOP) expenditures, *private insurance*, and *non-consumption* funds from such sources as donations and investment income.

The uses of funds are subdivided into the following categories:

1. hospitals;
2. other institutions, which include nursing homes and residential care facilities;
3. physicians;
4. other professionals, which include care primarily provided by dentists and denturists, optometrists and opticians, chiropractors, physiotherapists, and private-duty nurses; note that this category focuses on those professionals paid independently, as opposed to those already included in other budgets (e.g., most nurses tend to be included in other categories, including hospitals). In turn, other professionals are subdivided into dental care, vision care, and other;
5. drugs; this category excludes pharmaceuticals already included in other budgets, such as hospitals. Drugs are subdivided into prescribed drugs, over-the-counter (OTC) drugs, and personal health supplies;
6. capital;
7. public health, which CIHI defines as including expenditures for food and drug safety, health inspections, health-promotion activities, community mental health programs, public health nursing, measures to prevent the spread of communicable disease, and occupational health to promote and enhance health and safety at the workplace. Note that, as defined, this is entirely public sector spending and may not include some privately funded programs with similar objectives;
8. administration, which CIHI defines as including infrastructure costs to operate health departments and prepayment administration (the administrative expenses of providing health insurance by governments and private health insurance companies) but not the administrative expense of non-insured services; and

9. other health spending, which includes health research (but not research funded by pharmaceutical companies, which is included in the drugs category), medical transportation, hearing aids and appliances, voluntary health associations, and explicitly identified home care. CIHI subdivides this category into health research, other health care goods, and other health care services.

CIHI further notes that certain services that are identified by data sources as home care are included under the broad category of Other Health Spending. Private nursing care in the home would be included in the Other Professionals category. Home care programs provided by hospitals are included in the Hospitals category. Support services such as domestic maintenance and delivery of meals are considered to be social services within the current definition of home care and are removed when identified. Depending on the table, these subcategories may be collapsed in different ways.

Table 18.1 presents Canadian data for 2009 (the most recent audited data available at the time of writing), by category, for total expenditures (in $000,000), the percentage of total expenditures represented by each category, the estimated expenditure per capita, and the expenditures attributed to public and private sources (these should sum to the total expenditures). The final column indicates the percentage of spending for that category coming from private sector sources of funds.

Table 18.2 further examines the private expenditures by category. Beginning with the private expenditures (in $000,000) from Table 18.1, it divides this into how much was paid OOP, from private insurance, and how much was classified as non-consumption (and hence did not represent costs to patients). The next columns indicate what percentage of total spending for that category would be paid OOP, and from private insurance. The final two columns show the share each category is of total OOP, and of total private insurance spending. For example, only 1.7% of hospital costs were paid OOP, and another 2.4% through private insurance. Hospital costs accounted for 3.4% of all money spent OOP, and 5.8% of the money paid by private insurance. In contrast, 42.5% of dental care was paid OOP and 52% through private insurance. Of all OOP spending, 20.1% could be attributed to dental care. Similarly, 28.8% of private insurance spending went for dental care.

This CIHI data clarifies that about 70% of Canadian health expenditures are paid publicly; this has remained relatively stable for decades (Canadian Institute for Health Information, 2013). However this varies

Table 18.1. 2009 Health Expenditures, Canada, by Category

| Category | Expenditures ($ 000,000) | % of Total expenditures | Expenditure per capita | Public expenditures ($ 000,000) | Private expenditures ($ 000,000) | % private |
|---|---|---|---|---|---|---|
| 1 Hospitals | 52,949.5 | 29.1 | 1,570.3 | 48,098.7 | 4,850.8 | 9.2 |
| 2 Other institutions | 18,092.2 | 9.9 | 536.5 | 12,928.9 | 5,163.3 | 28.5 |
| 3 Physicians | 24,822.7 | 13.6 | 736.1 | 24,424.9 | 397.8 | 1.6 |
| 4 Other professionals, of which: | 19,173.2 | 10.5 | 568.6 | 1,564.2 | 17,609.1 | 91.8 |
| - Dental care | 12,136.9 | 6.7 | 359.9 | 660.0 | 11,477.0 | 94.6 |
| - Vision care | 4,221.4 | 2.3 | 125.2 | 293.6 | 3,927.8 | 93.0 |
| - Other | 2,814.9 | 1.5 | 83.5 | 610.6 | 2,204.3 | 78.3 |
| 5 Drugs, of which: | 29,563.7 | 16.2 | 876.7 | 11,528.2 | 18,035.5 | 61.0 |
| - Prescribed drugs | 24,807.3 | 13.6 | 735.7 | 11,528.2 | 13,279.0 | 53.5 |
| - OTC plus personal health supplies | 4,756.5 | 2.6 | 141.1 | 0 | 4,756.5 | 100.0 |
| 6 Capital | 8,761.9 | 4.8 | 259.8 | 7,244.9 | 1,517.0 | 17.3 |
| 7 Public health | 11,409.4 | 6.3 | 338.4 | 11,409.4 | 0 | 0.0 |
| 8 Administration | 5,831.8 | 3.2 | 172.9 | 2,528.5 | 3,303.3 | 56.6 |
| 9 Other, of which: | 11,508.2 | 6.3 | 341.3 | 9,361.6 | 2,146.6 | 18.7 |
| - Health research | 3,538.6 | 1.9 | 104.9 | 2,312.5 | 1,226.1 | 34.6 |
| - Other goods and services | 7,969.6 | 4.4 | 236.3 | 7,049.1 | 920.5 | 11.5 |
| Grand total | 182,112.7 | 100.0 | 5,400.7 | 129,089.4 | 53,023.3 | 29.1 |

*(Continued)*

Source: Canadian Institute for Health Information (2013).

Table 18.2. Distribution of Private Health Expenditures, Canada, 2009

| Category | Private expenditures ($ 000,000) | Of which: ($ 000,000) | | | % of category paid: | | Category share of total spending (%) | |
|---|---|---|---|---|---|---|---|---|
| | | Out-of-pocket (OOP) | Private insurance (PI) | Non-consumption | OOP | PI | OOP | PI |
| 1 Hospitals | 4,850.8 | 874.8 | 1,259.9 | 2,716.1 | 1.7 | 2.4 | 3.4 | 5.8 |
| 2 Other institutions | 5,163.3 | 5,163.3 | 0.0 | 0.0 | 28.5 | 0.0 | 20.1 | 0.0 |
| 3 Physicians | 397.8 | 390.3 | 7.5 | 0.0 | 1.6 | 0.0 | 1.5 | 0.0 |
| 4 Other professions, of which: | 17,609.1 | | | | | | | |
| - Dental care | 11,477.0 | 5,164.2 | 6,312.8 | 0.0 | 42.5 | 52.0 | 20.1 | 28.8 |
| - Vision Care | 3,927.8 | 3,136.0 | 791.8 | 0.0 | 74.3 | 18.8 | 12.2 | 3.6 |
| - Other | 2,204.3 | 1,274.1 | 930.2 | 0.0 | 45.3 | 33.0 | 5.0 | 4.3 |
| 5 Drugs, of which: | 18,035.5 | | | | | | | |
| - Prescribed drugs | 13,279.0 | 4,302.1 | 8,976.9 | 0.0 | 17.3 | 36.2 | 16.8 | 41.0 |
| - OTC plus personal health supplies | 4,756.5 | 4,756.4 | 0.0 | 0.0 | 100.0 | 0.0 | 18.5 | 0.0 |
| -of which: OTC only | | 2,704.0 | 0.0 | 0.0 | | | | |
| - Personal health supplies only | | 2,052.4 | 0.0 | 0.0 | | | | |
| 6 Capital | 1,517.0 | 0.0 | 0.0 | 1,517.0 | 0.0 | 0.0 | 0.0 | 0.0 |
| 7 Public health | – | | | | | | | |
| 8 Administration | 3,303.3 | 0.0 | 3,303.0 | 0.0 | 0.0 | 56.6 | 0.0 | 15.1 |

Table 18.2. (Continued)

| Category | Private expenditures ($ 000,000) | Of which: ($ 000,000) | | | % of category paid: | | Category share of total spending (%) | |
|---|---|---|---|---|---|---|---|---|
| | | Out-of-pocket (OOP) | Private insurance (PI) | Non-consumption | OOP | PI | OOP | PI |
| 9 Other, of which: | 2,146.6 | | | | | | | |
| - Health research | 1,226.1 | 0.0 | 0.0 | 1,226.1 | 0.0 | 0.0 | 0.0 | 0.0 |
| - Other goods and services | 920.5 | 620.3 | 300.2 | 0.0 | 7.8 | 3.8 | 2.4 | 1.4 |
| - of which: other goods | | 291.3 | 116.6 | 0.0 | | | | |
| - other services | | 329.0 | 183.6 | 0.0 | | | | |
| Grand total | 53,023.3 | 25,681.5 | 21,882.3 | 5,459.2 | 14.1 | 12.0 | 100.0 | 100.0 |

Source: Canadian Institute for Health Information (2013).

considerably by type of care. Note that these estimates indicate that about 99% of the cost of physician services and 90% of the cost of hospital services are paid for publicly. In contrast, a sizeable share of the costs is born privately for such categories as: "other professionals" (dental care, vision care, but also rehabilitation), outpatient prescribed drugs, outpatient over-the-counter drugs, personal health supplies and devices, long-term care, and home care. Diagnostic imaging presents a mixed picture; most services are given in hospitals, and must be publicly financed if deemed medically necessary, but some provinces are showing heavier reliance on private clinics (Canadian Institute for Health Information, 2006). Note that the social services associated with home care/long-term care are not included in this data, but also would be primarily paid for from private funds.

A recent survey by the Organisation for Economic Co-operation and Development (OECD) examined what they call "ten functions of care" and assessed the extent to which costs are publicly covered. Canada was placed at 100% coverage for: acute inpatient care, outpatient primary care physician contacts, outpatient specialist contacts, clinical laboratory tests, and diagnostic imaging. Pharmaceuticals are estimated at 51%–75% coverage. Services listed as "not covered" are: physiotherapist services, eyeglasses and/or contact lenses, dental care, and dental prostheses (Paris et al., 2010).

These tables can be used to compute rough estimates of where private spending is concentrated. In particular, the non-consumption private spending is less relevant to discussions of MSAs, since it primarily represents system-related costs (e.g., private funding for research or capital) rather than the sort of personal health expenditures that might be addressed by MSAs. Note also that some health-related costs (e.g., homeopathy) may or may not be captured by this data.

The private insurance category includes multiple models, with variations in what is covered and under what conditions. As noted by Deber and Lam (2011b), a possible source of confusion is a Canadian model called health spending accounts (or health care spending accounts), which has existed in Canada since 1986. This model does not meet the definition of MSAs, and is marketed as a tax savings device because it allows for payment of eligible health-related expenses with pre-tax dollars. These plans explicitly do not provide insurance coverage; they are intended only to reimburse certain costs. Any medical or dental expenses that would be eligible for deductions under the Income Tax Act can be paid for from these accounts. This includes any registered medical practitioners (including chiropractors, Christian Science practitioners, massage therapists, naturopaths, etc.), drugs, devices, acupuncture, cosmetic procedures, etc. Any unspent balance can be carried over for one year, but then reverts to the employer. However, some items are not covered; the University of Lethbridge Human Resources Frequently Asked Questions document gives as examples "drugs purchased without a prescription from a doctor or dentist, fitness club memberships, golf memberships and daycare" (University of Lethbridge, 2013). These plans are also advocated as a vehicle for increased consumer choice. As an online post titled "Why Are Health Spending Accounts a Necessity for Canadians?" noted, "One of the reasons why health spending accounts are a necessity for Canadians is because, unlike health insurance, HSAs allow you to choose any treatment you decide. Whether it is acupuncture or herbal medicine, HSAs leaves the health care choice to you. Even the little expenses such as pain killers and cough medicine can be funded by this service" (Clark, 2010). Because these accounts are "use it or lose it" models, they are usually designed to focus on subsidizing predictable and relatively small expenditures.

APPENDIX B: THE DISTRIBUTION OF HEALTH EXPENDITURES

A key variable in analysing health care financing models is the distribution of health expenditures. Although many models tend to assume that health care spending is normally distributed about the mean for a particular category, closer examination of the data does not back this up. In a series of influential studies, Berk and Monheit examined the distribution of expenditures for the US Medicare population (the government program which pays health costs, primarily for the elderly). They found that a rather small proportion of the population accounted for a large share of health expenditures; the lowest-spending 50% of the population accounted for only 3% of health expenditures (Berk & Monheit, 1992, 2001; Monheit, 2003). Similar findings obtain in most countries. As one example, the World Health Organization (WHO) sought to ascertain the degree to which individuals endure "financial catastrophe" (defined as having to spend in excess of 40% of family income on health expenditures) by examining survey data from 89 countries that collectively cover 89% of the world population. Its main finding was that 150 million people per year were at risk for such catastrophic expenditures, with the highest rates found in those countries relying on out-of-pocket payments, and the lowest rates found in models that pool financial risks. However, in all countries, the proportion of those actually confronting financial catastrophe was low (mean of 2.3%, median of 1.47%). In over half of the surveys, less than 2% of the population had to deal with catastrophic expenditures; just 18 countries had rates that were over 4% and even the highest rates did not exceed 10% (Xu et al., 2007). This skewing of health expenditures means that most people have relatively low expenditures. However, good health cannot be guaranteed; anyone might develop major health issues and incur the high costs that could accompany them.

Studies with Manitoba data also found the same patterns (Deber et al., 2004; Deber & Lam, 2009; Forget et al., 2002, 2008). For example, for the fiscal year 2005–6, if spending were evenly distributed, the highest 1% should account for 1% of expenditures, the bottom 50% for 50%, and half would fall below the mean. Instead, the highest 1% accounted for 35.06% of attributable spending for hospitals, physicians, and pharmaceuticals. The lowest 50% accounted for 2.27%, and approximately 85% of the population had health expenditures that fell below the mean (Deber & Lam, 2009). Such skewing was observed for each subcategory of expenditures, and in every age sex group. McGrail has found similar skewing in BC (McGrail, 2006, 2007, 2008; McGrail et al., 2000) There is also skewing in users of emergency departments in Alberta (associated with more complex chronic illness) (Fong, 2008).

## APPENDIX C: REFERENCES CITED AND FURTHER READINGS

Arrow, K.J. (1963). Uncertainty and the welfare economics of medical care. *American Economic Review, 53*(5), 941–73.

Baker, L., Bundorf, K., Royalty, A., Galvin, C., & McDonald, K. (2007). *Consumer-oriented strategies for improving health benefit design: An overview* (Technical Review 15). Stanford University-UCSF Evidence-based Practice Center, Agency for Healthcare Research and Quality. http://www.ncbi.nlm .nih.gov/books/NBK44061/pdf/TOC.pdf

Berk, M.L., & Monheit, A.C. (1992). The concentration of health expenditures: An update. *Health Affairs, 11*(4), 145–9. http://dx.doi.org/10.1377/ hlthaff.11.4.145

Berk, M.L., & Monheit, A.C. (2001). The concentration of health care expenditures, revisited. *Health Affairs, 20*(2), 9–18. http://dx.doi.org/10.1377/ hlthaff.20.2.9

Canadian Institute for Health Information. (2006). *Medical imaging technologies in Canada, 2006: Methodological notes*. https://secure.cihi.ca/estore/product Series.htm?pc=PCC211

Canadian Institute for Health Information. (2013). *National health expenditure trends, 1975–2011*. https://secure.cihi.ca/estore/productFamily.htm?pf= PFC2400&lang=en&media=0

Clark, N. (2010). *Why are health spending accounts a necessity for Canadians?* http://www.articlesbase.com/insurance-articles/health-spending-accounts-a-necessity-for-canadians-3322158.html

Deber, R., Forget, E., & Roos, L. (2004). Medical savings accounts in a universal system: Wishful thinking meets evidence. *Health Policy (Amsterdam)*, *70*(1), 49–66. http://dx.doi.org/10.1016/j.healthpol.2004.01.010

Deber, R., & Lam, K.C.K. (2009). *Handling the high spenders: Implications of the distribution of health expenditures for financing health care, 2009 Annual Meeting & Exhibition*. American Political Science Association. http://papers.ssrn .com/sol3/papers.cfm?abstract_id=1450788

Deber, R., & Lam, K.C.K. (2011a). *Experience with medical savings accounts in selected jurisdictions* (Paper 4). CHSRF Series of Reports on Financing Models. http://www.cfhi-fcass.ca/sf-docs/default-source/commissioned-research-reports/RAISA4_Experience_in_MSA_EN.pdf?sfvrsn=0

Deber, R., & Lam, K.C.K. (2011b). *Medical savings accounts in financing healthcare* (Paper 3). CHSRF Reports on Financing Models. http://www.cfhi-fcass.ca/ Libraries/Commissioned_Research_Reports/RAISA3-MedicalSAcc_EN .sflb.ashx

Fong, A.J. (2008). *Who are frequent users of the emergency department across different classification of ED use?* Calgary, AB: University of Calgary.

Forget, E.L., Deber, R., & Roos, L.L. (2002). Medical savings accounts: Will they reduce costs? *Canadian Medical Association Journal*, *167*(2), 143–7.

Forget, E.L., Roos, L., Deber, R., & Walld, R. (2008). Variations in lifetime healthcare costs across a population. *Health Policy (Amsterdam)*, *4*(1), 148–67.

Gabel, J.R., Lo Sasso, A.T., & Rice, T. (2002). Consumer-driven health plans: Are they more than talk now? *Health Affairs* (Supplement), w395–407.

Gauthier, A.K., & Clancy, C.M. (2004). Consumer-driven health care – Beyond rhetoric with research and experience. *Health Services Research*, *39*(4, Pt. 2), 1049–54. http://dx.doi.org/10.1111/j.1475-6773.2004.00272.x

Hurley, J.E., & Guindon, G.E. (2008). Medical savings accounts: Promises and pitfalls. In M. Lu & E. Jonsson (Eds.), *Financing health care: New ideas for a changing society* (pp. 125–47). Weinheim, Germany: Wiley-VCH Verlag GmbH, KGaA.

Mazankowski, D. (2001). *A framework for reform: Report of the Premier's Advisory Council on health.* http://www.assembly.ab.ca/lao/library/egovdocs/alpm/2001/132279.pdf

McGrail, K. (2007). Medicare financing and redistribution in British Columbia, 1992 and 2002. *Health Policy (Amsterdam), 2*(4), 123–37.

McGrail, K., Green, B., Barer, M.L., Evans, R.G., Hertzman, C., & Normand, C. (2000). Age, costs of acute and long-term care and proximity to death: Evidence for 1987–88 and 1994–95 in British Columbia. *Age and Ageing, 29*(3), 249–53. http://dx.doi.org/10.1093/ageing/29.3.249

McGrail, K.M. (2006). *Equity in health, health care services use and health care financing in British Columbia, 1992 and 2002.* Ph.D. Thesis. University of British Columbia: Vancouver, B.C. http://hdl.handle.net/2429/18515.

McGrail, K.M. (2008). Income-related inequities: Cross-sectional analyses of the use of Medicare services in British Columbia in 1992 and 2002. *Open Medicine, 2*(4), E3–10.

Monheit, A.C. (2003). Persistence in health expenditures in the short run: Prevalence and consequences. *Medical Care, 41*(7, Supplement), III-53–64. http://dx.doi.org/10.1097/00005650-200307001-00007

Paris, V., Devaux, M., & Wei, L. (2010). *Health systems institutional characteristics: A survey of 29 OECD countries* (OECD Health Working Paper No. 50). http://ideas.repec.org/p/oec/elsaad/50-en.html

Pauly, M.V. (1968). The economics of moral hazard [Comment]. *American Economic Review, 58*(3), 531–7.

Pauly, M.V. (2002). Insurance reimbursement. In A.J. Culyer & J.P. Newhouse (Eds.), *Handbook of health economics* (pp. 537–60). Amsterdam: Elsevier.

Shearer, G. (2004). Commentary: Defined contribution health plans: Attracting the healthy and well-off. *Health Services Research, 39*(4, Pt. 2), 1159–66. http://dx.doi.org/10.1111/j.1475-6773.2004.00280.x

University of Lethbridge. (2013). *Health spending account non-taxable: Frequently asked questions.* Human Resources Department. http://www.uleth.ca/hr/pension-and-benefits/sites/pension-and-benefits/files/FAQ%20HSA%20June%202013.pdf

Xu, K., Evans, D.B., Carrin, G., Aguilar-Rivera, A.M., Musgrove, P., & Evans, T. (2007). Protecting households from catastrophic health spending. *Health Affairs, 26*(4), 972–83. http://dx.doi.org/10.1377/hlthaff.26.4.972

# 19 Long-Term Care Reform in Ontario
## "The Long Delivery"

*PATRICIA BARANEK, JANE-ANNE CAMPBELL, KERRY KULUSKI,
CHRISTOPHER J. LONGO, FRANCES MORTON-CHANG, KAREN
SPALDING, CAROLYN STEELE GRAY, FERN TEPLITSKY, ROMY JOSEPH
THOMAS, JILLIAN WATKINS, ANNE WOJTAK, AND RAISA B. DEBER*

What services should be given to people who need assistance to remain in their home, and who should pay for them? A series of home care models have been proposed. What should the government do?

This case addresses several policy issues, including: alternative ways of financing and delivering care, public and private roles, definitions of medical necessity, and the impact of interests on policymaking.

**Appendices**

Appendix A: Long-term Care Services
Appendix B: Analyzing Home Care Models
Appendix C: Concerns Expressed during Procurement Review
Appendix D: References Cited and Further Reading

**The Case**

People who need some assistance in carrying out activities of daily living may benefit from receiving long-term care (LTC) services. Unlike acute care, which is required for a relatively short time, LTC services are often required on a sustained basis. LTC may be delivered within a specialized facility (e.g., nursing homes, homes for the aged) or in the community (e.g., in-home services, community support services, supportive housing). Most community-based LTC services, often referred to as "home care," are provided by family members, friends, and volunteers, but there is also a strong role for paid workers (Baranek et al., 2004).

A wide range of LTC services may be offered. One way of categorizing them is to distinguish between *health* and *social care*; another is to distinguish among *professional services* (provided by nurses, rehabilitation professionals, etc.), *personal care support* (often provided by unregulated health care workers), and *social support*. These categorizations may overlap, since those services classified as health care also tend to be clinical (e.g., medical care, nursing, and rehabilitation) and to be delivered by trained health care professionals and/or personnel under their supervision. Social care services include personal care, meals, day programs, transportation, and house maintenance services, as well as support groups and/or respite care to assist informal caregivers (family members and volunteers who provide care). Social care services are often delivered by less skilled workers and/or by volunteers. Depending upon needs, such non-clinical assistance as housing adaptations can also be helpful. Appendix A provides more details about the kinds of LTC services that might be provided.

How best to deliver such services is of concern internationally, particularly as the population ages, and technological advances allow care to shift outside of hospitals into home and community (Hollander & Prince, 2008; Williams, Challis, et al., 2009). Under ideal circumstances, this shift can improve both cost (if home care is cheaper than hospital-based care) and quality (if care in the community is what people prefer) (Baranek et al., 2004). However, if care is given to people who could have managed without it, the service may be an "add-on" (albeit a valued one), and total costs may increase. Conversely, if people's needs exceed the help they receive, care can be suboptimal, and caregivers can be under considerable stress (Williams, Challis, et al., 2009; Williams, Lum, et al., 2009). To the extent that community-based care relies on informal caregivers, problems can arise when family members do not live near the client, are in the workforce or otherwise unavailable, and/or do not exist at all. Getting the right balance is difficult.

Another variable is who should receive what, and who should pay. Potential clients range in age and needs, but usually include individuals of all ages who may have chronic illnesses, cognitive impairments, physical disabilities, and/or functional limitations. One common way of categorizing potential clients is by function: *acute care substitution* allows people to be safely discharged from acute hospitals; *long-term care substitution* serves those who might otherwise be in long-term care institutions, and *prevention/maintenance* keeps people healthy enough to remain out of institutions (Dumont-Lemasson et al., 1999). Those in the acute care substitution category are often referred to as *ALC* (alternate level of care) patients. Policymakers have repeatedly struggled with how to provide LTC, including the balance between facilities and community care, and how various services should be financed and delivered. A number of models have been put forth by different governments in different jurisdictions at different times. Suggested policy approaches have included various combinations of: expanding the definition of insured services to include publicly funded coverage for post-acute clients (as well as those needing end-of-life care), a tax credit / tax deduction for home care consumers, an insurance fund for home care, and/or benefits / job protection for family caregivers (Standing Senate Committee on Social Affairs Science and Technology, 2002). Policymakers have often focused on patients who occupy (publicly financed) hospital beds but might be cared for in other, less expensive settings. The care needs of ALC individuals are likely to be time-limited and hence easier to manage. Others have expressed concern that focusing only on the immediate needs of those requiring acute care substitution and ignoring the other categories of clients can be "penny wise and pound foolish." They point to studies suggesting that the prevention/maintenance services can be cost-saving in the long term, particularly by avoiding subsequent hospital, emergency, and LTC admissions (Hollander & Chappell, 2002). However, research has clarified that, even among the population that might benefit from LTC, the vast majority require relatively little care. Thus, although this care may be very much appreciated by the recipients and their families, if it is not carefully targeted, significant costs can be added without achieving those offsetting cost savings. Accordingly, a number of tools have been developed to try to identify the high-needs population.

One widely accepted approach classifies potential clients onto what is called the "Kaiser Permanente Triangle"; in this model, the base (most people) needs minimal help, while the few at the peak of the triangle require considerable resources. For example, the UK Department of Health found that 3%–5% of their home care clients used the most health and social care resources (Department of Health, 2005). Ongoing research has attempted to use one UK tool, the Balance of Care Model, to identify which Ontario seniors could be cost-effectively managed at home, which group would need more intensive services, and which group could manage with little support. These studies found that between 20% and 50% of those already on waiting lists for placement in

LTC facilities could be treated at home if the appropriate services were available (Williams, Challis, et al., 2009; Williams, Lum, et al., 2009).

As noted in Chapter 1, section 9.1 (Canadian Data), in Canada, about 70% of health expenditures come from public sources, but this varies considerably by subsector (Canadian Institute for Health Information, 2005, 2013). One reason is historical. The *Canada Health Act* (*CHA*) requires full coverage of insured persons for insured services (see Chapter 1, section 7.2). However, the comprehensiveness provisions of the *CHA* define insured services in terms of who provides them (physicians) and where they are provided (hospitals). In contrast, many LTC services fall within the category of "extended health care services," which are defined by the *CHA* as including: "(a) nursing home intermediate care service, (b) adult residential care service, (c) home care service, and (d) ambulatory health care service." These extended health care services do not fall within the *CHA* definition of comprehensiveness; provincial/territorial governments can still fund such services should they wish to do so, but are not required to. Depending on the jurisdiction, eligibility for, access to, and costs of community-based LTC may vary widely, as may the distribution of resulting costs between public and private sources. Some provinces base their coverage decisions on categories of services and/or categories of individuals (which in turn may be based on combinations of age, income, region, and/or diagnosis). In turn, this is related to the question of which services society believes should be publicly paid for (Deber & Gamble, 2007).

In practice, the way the *CHA* defines insured services often means that reorganization of care by shifting it from hospitals to home and community may mean moving services outside of the *CHA* funding guarantees (Baranek et al., 2004). The issue became more pronounced when concerted efforts to reduce health expenditures in the 1980s and 1990s led to the closure of many acute care beds, often on the assumption that home and community care could pick up the burden of care. A number of commissions have called for modernizing the legal basis of Canadian Medicare to ensure that necessary care is covered regardless of where it is provided (Commission on the Future of Health Care in Canada, 2002; Standing Senate Committee on Social Affairs Science and Technology, 2002), but this has not yet happened. However, many provinces have agreed to pay for care in the community for some services for some categories of people, although these arrangements are not entitlements and are subject to change with subsequent governments.

## Ontario's Multiple Strategies

Different models exist to finance and deliver home and community care. One way to categorize them is to analyze the public-private mix in how this care is financed, and how it is delivered (see Chapter 1, section 6.1, Dimensions of Health Care Systems). Between 1987 and 1995, five different home care delivery strategies were proposed by three different Ontario governments (see Appendix B, Analyzing Home Care Models). As described by Baranek et al. (2004), these proposed approaches used three different models; brokerage, quasi-public delivery, and managed competition.

In the *brokerage* model, a coordinating agency would offer coordinated assessment and case management services. All other services would be purchased by the agency from third-party providers, which could be for-profit (FP) or not-for-profit (NFP). Brokerage models were proposed by both the Peterson Liberal government (One-Stop Access and Service Access Organizations) and the Rae NDP government (Service Coordination Agency).

The *quasi-public delivery* model would amalgamate the majority of existing private provider organizations into a single organization, which would directly employ home care service providers. The Rae NDP government also proposed this model (Multi-Service Agency).

The *managed competition* model would set up geographically based NFP agencies to purchase services with public money from private providers, both FP and NFP, using a competitive bidding process. While this model still may include a coordinating agency that offers coordinated assessment and case management services, it differs from the brokerage model by requiring providers of the other services to compete for contracts, rather than be assured of continued contracts as long as their performance was seen as acceptable. This model was compatible with the "new public management" approaches, which sought to increase effectiveness of public service delivery (Osborne & Gaebler, 1992). This was the model implemented in Ontario by the Harris Conservative government in 1996, when they set up 43 geographically based purchasing agencies, which they called Community Care Access Centres (CCACs).

## Community Care Access Centres (CCACs)

CCACs are a series of regionally based, not-for-profit community agencies that were made responsible for the assessment, care planning, care coordination, and quality monitoring of publicly funded home-health services in Ontario. CCACs also provide information, referral, and navigation of community services. In addition, CCACs are the access points for long-term care home beds and, depending on the area of the province, for a variety of other community-based services, including convalescent care, adult day programs, and other support services. CCACs directly fund and arrange for delivery (via contracts) of a range of in-home services, including nursing, occupational therapy, physio-therapy, speech language pathology, social work, dietetic services, per-sonal support, and homemaking; CCACs may also purchase medical supplies and equipment on behalf of individuals living in the commu-nity. Their mandate includes assessment, authorization, and, for those meeting the eligibility criteria, arrangement for the provision of publicly funded home-based health and professional services, as well as school health support services. They also have responsibility for assessing and managing admissions to LTC facilities, including maintaining LTC wait lists. The CCACs are given a budget that is expected to cover both the case management services (directly provided by CCAC employees) and the contracts to external agencies to provide the CCAC-funded services. There are no age limitations for clients. One key difference between these community-based services and hospital and physician services, however, is that there is no entitlement to them; accordingly, clients may (and often do) privately purchase services from providers beyond the level that the CCAC will provide, and also pay for other services in the community, including some services that the CCACs will not cover but will connect them with.

One of the more controversial elements of the CCAC model was the requirement that contracts be awarded to the agencies that would ensure "the best quality for the best price." Consumer groups and pro-viders were concerned that this meant that service contracts would be awarded to providers who bid the lowest price, since there was very little experience in the LTC community sector in establishing outcome measures to ensure quality of service (Williams et al., 1999). In order to avoid placing some of the existing NFP service agencies (including the Red Cross and the Victorian Order of Nurses) at a competitive dis-advantage, the provincial government had promised to protect service volumes for existing providers until 1999. However, several studies con-cluded that the competitive model had destabilized the market for pro-viders. In some cases (including rehabilitation services), the new model had paradoxically increased costs, particularly when quasi-monopolies were created after already small/specialized groups of providers who had been unsuccessful in bidding for contracts were unable to remain in business to compete for future bids (Randall & Williams, 2006). Proponents of the competitive bidding process argued that, in the longer term, competition for contracts would improve quality by raising the bar for providers to win and maintain contracts with CCACs, and that providers with lower quality and/or higher administrative costs would eventually be driven out of the market.

In response to increasing provider costs and overall demand, the Ministry of Health and Long-Term Care (MOHLTC) froze CCAC funding for the 2001–2 and 2002–3 fiscal years at the 2000–1 levels. This was part of an overall attempt to control costs, which had also included hospital restructuring and budget freezes for many subsectors. As part of that effort, the provincial government informed CCACs that budgetary overruns would no longer be accepted; CCACs reacted by reducing service volumes and tightening eligibility criteria. The Auditor General of Ontario (2010) reported that homemaking hours had decreased by 30% and in-home nursing visits by 22% during 2001–2 and 2002–3.

### Enter the LHINS

In 2003, the Liberal party, under the leadership of Dalton McGuinty, formed the Ontario government. Their new governance model adopted the language of new public management, and spoke of "steering, not rowing." It spoke of moving the provincial government to a stewardship model rather than trying to directly manage service providers. One key approach was to move to a regionalized approach (see Chapter 1, section 2.2.4, Regional Authorities in Canada). Following a series of consultation workshops, in 2006 the government proclaimed the *Local Health System Integration Act*, which created 14 regional NFP corporations called Local Health Integration Networks (LHINs). Unlike the regional health authorities that had been established in other provinces, LHINs did not directly provide health services. Instead, they replaced the old District Health Councils (which had been involved in planning and coordination for their regions), and took on some functions from the provincial MOHLTC. The MOHLTC retained a stewardship role and overall responsibility for establishing strategic directions and provincial priorities for the health system, along with developing legislation, regulations, standards, policies, and directives to support those strategic directions (Ministry of Health and Long-Term Care, 2013). However, the LHINs were responsible at a local level to work with health providers and community members to best determine the health service priorities of their geographic regions, including planning, integrating, and funding of local health services. The services assigned to LHINs included: hospitals, Community Care Access Centres, community support services, long-term care, mental health and addictions services, and Community Health Centres (Ministry of Health and Long-Term Care, 2006). With the introduction of the LHINs, the CCAC boundaries were realigned and merged to fit the new LHIN boundaries. Whereas there had been 43 (and then 42), there were now 14. The CCACs were now funded both through their LHIN and, for some programs, directly through the MOHLTC. CCACs were still managed by community boards of directors. One potential problem for CCACs was that the LHIN boundaries did not fully match those of local governments, or of local catchment areas, although efforts had been made to base them on patterns of hospital patient visits.

In 2007 the MOHLTC allotted $700 million across the province to LHINs to allow them to address the community health needs of seniors in their respective regions. LHINs were expected to lead this initiative by identifying and providing funding for enhanced home care and community support services, as well as for innovative projects specific to the LHIN. In keeping with the theme of "rebuilding home care," Premier McGuinty increased CCAC funding to $1.3 billion (excluding dollars allocated to community support services) with a projected increase to $1.7 billion for 2007–8.

However, to answer concerns about the impact of competitive bidding on NFP providers and on costs, Premier McGuinty requested a review of the current competitive bidding/procurement process conducted in Ontario (see Appendix C for some concerns expressed). The review was chaired by former Minister of Health Elinor Caplan. Since the introduction of managed competition, the way services are procured and delivered had been a growing concern to clients, service providers, and CCACs. The mandate of the procurement review was to assess a number of areas, including quality of client care, mechanisms for selecting providers, effectiveness of current method of sourcing and delivery, level of stability in the home care workforce, and the role of the MOHLTC in supporting the delivery and procurement of home care delivery in Ontario (Caplan, 2005). Although the Caplan report's 70 recommendations for improving the CCAC procurement process did not recommend changing the overall CCAC procurement model, it did express some concerns (see Appendix C). One response to the recommendations came from Hugh McLeod, then an assistant deputy minister of health. In 2008, he put changes to the CCAC client services procurement process on hold until further notice while the Ministry reviewed the Caplan report's recommendations; he did allow procurement of medical supplies and equipment to continue.

In the interim, there have been suggestions that the CCACs have shifted their emphasis to helping acute care hospitals discharge ALC patients (a government priority), at the expense of those needing longer-term services or services to avoid nursing home placement. In his 2010 report, the Auditor General of Ontario (2010) was generally positive, but noted that there was considerable variability across CCACs, and that many people were waiting for services. In his June 2011 report, *Caring for Our Aging Population and Addressing Alternate Level of Care*, Dr. David Walker reinforced the emphasis on ALC; he suggested that, in order to address the growing issue of seniors waiting inappropriately for care in ALC hospital beds, there needed to be an integration of services across primary care, hospitals, and community care sectors in order to ensure that seniors could remain in their homes for as long as possible (Walker, 2011).

DECISION POINT

You are in a province that does not currently provide publicly funded home care services. You have been asked to examine Ontario's experience and suggest who should be covered, for what services, and using which model. What do you recommend?

SUGGESTED QUESTIONS FOR DISCUSSION

1. What is LTC and what types of services can it include? For whom?
2. Who should pay for what? How do the *Canada Health Act* definitions affect this? How does this relate to concepts of the proper role of the state?
3. How do these different models deal with financing and delivery of services?
4. What policy goals are being sought, and how do these different models relate to these goals? How can the effectiveness of LTC services be measured? Discuss the implications of the production characteristics of the various kinds of LTC services.

5. Who are the key interest groups, and what are their likely positions? How would different models of LTC affect other parts of the health care system?
6. How might local factors affect your answers (e.g., urban and rural areas)?


APPENDIX A: LONG-TERM CARE SERVICES

Long-term care (LTC) can be offered in facilities or in the community. There are several categories of LTC facilities, which vary in what they are called, in the types of clients they serve, and who pays for what. As noted, for the most part, LTC does not fall under the terms of the *Canada Health Act* (see Chapter 1, section 7.2, *Canada Health Act*). However, most provinces do pay a share of the costs of LTC in some categories of facilities, although residents may also have to pay a varying share of the bill.

The services that may be provided in LTC facilities include various mixes of medical, nursing, rehabilitative, attendant, activity, and social support services, as well as food and shelter. At the time of the case, Ontario had three main categories of LTC facilities:

*Retirement homes* can also be referred to by such terms as retirement residence, care home, assisted living, or rest home. These facilities were private and (at the time of the case) were not regulated. They received no government funding. They catered to individuals or couples wishing to live independently, but who would like/need light housekeeping, meals, low levels of personal care (usually from unregulated workers), and availability of staff on a 24-hour basis. The rooms ranged from shared living to apartments (bachelor or one or two bedrooms). They were owned and managed by private corporations (largely but not entirely FP). The cost per person for accommodation and care ranged from $1,500 to $5,000/month for a private room. Because these homes were considered to be private accommodation, they were covered by the same legislation applying to other rental housing (in Ontario, the *Tenant Protection Act*), but not otherwise regulated, although some municipalities may also have "care home" by-laws. However, some of these homes have voluntarily chosen to be accredited through the Ontario Residential Care Association. The CCACs were not involved with controlling access to retirement homes. Because retirement homes were considered residences, those living in Ontario retirement homes were eligible to receive home care services from the CCAC on the same conditions as those living in their own homes. A number of retirement homes advertise their services, including using television ads. They vary in their client mix, ranging from a focus on recreational activities for healthy seniors to providing supportive services for a sicker clientele.

*Supportive housing* may be called non-profit housing, social housing, or seniors' housing. This type of housing catered to individuals or couples who need daily personal care, 24-hour availability of a trained personal support worker, meal preparation, and/or homemaking to live independently. The rooms ranged from shared living to apartments (bachelor or one or two bedrooms). The type of building management varied, but services tended to be managed by NFP corporations. The costs per person were divided into rent and support services. The rental costs varied according to market rent in that location, but at the time of writing were in the range of $600 to $1,200/month, with rent subsidies available for some people in some locations. The support service costs were largely covered by MOHLTC. These facilities were also subject to the *Tenant Protection Act*. Service provision, however, fell under the *Long-Term Care Homes Act* and at the time was guided by the MOHLTC's policies. Supportive housing facilities could also seek voluntary accreditation through the Council on Health Services Accreditation. As was the case for retirement homes, the CCACs were not involved with access to supportive housing units, although clients in supportive housing might receive services from the CCAC.

*Long-term care homes* may be called homes, nursing homes, or homes for the aged. They catered to individuals who need higher levels of daily personal care, availability of 24-hour nursing care or supervision, and a secure environment. The rooms ranged from ward rooms (four people) to semi-private (two people) and private rooms (usually for an additional fee). For historical reasons, the term "homes for the aged" usually referred to facilities owned by municipal governments, whereas "nursing homes" may be owned by NFP corporations or private FP corporations. The costs of these facilities were also divided into those for accommodation and those for services. Because many residents were already receiving pension money (which in theory was expected to cover their costs for housing), there were varying co-payment rates charged to the resident. As of 1 July 2010, Ontario had set co-payment rates at $1,619.08/month for "standard or basic" accommodation; $1,862.41 for semi-private accommodation; and $2,166.58 for private accommodation. The provincial government might subsidize accommodation to the "basic or standard" rate for those who qualify for this subsidy, and it did pay for the nursing and support care provided in nursing homes. These facilities may be regulated under the *Homes for the Aged and Rest Homes Act*, the *Nursing Homes Act*, or the *Charitable Institutions Act*. They can seek voluntary accreditation through the Canadian Council for Health Services Accreditation. Unlike the other categories of facility care, people must apply via their local CCAC for placement in LTC homes. If eligible, they could designate their top five choices (except for short-stay respite care or if immediate admission is required due to a crisis). This has proven somewhat problematic, particularly for those wanting placement in facilities that seek to cater to members of particular ethnocultural groups. In many cases, their preferred LTC homes have had long wait lists (of up to 3–5 years); this has resulted in people waiting in expensive acute care beds, putting great pressure on the health care system to ensure that people are moved to the right place of care.

At the time of writing, operating revenue for all LTC facilities, both FP and NFP, came from four streams, which were labelled: Nursing and Personal Care (NPC), Program and Support Services (PSS), Accommodation Costs, and Extra Services. NPC and PSS funding came solely from the provincial government, but only for residents who were covered by the provincial health insurance plan (OHIP). The money allocated towards these services took into account the case mix index of the facility and had to be either spent on NPC and PSS or returned to the government at the end of the fiscal year. Accommodation costs included lodging, housekeeping, maintenance, dietary services, laundry services, administrative services, and raw food. Accommodation costs were shared between government and residents; the LTC facilities were permitted to keep surplus dollars from this revenue stream. The government share of the basic accommodation cost was means tested; government would pay the full cost of accommodation if the resident could not afford it, but did not subsidize the cost for "preferred accommodation" (e.g., private rooms) beyond the standard co-payment. Extra services for which the facilities could charge the clients included such items as cable television or hairdressing.

NFP nursing homes were eligible to receive capital grant funding from the provincial government related to construction and furnishing

of the facilities; most of these funds are channeled through Infrastructure Ontario.

*Community-based LTC* can be subdivided into the following three
components: in-home services, community support services, and supportive housing.

> *In-home services* (provided in-home by a paid worker) could be in
> turn subdivided into four sections. *Professional care* includes clini-
> cal services provided by regulated health professionals (e.g., nurs-
> ing, physiotherapy, occupational therapy, social work) in a person's
> home environment. *Personal support* includes support services pro-
> vided primarily by non-professional care providers (e.g., personal
> support workers, health care aides, community support workers)
> and involves provision of and/or assistance with and/or training
> to carry out personal activities of daily living (e.g., transferring,
> dressing, toileting, eating) and/or personal hygiene activities (e.g.,
> washing, mouth care, hair care, routine hand/foot care, changing
> dressings). *Homemaking* includes other support services provided in
> the home, such as light housecleaning, laundry, ironing, shopping,
> banking, paying bills, preparing meals, caring for children, super-
> vision, and/or assisting a person with any of the foregoing activi-
> ties. *Attendant care services* refers to provision of homemaking and
> personal support activities to people over 16 years of age who have
> permanent physical disabilities and require assistance with activities
> of daily living. Clients can also direct an attendant (often a personal
> support worker) to carry out predetermined tasks that they cannot
> physically do for themselves. Note that many of these services also
> can be, and often are, provided by unpaid caregivers, usually the
> family and friends of a person requiring such care.
>
> *Community support services* (CSS) refers to non-professional ser-
> vices provided to individuals in the community, both in their own
> homes and/or in other places in the community. Community support
> services might include transportation, meals on wheels, diners club,
> adult day service, home maintenance and repair, friendly visiting,
> security checks, caregiver support, respite care, home help, foot care,
> emergency response systems, life skills services, hospice, and inter-
> vention and assistance services. (Only some of these services were
> funded by the MOHLTC; most had shifted to the LHINs, with a sub-
> stantial proportion of their costs being met through fundraising and
> donations rather than public funding.) Community support services

can be provided by paid staff and/or volunteers. Increasingly, home-making services have been shifting from CCAC funding. Since provincial policy was that CCAC services were fully funded, but CSS services were not, this meant a shift in who paid for what.

*Supportive housing* (SH) refers to provision of case management and coordination and/or delivery of services to support individuals (primarily seniors) living in such facilities with activities of daily living (e.g., bathing, dressing, toileting) and instrumental activities of daily living (e.g., cooking, cleaning, shopping). SH was designed to help people who only need minimal to moderate care – such as homemaking or personal care and support – to live independently. SH accommodations usually consist of rental units within an apartment building, or in a small group residence. SH is intended to be available 24/7 and be sufficiently flexible to respond to increased service need when clients are not well, and decrease services as their health improves. SH can also work with other service providers to offer more intensive care on a short-term basis in palliative care situations, as resources and qualifications permit.

## APPENDIX B: ANALYZING HOME CARE MODELS

As noted in Chapter 1, section 6.1 (Dimensions of Health Care Systems), there are a number of ways to classify health care (Deber, 2000, 2004). One dimension is the public-private mix (see Chapter 1, section 6.1.1, Public and Private). The other is the distinction between who pays for what, and how care is delivered (see Chapter 1, section 6.1.2, Financing and Delivery). Payment can be public or private. Private payment, in turn, can come from private insurance or out-of-pocket expenditures. Delivery can be classified as public, NFP, FP private small business, or private FP corporations. Various combinations of financing and delivery are possible (see Chapter 1, section 6.1.3, Models of Health Systems).

### A Brief History of Home Care in Ontario

It has long been recognized that in-home services can be a cost-effective and humane alternative to facility care. A number of NFP agencies, including the Victorian Order of Nurses, the Saint Elizabeth Visiting Nurses Association, and the Red Cross, have long provided such services in various Canadian jurisdictions. In 1955, Ontario had already implemented the Special Home Care Program to allow payment to owners of private homes caring for seniors. In 1958, a provincial government-funded Homemakers and Nurses Services Program supported some visiting nursing care and homemaker services provided by the existing NFP agencies, funded in part by federal grants under the Canada Assistance Program. In 1974, Ontario had introduced the Acute Home Care program to treat individuals with acute health care needs at home instead of in hospitals. This program was followed by the Respite Care Program, to support informal caregivers. In 1975, a Chronic Home Care program was first piloted, with the aim of delaying institutionalization and maintaining elderly persons at home through the provision of such in-home support services as homemaking and assistance with activities of daily living. Unlike the Acute Home Care program, which had an established discharge date (based on predetermined treatment goals) and a maximum length of stay (LOS), the Chronic Home Care program could be used indefinitely. One policy dilemma was that, instead of replacing more expensive hospital care (as the acute home care had done), this newly funded program was often seen as an "add-on" to existing funded services.

In 1979, Ontario brought many of the NFP support services receiving government funding together under one umbrella structure called the Home Support Program for the Elderly. It included meals on wheels, wheels to meals (congregate dining), friendly visitors, security checks for the homebound, minor and seasonal home help, telephone reassurance, counselling and referral as they related to home support, day care for seniors, transportation, and other personal services. These community support services, often developed by charitable organizations, grew haphazardly, varying with the composition, culture, religion, and values of each community's existing charitable sector. Small, low-cost, and grass roots, the agencies which delivered these services were run, in part, by volunteers and supported by a combination of user fees, local government, corporate programs, and charitable donations, including some funds from the provincial Ministry of Community and Social Services. At the same time, the province implemented a Placement Coordination Service.

With increased demand on programs, as a result of a growing population of seniors and developing technology, LTC costs soared. By the early 1980s there was increasing recognition that LTC services were seriously in need of reform. Services were fragmented; there was no overall framework for LTC. At the provincial government level, responsibility for LTC was spread across several ministries (health, social services). Some services were funded at the municipal level, others at the provincial and federal level. There was no logic to the eligibility criteria. Most of the services were concentrated in Southern Ontario, which had more voluntary organizations, leaving individuals in the more rural and remote regions underserviced. In 1981, the Conservative government had promised to establish an Office on Aging, and to review, develop, and pilot new strategies for delivering LTC services.

In 1985, the Ontario Liberal party was elected with a minority government (in partnership with the New Democratic Party), ending a 40-year Conservative party reign. Following up on the initiatives begun by its predecessor, this government also identified LTC reform as a key issue. Soon after the election, a Minister without Portfolio responsible for senior citizens affairs was appointed; he immediately undertook a consultation tour across the province to garner public input on seniors' issues. The consultation identified lack of coordination and fragmentation of services as two key concerns. Within a year, the new government had introduced phase I of the Integrated Homemaker Program. This program did not require medical referral; the intent was to deliver fully funded homemaking and personal care services to frail elderly persons and adults with physical disabilities to help them remain in the community. By 1993, it existed across the province (in 38 sites). Indeed, the One Stop Access pilot project, described briefly below, was intended to provide a single point of access to community-based services for these same target populations through an integrated assessment and case management approach. This model had emerged from a public consultation process that had also produced a white paper. Although the model itself was repeatedly placed on hold, and was never really implemented, in large part because of difficulties in coordinating among the various government departments with responsibility for these programs, the process of developing it had mobilized participants, most with concentrated interests in long-term care (see Chapter 1, section 4.1, Concentrated/Diffuse Interests). These included providers of LTC services, consumers, and their families. In the process the "scope of conflict" (see Chapter 1, section 4.3) had broadened (Deber & Williams, 1995).

Over the next decade, a number of other care models were proposed but never really implemented (Baranek et al., 2004). They could be summarized in terms of their approaches to financing and delivery as follows.

Three of the proposed models could be classified as *brokerage* models.

The *One-Stop Shopping/Access* model noted above, proposed by the Liberal government in 1987, would have used mixed funding, with in-home professional and homemaking services fully funded for those deemed eligible by a physician, and community support services (CSS) partially covered by the Ontario Ministry of Community and Social Services (MOHSS) on a means-tested basis and partially privately financed (since CSS was not considered to be a universal entitlement). Delivery would have remained private, with a mix of FP and NFP providers (but NFP preference). The model would provide a single point of access for service assessment and coordination. In-home professional and personal support would be purchased for the consumer by the brokerage agency. It was never implemented.

The *Service Access Organization (SAO)* model, proposed by the Liberal government in 1990, would also employ mixed funding. The public funding would include LTC placement coordination, administration costs of SAOs, and service coordination; government would also directly fund some CSS services. No user fees would be charged for in-home professional and personal support, but there would be user fees for homemaking and CSS services, based on income. This proposed model would introduce regional funding envelopes, with some expectation that costs for home care would eventually be taken from the publicly funded physician (OHIP) funding envelope. Delivery would be private; the SAOs would use their government funds to purchase in-home professional and homemaking services. SAOs resembled the unimplemented One Stop Access model; they would assess clients and purchase services on their behalf, and act as a single access point to the LTC system, "combining information, referral, service co-ordination and service provision on a case-managed basis" (Deber & Williams, 1995). The goal of the SAO was to provide services at the lowest care level possible, treat institutionalization as a last resort, and rely instead on community based services. SAOs would report to 14 regional management offices, which would allow the province to preserve much of the existing LTC system and still try to meet individual and regional needs. Each regional office was to have a "funding envelope" that would be used to fund the operational and capital expenses of all institutional and community-based long-term care services in a region. (The regionalization model followed the MCSS example of regional area offices, but was foreign to the Ministry of Health's tradition of centralized management. As such, it was perceived with some scepticism by those in the health sector.) While the consultation process was underway, the Liberal government was defeated in 1991. The new NDP government had different proposals.

The *Service Coordination Agency (SCA)* model proposed by the NDP government in 1991 was basically the same as the SAO model. It would also use mixed funding, with government paying for an integrated health and personal support program. Access to non-professional services would no longer be dependent on having physician referral for in-home professional and personal support. There would be increased funding for CSS; user fees would be based on income. Delivery would be private. The intent was to establish 40 SCAs across the province to provide LTC placement and service coordination for professional and personal support; CSS would be accessed directly by the client. The model incorporated a preference for NFP providers, an increase for homemaker wages, and pay equity requirements for community-based providers. The model also would have provided for a pilot project giving direct funding to persons with disabilities to purchase their own care.

Following a series of consultations, the NDP dropped that model, and recommended a new approach, which would rely on *quasi-public delivery*. In 1994, the NDP government suggested a *Multi-Service Agency (MSA)* model. Public funding would include in-home professional and personal support services. A dedicated funding envelope would allow the province to determine how much they wished to spend on these services. A major change was that the MSA would be responsible for both budgeting and providing service. Up to 20% of the budget could be used for external purchasing of services from NFP or FP agencies, but at least 80% of services were to be provided by agencies that were part of the MSA umbrella system. Government would determine which organizations would be part of the MSA, and would determine the MSA budgets. This would require that the over 1,200 existing community agencies be merged (and that those organizations that were located in multiple geographical areas be subdivided to match the MSA boundaries); not surprisingly, this generated considerable opposition from most key stakeholders.

The models actually implemented used *managed competition*. Introduced by the Conservatives and continued by the Liberal government, *Community Care Access Centres* (CCACs) used mixed funding, with capped budgets provided by the province. Within these budgets, each CCAC would determine eligibility for professional and personal support, and homemaking services. No user fees were to be charged for the professional and personal support services provided by CCACs; however, the model guaranteed only that clients would receive an assessment, not that they would actually receive services. Neither did it prohibit clients from purchasing services with their own money. The model, in theory, served a number of populations with LTC needs, but in an era of fiscal restraint, service limits and stricter eligibility were not uncommon. Delivery was private, with CCACs purchasing services from outside agencies based on a competitive bidding process, seeking the "best quality for the lowest price." However, the program giving direct public funding to some persons with disabilities to allow them to purchase services continued.

CCACs operated within a regional model. At the time of writing, the 14 geographically based Local Health Integration Networks (LHINs) received funds from the provincial MOHLTC, and were responsible for planning, funding, and monitoring a specified range of providers and services for their region. LHINS employed a public contracting model; the providers remained private but received public funds through the LHINs to cover for the specified services. Governance involved two sets of accountability arrangements – between the LHINS and the province and between the LHINS and the local providers. Responsibility for certain services remained at the provincial level, but, as noted above, the LHINS were given responsibility for hospitals, CCAC home care services, community support services, community-based mental health and addiction (MHA) services, and LTC institutions (themselves a mix of FP and NFP facilities). LHINS were not responsible for (and did not fund) all publicly funded services; among the activities not in their mandate were physician services paid by the provincial health insurance plan, publicly funded outpatient drugs for specific populations, and public health.

APPENDIX C: CONCERNS EXPRESSED
DURING PROCUREMENT REVIEW

In 2005, the OMOHLTC commissioned a former Minister of Health, the Honourable Elinor Caplan, to investigate concerns regarding the CCAC procurement process. Caplan travelled through the province for six months, meeting with 37 of the 42 CCACs, and with provider groups, health care workers, clients and their family members, researchers, suppliers, information technologists, and quality management experts. A variety of venues were used, including roundtable discussions, private meetings, and solicitation of letters and papers. In addition, a survey of 1,000 members of the general public, 500 home care clients, and 200 home care workers was conducted (Caplan, 2005). The issues raised included the following:

*Contracting Issues*
 – Clients and workers are dissatisfied with length of contracts (too short);
 – Each CCAC has different pre-qualification criteria for service providers;
 – No consistent mechanisms of monitoring contracts (activities and results of service providers);
 – No incentives in place for service providers (e.g., volume allocation is inconsistent);
 – Service prices are high;
 – Not-for-profit service agencies are losing CCAC contracts;
 – No incentive to create partnerships;
 – No incentive to foster innovation;
 – Standards for purchasing medical/surgical supplies vary in quality and vary by CCAC;
 – High cost of supplies a concern in light of short-term contracts;
 – Suppliers of medical equipment lack important information (supply and equipment rates, expected volumes, and geographical distribution of clients);
 – Discrepancies in the basket of services across CCACs;
 – Discrepancies across CCAC boards (some micromanage while others are considered more "hands off"); and
 – Accreditation (not all CCACs are accredited by the Canadian Council on Health Services Accreditation).

*Reporting Issues*
 – No consistent mechanism to report on client outcomes;
 – Variability in RFP evaluation between CCACs;
 – Difficult to measure quality and performance across CCACs; and
 – More training needed to apply new measurement tools.

*Worker Issues*
 – Rewards for good employment are lacking; and
 – Educational barriers for personal support workers.

*Client Issues*
- Clients want to have a voice in decision making;
- Clients want continuity of care;
- Access issues (increasing prices = lower service volumes = stricter eligibility = consumers have insufficient access);
- CCACs need to communicate more with the public to increase awareness of their services;
- No effective process in dealing with complaints; and
- Blurry roles between case managers and service providers (role in assessing clients is unclear; service providers feel they should have input into care plan).

The report made 70 recommendations, focusing on the need for better quality and value for money (Caplan, 2005).

APPENDIX D: REFERENCES CITED AND FURTHER READING

Auditor General of Ontario. (2010). Home care services. In *Annual Report of the Office of the Auditor General of Ontario* (Chapter 3, section 3.04, pp. 113–31). Toronto: Office of the Auditor General of Ontario. http://www.auditor.on.ca/en/reports_en/en10/2010ar_en.pdf

Baranek, P.M., Deber, R., & Williams, A.P. (2004). *Almost home: Reforming home and community care in Ontario*. Toronto: University of Toronto Press.

Canadian Institute for Health Information. (2005). *Exploring the 70/30 split: How Canada's health care system is financed*. https://secure.cihi.ca/estore/productSeries.htm?pc=PCC292

Canadian Institute for Health Information. (2013). *National health expenditure trends, 1975–2013*. https://secure.cihi.ca/estore/productFamily.htm?pf=PFC2400&lang=en&media=0

Caplan, E. (2005). *Realizing the potential of home care: Competing for excellence by rewarding results*. CCAC Procurement Review. http://www.health.gov.on.ca/en/common/ministry/publications/reports/ccac_05/ccac_05.pdf

Commission on the Future of Health Care in Canada. (2002). *Building on values: The future of health care in Canada*. http://publications.gc.ca/collections/Collection/CP32-85-2002E.pdf

Deber, R. (2000). Getting what we pay for: Myths and realities about financing Canada's health care system. *Health Law in Canada, 21*(2), 9–56.

Deber, R. (2004). Delivering health care services: Public, not-for-profit, or private? In G.P. Marchildon, T. McIntosh, & P.-G. Forest (Eds.), *The fiscal sustainability of health care in Canada: Romanow papers* (Vol. 1, pp. 233–96). Toronto: University of Toronto Press.

Deber, R., & Gamble, B. (2007). What's in, what's out: Stakeholders' views about the boundaries of Medicare. *Healthcare Quarterly, 10*(4), 97–105. http://dx.doi.org/10.12927/hcq.2013.19339

Deber, R., & Williams, A.P. (1995). Policy, payment and participation: Long-term care reform in Ontario. *Canadian Journal on Aging, 14*(2), 294–318. http://dx.doi.org/10.1017/S0714980800011855

Department of Health. (2005). *Supporting people with long-term conditions: An NHS and social care model to support local innovation and integration.* http://web archive.nationalarchives.gov.uk/+/dh.gov.uk/en/publicationsandstatistics/ publications/publicationspolicyandguidance/dh_4100252

Dumont-Lemasson, M., Donovan, C., & Wylie, M. (1999). *Provincial and territorial home care programs: A synthesis for Canada.* Minister of Public Works and Government Services Canada. Health Canada. http://www.hc-sc.gc.ca/ hcs-sss/pubs/home-domicile/1999-pt-synthes/index-eng.php

Hollander, M., & Prince, M. (2008). Organizing health care delivery systems for persons with ongoing care needs and their families: A best practices framework. *Healthcare Quarterly, 11*(1), 44–54. http://dx.doi.org/10.12927/ hcq.2013.19497

Hollander, M.J., & Chappell, N. (2002). *Synthesis report: Final report on the national evaluation of the cost-effectiveness of home care.* Health Transition Fund. Health Canada. http://www.coag.uvic.ca/documents/research_reports/ hollander_synthesis.pdf

Ministry of Health and Long-Term Care. (2006). *Local health integration networks: Building a true system.* Ontario Ministry of Health and Long-Term Care. http:// www.ontla.on.ca/library/repository/ser/247449/2006/2006no21.pdf

Ministry of Health and Long-Term Care. (2013). *About the ministry.* http://www .health.gov.on.ca/en/ministry/default.aspx

Osborne, D.E., & Gaebler, T. (1992). *Reinventing government: How the entrepreneurial spirit is transforming the public sector.* Reading, MA: Addison-Wesley.

Randall, G.E., & Williams, A.P. (2006). Exploring limits to market-based reform: Managed competition and rehabilitation home care services in Ontario. *Social Science & Medicine, 62*(7), 1594–604. http://dx.doi.org/10.1016/j.socsci med.2005.08.042

Standing Senate Committee on Social Affairs Science and Technology. (2002). *The health of Canadians: The federal role, final report: Vol. 6. Recommendations for reform.* Parliament of Canada. http://www.parl.gc.ca/Content/SEN/Com mittee/372/SOCI/rep/repoct02vol6-e.htm

Walker, D. (2011). *Caring for our aging population and addressing alternate level of care*. Ministry of Health and Long-Term Care. http://www.ryerson.ca/crncc/knowledge/related_reports/pdf/walker_2011.pdf

Williams, A.P., Barnsley, J., Leggat, S., Deber, R., & Baranek, P. (1999). Long-term care goes to market: Managed competition and Ontario's reform of community-based services. *Canadian Journal on Aging, 18*(2), 125–53. http://dx.doi.org/10.1017/S0714980800009752

Williams, A.P., Challis, D., Deber, R., Watkins, J., Kuluski, K., Lum, J.M., et al. (2009). Balancing institutional and community-based care: Why some older persons can age successfully at home while others require residential long-term care. *Healthcare Quarterly, 12*(2), 95–105. http://dx.doi.org/10.12927/hcq.2009.3974

Williams, A.P., Lum, J.M., Deber, R., Montgomery, R., Kuluski, K., Peckham, A., et al. (2009). Aging at home: Integrating community-based care for older persons. *Healthcare Papers, 10*(1), 8–21. http://dx.doi.org/10.12927/hcpap.2009.21218

The following website may also be helpful:

Ontario Ministry of Health and Long-Term Care, Home, Community and Residential Care Services, http://www.health.gov.on.ca/en/public/programs/ltc/

# 20 Depending on How You Cut It

## Resource Allocation by a Community Care Access Centre

*JANE-ANNE CAMPBELL, HEATHER CHAPPELL, JOANNE GRECO,*
*JEFF HOHENKERK, JOSHUA KLINE, SHANNON L. SIBBALD,*
*KAREN SPALDING, FERN TEPLITSKY, ANNE WOJTAK, AND*
*RAISA B. DEBER*

The board of a Community Care Access Centre must decide how to use their home care resources. Their budget is already insufficient to meet all current demand. A group of parents of children with disabilities have requested increased support. The board has been asked to develop a framework for allocating their budget. This case can also be taught as a role play exercise.

This case addresses several policy issues, including resource allocation ethics and street-level bureaucracy.

**Note:** The Montgomery Region CCAC and the people living there are fictitious. While effort was made to provide enough information to describe the policy issues presented in this case study, and for this information to be "typical" of a CCAC, resemblance of information or issues to any particular CCAC is entirely coincidental. Many thanks to Mr. Steven Handler, Mr. Bill Innes, and Ms. Tracey McGillivray, for their generous assistance in the development of this case study.

**Appendices**

Appendix A: CCACs
Appendix B: Demographics of the Montgomery Region and the CCAC
Appendix C: References Cited and Further Reading

**The Case**

As described in Chapter 19 (Long-Term Care Reform in Ontario), home and community-based long-term care (LTC) can encompass a variety of services, including: *professional services* provided by nurses, rehabilitation professionals, etc.; *personal care support*, often provided by unregulated health care workers, including personal support workers (PSWs); and *social support* through such services as meal delivery and dining programs, homemaking, transportation services, and/or friendly visiting, often provided by volunteers. Community-based LTC can be subdivided into *acute care substitution* (which allows people to be discharged from acute hospitals), *long-term care substitution* (which serves those who might otherwise be in long-term care institutions), and *prevention/maintenance* (which keeps people healthy enough to remain out of institutions) (Dumont-Lemasson et al., 1999).

In Ontario, access to publicly subsidized LTC has been coordinated by a series of geographically based Community Care Access Centres (CCACs). At the time of the case, there were 14 CCACs. Through their case management role, CCACs worked with clients and their families to develop care plans and coordinate a range of home and community-based services, but, with a few exceptions, did not directly provide them. The care plans could include a combination of services paid for by the CCACs, plus other services that clients would have to pay for. The CCAC-funded services were largely delivered by private providers (both for-profit and not-for-profit organizations) who had been awarded contracts via a competitive request for proposal (RFP) process. Those in-home services delivered by providers through CCAC contracts were 100% funded through the provincial Ministry of Health and Long-Term Care (MOHLTC) and/or the regional Local Health Integration Networks (LHINs) (see Chapter 1, section 2.2.4, Regional Authorities in Canada). Such services could include personal care, homemaking, nursing, physiotherapy, occupational therapy, speech-language pathology, social work, dietetics services, medical supplies, medical equipment and laboratory tests, as well as prescription drug coverage for those eligible for the Ontario Drug Benefit Plan. As noted, individuals and their families were free to purchase additional services, should they wish (and be able to afford) to do so; in that case, they were not restricted to agencies holding CCAC contracts, although they could choose to use them. As noted in Appendix A, CCACs also managed placement into publicly funded LTC homes and convalescent care, provided school health support services, and coordinated transitions for clients moving between different health care providers in their specified geographic areas (see also Chapter 19, Long-Term Care Reform in Canada). In general, social support services were paid for by the clients, although public subsidies could be available. The Ontario government had also set service maximums, which were followed by all CCACs. These rules specified that a client could receive up to 80 hours of personal support in the first 30 days, and up to 60 hours in any subsequent 30-day period. (The maximums could be exceeded for up to 30 days if the CCAC determined that this was justified by extraordinary circumstances.) Nursing maximums were set for seven-day periods; in each, a client could receive any one of the following: up to 28 visits from a registered nurse (RN) or registered practical nurse (RPN); 43 hours of RN service; 53 hours of RPN service; or 48 hours of a mix of RN and RPN service. There were no legislated maximums for other services.

## Montgomery CCAC

The Montgomery Region CCAC serves a suburban fringe community, including several "bedroom" developments, as well as rural and semirural areas. The total population of Montgomery Region is 344,000, but most of the employed adults work in a large city 30 km away. The community is characterized by a rapidly growing population. (A more detailed description of the population and the services provided to them is included in Appendix B.) Other resources in the area include an acute care hospital with 200 beds, 10 LTC facilities serving adults (primarily seniors), and agencies providing community mental health services, community support services, and other health and social services. The CCAC has come under increased pressure to assist the local hospital in reducing its ALC (alternate level of care) patient load by ensuring short-term care for those discharged from the hospital. (The term ALC refers to patients who are occupying a bed in a hospital but do not require the intensity of resources/services provided in that care setting, and who thus should be transferred to a more appropriate – and more cost-effective – setting.)

The Montgomery Region CCAC's budget for 2008–9 was $48 million, including a $3 million increase from the previous year. Given the fiscal environment, it was expected to remain within its budget. Analysis of its activities showed that, in 2007–8, it served approximately 6,300 individuals; this was expected to increase by about 33% in 2008–9. About two-thirds of its clients were women. The average age of clients was about 58 years; the distribution showed that 56% were 65 years of age or older, 32% were aged 20 to 64, and 12% were under age 20. Closer examination of the clients less than age 20 showed that 50% were children who required assistance (primarily nursing and rehabilitation therapies) to attend school, and 40% were children and youth receiving services following an acute care admission for treatment of cancer, cardiovascular conditions, and other conditions. (These figures did not include postnatal health visit services to newborns and their parents, which were provided by public health rather than by the CCAC.) The remaining 10% (38 children) were receiving long-term in-home services because of severe disability and/or chronic illnesses. These services often involved complex nursing and related services; even though there are only 168 hours in a week, because more than one provider could be involved at a given time, these children could be receiving up to 184 hours of services per week.

Further examination found that a number of different services offered by other organizations were available for children. The Healthy Babies Healthy Children program, run out of the local Public Health Department, offered information on parenting and child development to all families with new babies, and some additional help and support (largely through referrals) to those families who would benefit. That program did not serve children older than age six. Preschool-age children facing physical, communication, and/or developmental challenges could receive speech and language services through local children's treatment centres. The Special Services at Home program, funded and managed by the provincial Ministry of Community and Social Services, helped families who were caring for a child with a developmental or physical disability, as well as adults with a developmental disability, to pay for special services in or outside the family home as long as the child was not receiving support from a residential program. Such services could include hiring people to help the child learn new skills, or to provide respite support to the family.

However, the main responsibility for coordinating and providing services still rested with the CCAC. Through the School Health Support Services, which also supported children being home schooled, it coordinated and provided speech and language services (for children of school age), and nursing and rehabilitation services (for children of all ages). Such services could be provided in the home and school settings for children with acute or chronic health care needs. Children were defined as being under age 21; as long as the child was in school, he/she remained eligible for receiving services under that program. The goal was to use a family-centred approach, recognizing the unique needs of each family, and to provide care coordination by professionals dedicated to working with children and their families.

## Governance and Organizational Structure

The CCAC had a voluntary 10-member community Board of Directors; at the time of the case, it consisted of local business leaders, accountants, a lawyer, and a consumer. The CCAC had an executive director and a staff of 150 full-time equivalents (FTEs), most of whom were case managers (also known as care coordinators). The corporate services staff managed finances, information systems, and the contracts with service provider agencies (at the time of the case, there were 30 such contracts). The CCAC was fully computerized, with an electronic health record for all clients.

Client services used to be provided by four geographically based teams, but the model had shifted to one based on the following defined populations:

*Children*:
Support for children to get health care in schools; this included both children who have complex medical needs and children with short-term support needs.

*End-of-life*:
Supporting clients to die at home with dignity.

*Adults*:
Supporting adults to manage long-term chronic conditions and disabilities.

*Post-acute / short-term support*:
Assisting clients who have short-term medical and rehabilitation needs.

*Frail seniors*:
Providing seniors and caregivers with intensive seniors-focused care support so that they could remain at home with dignity.

*Community independence*:
Coordinating access to services for higher-functioning seniors so that they could remain independent in the community.

The CCAC divided its teams by client population, with each case manager assigned to a team that served a particular client population within their geographical area (e.g., the end-of-life team). These teams strived to meet the particular needs of their different client populations. Each team consisted of a director, managers, case managers, and clerical staff. The case managers had caseloads that varied in size, depending on the population of clients they served. For example, case managers serving clients who needed palliative care, or who had highly complex medical needs, would have lower caseloads and provide more intensive case management support than would those supporting client groups seen as requiring lighter levels of care (e.g., school health support, post-acute, community independence).

### Case Management

Referrals for clients were received from the community (often through the client's physician) or when clients were discharged from hospital to home. The case managers assessed the needs of clients and worked with the client to determine a service plan for CCAC or other paid community services. Home visits were completed to ensure that the client's needs were assessed in his or her home environment. Clients being discharged from hospital met with a CCAC case manager in the hospital before going home. Services were provided to meet the client's individual care needs by the most appropriate contracted service provider (e.g., nursing, physiotherapy, personal support); clients were also linked to other community services not necessarily funded by the CCAC, including community support (which could include such services as meals programs, adult day programs, transportation, and housecleaning).

For each service, a review date was determined to reassess the client's needs for ongoing service. The case manager conferred with the provider and client to determine if services needed to be adjusted, continued, or discontinued. There was an appeals process if clients disagreed with such decisions.

### The Budget Crunch

As the province put pressure on the system to reduce hospital lengths of stay, reduce the number of people in acute care who were waiting for an alternate level of care, and reduce emergency department visits,

Montgomery CCAC was experiencing a surge in referrals from its own local hospital and adjacent hospitals. In particular, Montgomery CCAC was seeing a growth in the number of new clients with higher, more complex health care needs, who would fall into the higher-cost category. As a suburban area, Montgomery was also experiencing population growth. The board's primary challenge was to review the demand for services while balancing the budget. They were concerned that their budget of $48 million might not be sufficient to meet all client and provider demands. The Montgomery Region CCAC was at risk of going over budget unless the board revised their system of allocating resources. The budget had been determined by the Local Health Integration Network (LHIN) based on previous utilization, and already included an increase of $3 million because of increased demand for services related to growing population in the region.

### The Parents of Children with Special Needs

As noted above, 38 families were receiving long-term services for their children with severe disabilities; the children who were receiving some school health support services were also receiving support from the CCAC to enable nurses or PSWs to accompany these children to school. All of the children with long-term needs were receiving at least one, and often two or three, forms of therapy in the school setting. The families of the school-aged children, as well as those of the preschool aged children, were also receiving varying levels of in-home support. However, even these supports were not always sufficient to meet the high needs of these children. A group of parents of children with disabilities, who had begun to meet together, sent a petition to the board of the CCAC; they argued that they needed a 25% increase in the hours of nursing care that they were receiving, and that they planned to go directly to the MOHLTC if their concerns were not addressed. They also made the following points:

- Society supports saving the lives of children with disabilities, but is not accepting responsibility for their ongoing support.
- Increasing use of technology means that many children, such as those on ventilators, require 24-hour care.
- Care in the home is more cost-effective than care in an institutional setting.
- Children belong in the home with their families.

- With the deinstitutionalization movement, government is providing fewer and fewer out-of-home placements.
- The visible and hidden costs of raising a child with a severe disability are exorbitant.
- Mothers with children with disabilities should not be forced to give up their careers to stay home and care for their children. Besides the detrimental effects on the mother's career and the family's income, forcing mothers to stay at home has a negative effect on the economy.
- Single fathers are given more in-home support than single mothers, which seems unfair.
- Parents of very young children with disabilities should have access to in-home support during the day if appropriate day care is unavailable.
- Parents require additional in-home support beyond the work day in order to have respite from their caregiving responsibilities when not at work.

To illustrate their points, the parents enclosed the following case study in their submission to the board.

Ms. Thomas is a 27-year-old mother of 3-year-old twins named Cathy and Tim. These children have severe cerebral palsy resulting from birth asphyxia. Cathy has a tracheostomy to enable her airway to be cleared of mucous through suctioning. She needs to be "tip" suctioned every 15 minutes. Every two hours or so, she needs to be 'deep' suctioned into her trachea with a catheter. She requires oxygen intermittently. Both children are fed through gastrostomy tubes. Cathy tends to have problems with vomiting during feedings. Both children take several medications, including anticonvulsants to prevent seizuring, bronchodilators to prevent respiratory difficulties, and medications to improve their gastric motility.

Cathy has severe cognitive disabilities, and is unable to speak, hear, or see. Her teachers are attempting to assist her to develop some ability to communicate. Tim is learning to communicate using computerized equipment specially adapted to respond to his visual cues. Both children attend a Children's Treatment Centre education program for children with special needs three mornings a week, accompanied by their mother and a nurse.

Both children require almost constant monitoring. Ms. Thomas is currently receiving 90 hours of support per week from the CCAC, and is also receiving an additional eight hours a week of respite through Special Services at Home, a program provided by the Ministry of Children & Youth Services. Ms. Thomas, a single parent, has not returned to work as an office clerk since her children were born. She now wants to return to school to become a registered nurse. She feels that she would require far more support from the CCAC for this to be possible.

The Board of Directors took the concerns of these parents very seriously, but it was unsure how best to address them. It had recently developed mission, values, and vision statements. The values statement included the following: fairness, timeliness and consistency in service delivery; sensitivity to diversity; respect for individuals, and support for their right to make informed decisions; open and honest communication; responsibility and accountability; and commitment to excellence and quality improvement. The board believed that the parents' request needed to be put in the broader context of resource allocation by the CCAC, knowing that other groups of clients also had high needs. In addition, the board was aware that there were many other potential clients in the community who did not yet know what was offered by the CCAC, but had the potential to require services.

In discussions with the CCAC management, the Board of Directors produced a list of 15 possible strategies to deal with the discrepancy between demand for service and available resources. Some focused on increasing revenue, others on reducing demand, others on reducing costs, and others on protecting certain populations. The board recognized that these strategies were not mutually exclusive. They included the following:

1. Limit client access to some services, based on their incomes (i.e., means testing). Management pointed out that it didn't seem fair that wealthy clients were obtaining housecleaning services from the CCAC that they could pay for themselves.
2. Begin to implement user fees for some services (e.g., homemaking services) for clients who are able to pay. The board recognized that this would require agreeing on a policy about who would be classified as able to pay, and determining which share of the fees would go to the CCAC and which to the agency providing that care.
3. Negotiate transfer of funds from the acute care hospital to the CCAC to support an early discharge program.

4. Lobby government for additional funds, backed up with demographic data and data about the needs of particular groups, which might include parents of children with severe disabilities.
5. Approach charitable organizations or do their own fundraising to establish a fund for clients who had extraordinary needs.
6. Delay services by establishing wait lists for any new client (which might involve giving lower priority to those in the least complex needs categories). Those not being served could be referred to community services (which would be paid for by the client, not by the CCAC).
7. Cap the maximum number of hours of service per month each client can receive, and recommend institutional care for people who require more extensive support.
8. Cut the amount of service provided to all clients by 5% in order to be able to serve more clients in the community.
9. Examine alternatives for establishing community-based respite programs to reduce the dependence on more costly in-home support.
10. Stop all of the current community relations strategies "advertising" the CCACs services. This not only would save money but also would prevent any more people from finding out what the CCAC had to offer.
11. Make cost a priority in the RFP process, so that more service could be provided at less cost, by using less skilled workers to provide some services and/or reducing the wages paid to existing workers. Another possibility would be to invest in more efficient delivery models, including telehomecare.
12. Contract with as few providers as possible, in order to reduce costs associated with internal administration, and reinvest these resources in services for clients.
13. Create protected budgets for certain programs that have less powerful political support, so they do not have to compete against politically powerful programs.
14. Cap the dollars per client, and consider moving to a self-directed model where those clients would receive that money and be allowed to decide how best to provide the care they require. The board noted that a similar model was being used by adults with disabilities.
15. Working within the population-based model, discuss which populations to invest in, and which should have their funding and services reduced.

DECISION POINT

You are the chair of the Board of Directors of the CCAC. Your board must develop a framework for resource allocation. In doing so, they must consider what approaches to resource allocation are open to them, and the pros and cons of the proposed strategies, as well as the process they should use to decide among them. They must also consider the potential impacts of CCAC funding decisions on other parts of the health care system (including hospitals, community support, primary care, and long-term care facilities). What should they do in responding to the families of these children?

SUGGESTED QUESTIONS FOR DISCUSSION

1. What services should be provided, and to whom? Who should pay for what? What are the roles of individuals, families, charity, and government?
2. Resource allocation decisions take place at many levels, including macro, meso, and micro. How should these decisions be made? Who should make them? How much variation across CCACs is appropriate? What is a fair distribution?
3. Discuss the role of interests.
4. How does street-level bureaucracy affect the decision of the CCAC board?
5. Discuss the options available to the board, and their strengths and weaknesses.

APPENDIX A: CCACs

In 2001, the CCACs became incorporated with the introduction of the *Community Care Access Corporations Act (2001)*. This *Act* outlined the main responsibilities of CCACs as the following:

1. To provide, directly or indirectly, health and related social services and supplies and equipment for the care of persons.
2. To provide, directly or indirectly, goods and services to assist relatives, friends, and others in the provision of care for such persons.
3. To manage the placement of persons into long-term care facilities.

4. To provide information to the public about community-based services, long-term care facilities, and related health and social services.
5. To cooperate with other organizations that have similar objects.

In 2009, the *Community Care Access Corporations Act (2001)* was amended to expand the case management function of CCACs. These changes expanded the role of CCACs to include managing the placement of persons into: adult day programs provided under the *Long-Term Care Act, 1994*, supportive housing programs funded by the MOHLTC or by a LHIN, and chronic care and rehabilitation beds in public hospitals. These changes enabled CCACs to expand their role as a systems navigator, leveraging their expertise in case management to improve both client service and health system efficiency. Effective April 1, 2009, additional amendments were made to the *CCAC Act* that modified the governance structure. These changes changed the classification of CCACs from government agencies and returned them to their former status as non-profit organizations with non-government appointed boards.

The regulations relating to the provision of home care services were consolidated and updated under the *Long-Term Care Act* of 1994; new provisions were added to allow CCACs to provide additional services and service choices to their clients, including amendments that would allow home care clients to access the following.

*New venues for service.* The amendments provided CCACs with a new venue for delivering professional services to clients other than in their homes – that is, a congregate or group setting. The following services could be offered in this new venue: nursing, occupational therapy, speech-language pathology, dietetics, social work, social service work, respiratory therapy, training, diagnostic and laboratory services, and medical supplies and equipment. Physiotherapy services could also be provided in a congregate or group setting provided that the client satisfied certain eligibility criteria.

*New specialized services.* The amendments enabled CCACs to provide their clients with three new professional services: *respiratory therapy services* for eligible clients in their home, in a congregate or group setting, or in a long-term care home; *pharmacy services* for eligible clients in their home; and *social service work services* for home care clients in their home, or in a congregate or group setting. Specific eligibility criteria were listed for receiving respiratory therapy services and pharmacy services.

*New services to long-term care home clients.* The amendments to the regulations also authorized CCACs to provide additional professional services in long-term care homes. CCACs could provide residents of long-term care homes with: nursing services in the context of the MOHLTC Outreach Team initiative; training to provide nursing services; and respiratory therapy services if the resident satisfied the eligibility criteria for receipt of this service. These new services complemented the physiotherapy, occupational therapy, and speech-language pathology services already being provided to residents of long-term care homes through CCACs.

The CCACs continued to be funded by their local LHINs through line-by-line budgeting. As noted in Chapter 1, section 2.2.4 (Regional Authorities in Canada), LHINs are funded by the MOHLTC. CCACs must receive permission to move funding between lines for any amount greater than 5%. Every year, each CCAC submitted a plan, including budget and service needs in its geographic area, for approval to its LHIN. Each CCAC completed and signed a CCAC/LHIN accountability agreement that confirms obligations of performance; these were tied to funding. The CCACs had their own structures in place for making decisions around home care services, but had to abide by the service maximums for personal care and nursing, as noted in the case. The accountability agreement with the LHIN also specified that the CCACs could not exceed their budget. (Historically, prior to the LHINs, CCACs had regularly gone over budget if clients' requirements exceeded expectations.)

APPENDIX B: DEMOGRAPHICS OF THE
MONTGOMERY REGION AND THE CCAC

At the time of the case, the Montgomery Region was 900 square km, with a population of 344,000. The average income was $70,000, and the proportion with university education was higher than the provincial average. About one-third of the population were immigrants to Canada, of whom 17% did not speak English or French. The region was ethnically diverse, with 5% of Asian background, and 4% Italian. The Montgomery Region contained at least five distinct communities, each with a different socioeconomic and ethnocultural profile. There was one small First Nations community.

The Montgomery Region was one of the fastest growing regions in Ontario. In 2021, it was projected to represent 16% of the province's population, compared to the current 8%. The seniors population had grown by 5% over the past five years. There were 106,000 people under the age of 19 years. In the past year, about 1.8% of the population had received some services from the CCAC; this was expected to rise as people learned about the CCAC services.

**Facts about the Montgomery CCAC**

Annual operating budget 2007/2008: $45 million
Annual operating budget 2008/2009: $48 million
Number of staff: 150 full-time equivalents (FTEs)
Individuals served in 2006/2007: 5,500
Individuals served in 2007/2008: 6,300 (projected)
Expected increase for 2008/2009: An additional 33%
Average age of clients: 58

*Direct Services Arranged and Funded by the CCAC,*
*# of visits per year*

Homemaking/personal support: 237,163
Nursing: 88,611
Physiotherapy: 7,379
Speech therapy: 3,217
Occupational therapy: 2,805
Social work: 1,428
Dietitian services: 434

*Client Turnover*

Approximately 50% of clients received services for less than one
    month.
Approximately 10% of clients received services for more than one
    year.

## Long-Term Care (LTC) Placement Services (# per year)

LTC Placement within Montgomery Region: 417
LTC Placement in other parts of Ontario: 115

## Referral Sources

33% from the community
33% from adjacent large city hospitals
34% from the Montgomery Regional hospital

APPENDIX C: REFERENCES CITED AND FURTHER READING

Dumont-Lemasson, M., Donovan, C., & Wylie, M. (1999). *Provincial and territorial home care programs: A synthesis for Canada*. Minister of Public Works and Government Services Canada. Health Canada. http://www.hc-sc.gc.ca/hcs-sss/pubs/home-domicile/1999-pt-synthes/index-eng.php

Peter, E., Spalding, K., Kenny, N., Conrad, P., McKeever, P., & Macfarlane, A. (2007). Neither seen nor heard: Children and homecare policy in Canada. *Social Science & Medicine, 64*(8), 1624–35. http://dx.doi.org/10.1016/j.socscimed.2006.12.002

Spalding, K., & Salib, D. (2008). *Children and youth home care in Canada*. Canadian Research Network for Care in the Community. http://www.crncc.ca/knowledge/factsheets/pdf/In_Focus_Children_and_Youth_Homecare_FINAL.pdf

Williams, A.P., Challis, D., Deber, R., Watkins, J., Kuluski, K., Lum, J.M., et al. (2009). Balancing institutional and community-based care: Why some older persons can age successfully at home while others require residential long-term care. *Healthcare Quarterly, 12*(2), 95–105. http://dx.doi.org/10.12927/hcq.2009.3974

# 21 Shoot and Tell

## Mandatory Gunshot Wound Reporting by Physicians

*CARRIE-LYNN HAINES, JULIE HOLMES, PAUL MILLER, SHARON VANIN, AND RAISA B. DEBER*

In September 2005, the *Mandatory Gunshot Wounds Reporting Act* was proclaimed in Ontario. It required public hospitals to report the name and location of anyone being treated for a gunshot wound. Representatives of health professions expressed concern that this might damage their duty to patients, while others wondered whether similar reporting requirements should apply to other violent injuries.

This case addresses several policy issues including: balancing societal needs for protection with patients' right to privacy, the ethical basis of the physician-patient relationship, and framing of policy issues.

### Appendices

Appendix A: *Ontario Mandatory Gunshot Wounds Reporting Act, 2005*
Appendix B: Ontario Mandatory Reporting Requirements and
  Exceptions
Appendix C: References Cited and Further Reading

### The Case

Gun violence not only poses a health and safety risk to those immediately affected by the injury but also can pose a health and safety risk to the public at large. In 2005, Ontario was the first province to enact legislation mandating reporting to the police of all gunshot wounds treated in designated health care facilities. A handful of other provinces have since followed suit. The rationale for the legislation is that reporting provides the police with information needed to investigate gun violence, which can also help prevent future assaults. The *Mandatory*

*Gunshot Wounds Reporting Act, 2005* had the potential to conflict with other legislation which required health care facilities to protect personal health information. Both the *Regulated Health Professions Act* and the *Personal Health Information Protection Act* required that all regulated health care providers in Ontario had a fiduciary duty to respect patient confidentiality unless the individual consented to disclosure or unless disclosure was permitted in limited circumstances established by law as being in the public interest. Breaching these obligations could amount to a finding of professional misconduct. Mandatory gunshot wound reporting legislation was written to fall under this public interest exemption to the confidentiality requirements.

Advocates of the legislation emphasized the role of health care providers in making communities safer and providing police with the tools necessary to protect the public from violence, injury, or death resulting from firearms. Others disagreed, on a variety of grounds. Some were uncomfortable with having such a close involvement between health care providers and the criminal justice system, and were concerned that people with gunshot wounds might delay in getting medical help. They also noted that, without an expectation of privacy, patients might be less likely to disclose sensitive personal information that might be crucial to their treatment. Others were concerned that, should health care facilities be seen as reporting to the police, violent offenders might seek to threaten providers. Some felt that patient rights to privacy should not be easily overridden. Others wondered where the line should be drawn; particularly since many injuries were not gunshot-related, should providers also be forced to report on other human behaviours that might also pose a threat to the public?

**Violent Crime in Canada**

Violent crime is defined as murders, sexual assaults, common assaults, assaults with a weapon, and robberies. There are three levels of assaults as defined by the Canadian *Criminal Code*. Level 1, or common assault, is the least serious form, and includes pushing, slapping, punching, or threats. Level 2 assaults are assaults with a weapon or causing bodily harm. Level 3 assaults, also called aggravated assaults, are associated with events more likely to cause greater bodily harm than are associated with Level 2 assaults. According to Statistics Canada, Canada's violent crime rate is relatively low, and has been falling (Brennan & Dauvergne, 2011). National statistics indicated that police reported just over 437,000 violent incidents in 2010, about 7,200 fewer than in the previous year. Violent crimes accounted for just over one in five offences, and homicides made up less than 1% of violent crimes. The violent Crime Severity Index has also been decreasing over time. By 2010, the number of homicides had declined to 554, and the rate to 1.62 per 100,000 population, the lowest since 1966. The number of attempted murders also declined, from 801 in 2009 to 693 in 2010. This resulted in the lowest rate for this offence in over 30 years. Serious assaults also dropped slightly. The volume and severity of crime fell or remained stable in virtually all of Canada's largest metropolitan areas. The robbery rate in Canada has also been gradually decreasing; about 15% of robberies involved a firearm.

Homicide victims in Canada were most likely to be stabbed or shot, with each method accounting for about one-third of all homicides. A further 20% of victims were beaten, 7% were strangled or suffocated, and the remaining 7% were killed by other methods. More than half of all homicides committed with a firearm in 2009 were gang-related.

### Violent Crime as a Public Health Issue

Violent crime can be seen as a public health issue whose impact is especially profound among youth and other vulnerable populations. Adopting that viewpoint stresses the need for good data to help design and implement prevention programs. The National Crime Prevention Council specifically identifies violence as a determinant of health; similar views have been expressed by other public health groups, including the Ontario Public Health Association (OPHA), which formally recognized violence as a public health issue in 1997, and the Public Health Agency of Canada (PHAC). These groups have stressed that violence particularly affects youth. Firearm deaths were the third leading cause of death among young people aged 15–24. Among 26 industrialized countries, Canada ranked fifth in the world, with the fifth highest rate of firearms deaths among children under the age of 14 years. In 2006, Canadian police services reported a rate of over three youths per day (1,287 youth in total) accused of a firearm-related violent offence; this rate increased by 32% between 2002 and 2006 (Dauvergne & De Socio, 2008).

In the city of Toronto in an average year, a person was taken to the emergency department every other day due to a firearm injury, either intentional or unintentional. More of these visits were for unintentional firearm injuries, in which the person discharging the firearm did not intend to hit anyone, than for intentional injuries, such as assault. Some researchers thus suggest that the public safety threat from firearms does not depend on the intent of the user, but is related to the presence of the firearm itself. Others disagree. Gun ownership is contentious, and there are ongoing debates as to the appropriate role of the state in regulating it. Some argue that that hunting and gun ownership are intrinsic parts of their chosen lifestyle, and that government has no right to interfere, as long as these firearms are used for lawful purposes. Others argue that cars must be licensed, and guns should be treated similarly. Others argue that guns should not be permitted at all. The debate often pits those living in more rural/remote communities against those living in cities. In the United States, gun rights have become particularly symbolic, with many politicians interpreting the Constitutional protection of the right to bear arms as extending to the rights to carry concealed weapons in most locations. Some of this debate has spilled over the border to Canada.

## Legal and Regulatory Frameworks

The federal *Firearms Act* was intended to reduce the number of firearm-related deaths and injuries; it requires individuals to obtain a license to purchase a firearm and/or ammunition. The license must be renewed every five years. Individuals with histories of violence were prohibited from obtaining a license. Between 1999 and 2008, 22,523 licenses were refused or revoked from individuals deemed a potential risk to themselves or others. The *Act* also outlines the requirements for firearms and ammunition storage. Another provision of the *Act* (introduced in 2003) required firearms to be registered with a national gun registry. However, the federal government of Stephen Harper believed that such requirements were both unnecessary and a violation of the rights of firearm owners. Following several years when this provision was not enforced, legislation was passed in 2012 to eliminate the long gun registry and destroy the records (except in Quebec, which has challenged this provision in the courts).

Illegal firearms make their way into the hands of perpetrators, with major sources of illegal firearms in Canada being smuggling and theft. For example, it has been estimated that approximately two-thirds of guns apprehended by the Toronto Police Service entered Canada illegally across the Canada-US border, with the rest coming from domestic sources.

## Provincial Mandatory Gunshot and Stab Wound Reporting Legislation

Many US states require health care facilities to report gunshot wounds to the police. In 2005, Ontario became the first Canadian jurisdiction to introduce this type of legislation through the *Mandatory Gunshot Wound Reporting Act* (see Appendix A). Other provinces have followed. The information below summarizes the laws at the time of writing by province, indicating what had to be reported and by whom. Note that there was a high degree of similarity in these provisions, although most provinces (but not Ontario) have expanded their legislation to mandate reporting of stab wounds in addition to gunshot wounds.

### Alberta:
The *Gunshot and Stab Wound Mandatory Disclosure Act, 2010* requires reporting on gunshot and stab wounds by facilities that provide health care services (hospitals, medical centres, medical clinics, and doctors' offices) as well as by ambulance personnel. Reporting includes person's name, if known; the fact that he or she is being treated for a gunshot or stab wound; and name of reporting health facility.

### British Columbia:
The *Gunshot and Stab Wound Disclosure Act, 2010* requires reporting on gunshot and stab wounds by: those facilities operated by a regional health board designated under the *Health Authorities Act* (including hospitals and provincial mental health facilities); an organization or institution that provides health care services; a clinic that provides health care services; the office of a medical practitioner; and/or a prescribed facility, as well as by emergency medical assistants as defined in the *Emergency and Health Services Act*. Reporting includes person's name, if known; the fact that he or she is being treated for a gunshot or stab wound; in the case of treatment by a health care facility, the name and location of the health care facility; and in the case of treatment by an emergency medical assistant, the location where treatment occurs.

### Manitoba:
The *Gunshot and Stab Wounds Mandatory Reporting Act, 2008* requires reporting gunshot and stab wounds by hospitals and other prescribed health care facilities. Reporting includes person's name, if known; the

fact that he or she is being treated for a gunshot or stab wound; and name and location of the health care facility.

### Nova Scotia:

The *Gunshot and Stab Wounds Mandatory Reporting Act, 2007* requires reporting gunshot and stab wounds by hospitals; health facilities; emergency ambulance, health, fire, or medical service. Reporting includes person's name, if known; the fact that he or she is being treated for a gunshot or stab wound; and the name and location of the hospital, facility, or service.

### Ontario:

The *Mandatory Gunshot Wounds Reporting Act, 2005* requires reporting gunshot wounds by hospitals, and prescribed organizations and institutions providing health care services. Reporting includes person's name, if known; the fact that he or she is being treated for a gunshot wound; and the name and location of the facility.

### Saskatchewan:

The *Gunshot and Stab Wounds Mandatory Reporting Act, 2007* requires reporting gunshot and stab wounds by hospitals and facilities by the CEO (or delegate) of the regional health authority responsible for either the hospital or facility where the person is being treated. Reporting includes person's name, if known; the fact that he or she is being treated for a gunshot or stab wound; and name and location of the hospital or facility.

### What Else Must Be Reported?

In addition to gunshot wounds, physicians in Ontario were required by law to report 17 other particular events or conditions to the appropriate government or regulatory agency. This included child abuse and health conditions that would make it dangerous for an individual to drive. Other provinces have similar requirements. The rationale for such requirements is that they are in the public interest, because the enumerated events or conditions pose a threat to members of the public, often vulnerable members, which will necessitate intervention by the relevant authority (see Appendix B).

### Professional and Ethical Duties

Prior to the introduction of mandatory reporting legislation, physicians and other health care professionals were allowed to use their professional judgment to decide when it was in the public interest to report certain conditions and events (see Chapter 1, section 6.4, Professionalism). Accordingly, the provincial regulatory body for physicians, the College of Physicians and Surgeons of Ontario (CPSO), requires physicians to abide by its regulatory policies, which serve to establish the standards of professional conduct. The CPSO's *Mandatory Reporting Policy* reaffirms that physicians must comply with all mandatory reporting obligations, which includes reporting gunshot wounds to the police. Mandatory reporting raises issues related to certain professional duties of physicians and the rights of patients. The duties discussed below are rooted in case law and codified in the *Regulated Health Professions Act*, which all regulated health professionals in Ontario must abide by. A breach of the *Act* can be considered grounds for professional misconduct. Physicians' professional and ethical duties are also codified in the Canadian Medical Association *Code of Ethics*. (Note that this code of conduct is neither legislation nor a document produced by a regulatory body, and as such is not enforceable by the courts or the professional colleges, but it is widely regarded as the gold standard for ethical conduct by physicians.) These ethical duties include the following.

*Confidentiality:*
Physicians owe patients a legal, ethical, and professional duty not to disclose personal health information except in limited circumstances. In the context of the physician-patient relationship, confidentiality is a *prima facie* right.

*Fiduciary duty:*
The duty of confidentiality stems from the fiduciary duty which physicians owe their patients. The fiduciary duty is the highest standard of care at law. It requires physicians to act in good faith for the sole benefit and best interest of their patients.

*Autonomy:*
Patients have a right to make decisions about their care without the influence of their physician. The physician may provide information to help educate the patient, but he/she should refrain from making the

decision on the patient's behalf. Autonomy respects the right of individuals to self-determination, which is rooted in society's recognition that individuals should have the right to make decisions about personal matters.

## Personal Health Information Protection Act, 2004

Ontario's *Personal Health Information Protection Act, 2004* specifically protects personal health information from being disclosed to third parties unless the patient consents, or unless it is permitted by other legislation. However, under certain circumstances, this legislation permits disclosure of personal health information by physicians, without risk that they might breach their professional duties (and thus be found liable for professional misconduct), when the duty to protect vulnerable individuals and/or the public at large is thought to trump the individual's right to confidentiality under the circumstances. Reporting gunshot wounds is thus included under that duty to protect provision.

In addition to specific legislation that permits disclosure of personal health information, there are additional common law exceptions to the strictures placed on confidentiality. One of these common law exceptions is known as the *duty to warn*. It applies to circumstances where there is a known risk to people or property. A number of court decisions, including from the Supreme Courts of Canada and of California, have held that there is a duty to warn any person in danger where such a known risk exists, and that failure to do so could constitute a breach of professional obligations. However, the mandatory gunshot reporting would not appear to fall under that exception, since it requires disclosure to the police, not to those who may be at risk.

## Stakeholder Views on Mandatory Gunshot Wound Reporting Legislation

The *Canadian Association of Emergency Physicians (CAEP)* supported legislation mandating that health care facilities report gunshot wounds, but not knife injuries or other violent injuries. (It also recommended continued support for the federal gun control law and the firearms registry.) It advocated for the implementation by the government of a nationwide surveillance system for firearm-related injury and mortality. In particular, it urged the expansion of programs focused on the prevention of suicide, intimate partner violence, and gang-related violence.

It also advocated for continued support for research into firearm-related injuries and deaths in order to guide further public policy development and future legislation.

The *Ontario Medical Association (OMA)* Section on Emergency Medicine argued that whenever a patient is intentionally or unintentionally injured by a firearm, a violation of safe storage or handling practice has occurred. The potential for future harm supports the concept that this is a public health issue. However, it also argued that the reporting law might have limited usefulness as a public health strategy in that the potential for further harm due to crimes of retribution, or from further accidents or suicide attempts, is difficult for the emergency physician to assess, as it is based solely on a victim's self-report of the circumstances. The OMA did not support mandatory stab wound reporting. It felt that gunshot injuries were inherently different from other violent injuries, such as stabbings; guns were more likely to be lethal, including lethality at a distance, and hence gunshot wounds could be a public health risk to people in the vicinity when the trigger is pulled. It argued that the huge burden that knife wound reporting would place on health care workers and police was disproportionate to the minimal potential health benefit (Ovens, 2004).

The *College of Nurses of Ontario (CNO)* felt that the law would take away the ability of competent health care professionals to independently exercise judgment and make decisions. Besides the potential threat to confidentiality and trust in the patient-provider relationship, the CNO was particularly concerned that nurses and physicians should not be perceived as extensions of the police force.

The *Registered Nurses Association of Ontario (RNAO)* did not support the legislation. RNAO believed that placing an additional obligation on health care professionals to report to police would have a negative impact on the confidentiality of the therapeutic relationship between registered nurses and patients. The RNAO was concerned that mandatory reporting of gunshot wounds could deter people with such injuries from seeking treatment, and thereby jeopardize the safety of such individuals as abused women, families and their children, and teens.

The *Ontario Hospital Association* (OHA) believed that any mandated reporting must also include physician offices, after-hours clinics, and other community care centres. The Association argued that restricting reporting to hospital-based occurrences might inadvertently encourage injured patients to seek care at inappropriate venues. The OHA also supported broadening the definition of violent crime to include stab wounds. In order to clarify responsibilities and liabilities the OHA felt that the attending physician should be the individual responsible for making the report, with the ability to delegate to another health care professional, as required. The OHA also felt that there were valid concerns about retention and disclosure of information held by the police as a result of a report. Appropriate safeguards should be considered to protect this information that may still be considered part of the "health information record" with due legal protection beyond that of the standard police file.

The *Ontario Association of Chiefs of Police (OCAP)* had called on the government in 2000 to enact legislation to permit medical professionals in hospitals to disclose personal health information for the purpose of reporting a crime if there were reasonable grounds to believe that a crime had been committed. The OACP lobbied for inclusion of an amendment to the *Personal Health Information Protection Act* that would have allowed disclosure of personal information for the express purpose of reporting a crime, although such an amendment was never introduced into the legislature. The OCAP argued in favour of a more extensive list of reportable conditions to assist in their efforts to maintain public safety.

The *Family Violence Prevention Fund (FVPF)* was opposed to the law. It noted that the goals potentially served by mandatory reporting included enhancing patient safety, improving health care providers' response to domestic violence, holding batterers accountable, and improving domestic violence data collection and documentation. The FVPV argued that mandatory reporting would not necessarily accomplish these goals. Further, the implications of mandatory reporting for patient health and safety, as well as ethical concerns raised by such a law, argued against its general application. The FVPV also argued that the law could deter patients from seeking care; it could create a risk of retaliation by perpetrators of crime, which could threaten health care providers; and it could have negative consequences for patient autonomy.


DECISION POINT

You have been asked to advise the government of your province as to whether it should enact a similar law, and if so, what should be required to be disclosed.

SUGGESTED QUESTIONS FOR DISCUSSION

1. What kind of a public health risk does violent crime pose? How does this risk compare to child abuse? Spousal abuse? Infectious diseases?
2. How should violence be defined for the purposes of reporting? Should it apply to gunshots only? Stab wounds? Should it matter whether these were intentional or unintentional?
3. What are the ethical issues involved? How would this be affected by how the question is framed (including the appropriate balance between societal protection and confidentiality when confronted with a violent crime)?
4. Who should be responsible for reporting? To whom should that report go? What are the options? Are there trade-offs that need to be considered?
5. What policy options might help reduce the risk of violent crimes?

APPENDIX A: ONTARIO MANDATORY GUNSHOT WOUNDS REPORTING ACT, 2005

*Preamble*

The people of Ontario recognize that gunfire poses serious risks to public safety and that mandatory reporting of gunshot wounds will enable police to take immediate steps to prevent further violence, injury or death.

Therefore, Her Majesty, by and with the advice and consent of the Legislative Assembly of the Province of Ontario, enacts as follows:

*Definition*

1. In this Act, "facility" means,
    (a) a hospital as defined in the *Public Hospitals Act*,
    (b) an organization or institution that provides health care services and belongs to a prescribed class,
    (c) if a regulation is made under clause 5 (b), a clinic that provides health care services, or
    (d) if a regulation is made under clause 5 (c), a medical doctor's office.

*Mandatory disclosure of gunshot wounds*

2. (1) Every facility that treats a person for a gunshot wound shall disclose to the local municipal or regional police force or the local Ontario Provincial Police detachment the fact that a person is being treated for a gunshot wound, the person's name, if known, and the name and location of the facility.

*Manner and timing of disclosure*

(2) The disclosure must be made orally and as soon as it is reasonably practicable to do so without interfering with the person's treatment or disrupting the regular activities of the facility.

*Other obligations not affected*

3. Nothing in this Act shall prevent a facility from disclosing information to a municipal or regional police force or the Ontario Provincial Police that the facility is otherwise by law permitted or authorized to disclose.

*Protection from liability*

4. No action or other proceeding for damages shall be instituted against a facility, a director, officer or employee of a facility or a health care practitioner for any act done in good faith in the execution or intended execution of a duty under this Act or for any alleged neglect or default in the execution in good faith of that duty.

*Regulations*

5. The Lieutenant Governor in Council may make regulations,

(a) prescribing organizations and institutions that provide health care services, or classes of them, that are facilities for the purposes of this Act;

(b) adding a clinic that provides health care services to the definition of "facility" in section 1;

(c) adding a medical doctor's office to the definition of "facility" in section 1;

(d) exempting facilities or classes of facilities and persons or classes of persons from any provision of this Act or of a regulation made under this Act and prescribing circumstances and conditions for any such exemption;

(e) governing the requirements in section 2 respecting the manner and timing for the disclosure under that section, including prescribing the persons responsible for making

the disclosure on behalf of the facility, and prescribing
additional requirements;

(f) defining, for the purposes of this Act, any word or expression used in this Act that has not already been expressly
defined in this Act;

(g) respecting any matter that the Lieutenant Governor in
Council considers necessary or advisable to carry out effectively the purposes of this Act.

(Government of Ontario, 2005)

APPENDIX B: ONTARIO MANDATORY REPORTING
REQUIREMENTS AND EXCEPTIONS

In addition to the requirements to report gunshot wounds (*Mandatory Gunshot Wounds Reporting Act*), Ontario physicians are required
by other pieces of legislation to report a series of things, including:
(1) child abuse or neglect (*Child and Family Services Act*); (2) suspected
elder abuse or death in nursing homes (*Nursing Homes Act*); (3) health
conditions that make it dangerous for an individual to drive (*Highway
Traffic Act*); (4) health conditions that make it dangerous to fly an airplane or perform the duties of an air traffic controller (*Aeronautics Act*);
(5) health conditions that make it difficult to operate railway equipment
(*Railway Safety Act*); (6) births, stillbirths, and deaths (*Vital Statistics
Act*); (7) communicable diseases, or adverse reactions to immunizations (*Health Protection and Promotion Act*); (8) health card fraud (*Health
Insurance Act* and the *Health Fraud Regulations*); and (9) sexual abuse
by a health professional (*Health Professions Procedural Code; Regulated
Health Professions Act*).

If they are facility operators, they also have a duty to report incapac-
ity, incompetence, or sexual abuse (*Health Professions Procedural Code;
Regulated Health Professions Act*), and the termination of employment
of a health professional due to incapacity or incompetence (*Regulated
Health Professions Act; Public Hospitals Act*). There are also reporting
requirements related to treatment of inmates in a correctional facility
(*Youth Criminal Justice Act*), theft of controlled drugs and substances
(*Controlled Drugs and Substances Act*), and other reporting duties under
the *Mental Health Act*, as well as preferential treatment (queue jump-
ing) (*Commitment to the Future of Medicare Act*). Additional provisions

relating to occupational health and safety (*Occupational Health and Safety Act*) exist, including for such populations as merchant seamen (*Merchant Seamen Compensation Act*).

Exceptions to the duty of confidentiality include: *patient consent*, the *duty to warn* when a health care provider reasonably believes that a patient poses a foreseeable risk to an identifiable third party (usually by reporting to the police), and a *public safety exception* if there is a clear, serious, and imminent threat of physical or psychological harm. Legislation offers protection for health care professionals who act in good faith under the law.

Most other provinces have similar provisions in their legislation.

## APPENDIX C: REFERENCES CITED AND FURTHER READING

Brennan, S., & Dauvergne, M. (2011). *Police-reported crime statistics in Canada, 2010*. Statistics Canada. http://www.statcan.gc.ca/pub/85-002-x/2011001/article/11523-eng.pdf

Dauvergne, M., & De Socio, L. (2008). Firearms and violent crime. *Juristat, 28*(2), 1–13.

Government of Ontario. (2005). *Mandatory Gunshot Wounds Reporting Act*. S.O. 2005. Chapter 9. http://www.e-laws.gov.on.ca/html/statutes/english/elaws_statutes_05m09_e.htm

Mackay, B. (2004). Gunshot wounds: The new public health issue. *Canadian Medical Association Journal, 170*(5), 780. http://dx.doi.org/10.1503/cmaj.1040239

Macpherson, A.K. (2007). Penetrating trauma in Ontario emergency departments: A population-based study. *Canadian Journal of Emergency Medicine, 9*(1), 16–20.

Ovens, H. (2004). Why mandatory reporting of gunshot wounds is necessary: A response from the OMA's Executive of the Section on Emergency Medicine. *Canadian Medical Association Journal, 170*(8), 1256–7. http://dx.doi.org/10.1503/cmaj.1040464

Pauls, M.A., & Downie, J. (2004). Shooting ourselves in the foot: Why mandatory reporting of gunshot wounds is a bad idea. *Canadian Medical Association Journal, 170*(8), 1255–6. http://dx.doi.org/10.1503/cmaj.1040416

The following websites may also be helpful:

College of Physicians and Surgeons of Ontario, Mandatory and Permissive Reporting, http://www.cpso.on.ca/policies/policies/default.aspx?ID=1860

Ontario Public Health Association, Violence Prevention, http://opha
    .on.ca/Resources/Browse-by-Category.aspx?categoryname=Violen
    cePrevention
Public Safety Canada, Crime Prevention, http://www.publicsafety
    .gc.ca/cnt/cntrng-crm/crm-prvntn/index-eng.aspx

# 22 Dying to Die

## Euthanasia and (Physician-) Assisted Suicide

*CHRISTOPHER A. KLINGER, JOE SLACK,*
*AND RAISA B. DEBER*

What is a good death, and how does one balance individual preferences against societal values? What is the role of physicians? A number of highly publicized cases have highlighted the dilemmas and reignited the debate on euthanasia and (physician-) assisted suicide in Canada. What should the legislature and the courts do?

This case addresses several policy issues, including: roles of legislature/courts; scope of conflict; roles of interest groups and media; and ethical frameworks.

### Appendices

Appendix A: Amyotrophic Lateral Sclerosis (ALS)
Appendix B: Excerpts from Relevant Laws and Bills
Appendix C: Previous Attempts to Change Euthanasia Law in the
  Canadian Parliament
Appendix D: Euthanasia and Assisted Suicide in Other Jurisdictions
Appendix E: References Cited and Further Reading

### The Case

The concept of a good death depends in part on one's values. A number of related issues arise. Who should decide what treatment(s) a person should receive, and when treatment should be stopped? What is the appropriate role in making such decisions for patients, their families, individual health care providers, health care institutions, governments, and the courts? To what extent should decisions depend upon whether the person is deemed to be mentally competent, and/or his or her clinical outlook?

In most countries, there has been a heated debate about issues of euthanasia and (physician-) assisted suicide for patients with a terminal illness or suffering from a debilitating disease. In Canada, some of this has been fought out in the courts. In particular, the case of Sue Rodriguez highlighted some of the issues.

### The Rodriguez Case

Sue Rodriguez, born Sue Shipley on August 2, 1950, was diagnosed with amyotrophic lateral sclerosis (ALS; see Appendix A) in 1992. This mother from Victoria, BC, suffering from this rapidly debilitating disease, soon demanded the right to be allowed to end her own life through technological means under the supervision of a qualified physician. She based this demand on her rights under Sections 7, 12, and 15(1) of the Canadian *Charter of Rights and Freedoms* (see Appendix B and Chapter 1, section 2.2.2). Her lawsuit urged the Supreme Court of Canada to strike down Section 241(b) of the Criminal Code, which prohibited the giving of assistance to commit suicide. Observers noted that it was likely that many Canadians illegally ended their lives each year through assisted suicide, but did so quietly. Sue Rodriguez was determined to challenge these laws.

In a 5 to 4 decision, the Supreme Court of Canada rejected Mrs. Rodriguez's arguments. Instead, it stressed society's obligation to preserve life and protect vulnerable populations, grounded in the belief that "human life should not be depreciated by allowing life to be taken." The judges concluded that a person's wishes need to be considered in light of all the principles mentioned in Section 7 of the *Charter of Rights and Freedoms* (see Chapter 1, sections 2.2.1, Federalism in Canada, and 2.2.2, *Charter of Rights and Freedoms*).

The court's majority also rejected her Section 12 argument, writing that Section 241(b) of the Criminal Code did not subject Mrs. Rodriguez to any cruel treatment or punishment, because a mere prohibition of an action by the state does not constitute "treatment" under this section. The dissenting judges, however, suggested that Section 241(b) did infringe on the principle of autonomy, inasmuch as Parliament "has put into force a legislative scheme which makes suicide lawful but assisted suicide unlawful. The effect of this distinction is to deny to some people the choice of ending their lives solely because they are physically unable to do so, preventing them from experiencing the autonomy over their bodies available to other people." They concluded that this amounted to a limit to the right to security of the person, and hence did violate the principles of fundamental justice.

Subsequently, in February 1994, Mrs. Rodriguez took her life with the help of an anonymous physician. The policy debate, however, continued.

### Trying to Change the Law

Determining what to do about medically assisted death has evoked considerable passion. One question is whether to distinguish between voluntary and non-voluntary forms; the "slippery-slope" argument focuses on how to manage individuals who appear to be suffering but are no longer able to ask for help (Stingl, 2010). Decisions have variously involved legislatures, courts, patients, and providers. For example, the Netherlands and the US states of Oregon (since 1998) and Washington (since 2009) legally permit physician-assisted suicide (see also Appendix D).

In 1972, Canada had decriminalized suicide and attempted suicide. The legal right for mentally competent persons to turn down medical treatment was also clarified. The Canadian Senate struck a Special Committee on Euthanasia and Assisted Suicide in 1995; its report was titled *On Life and Death* (Special Senate Committee on Euthanasia and Assisted Suicide, 1995). Other committees were struck by provincial governments and by physician groups, including several in Quebec.

In the interim, several celebrated cases resulted when police laid homicide charges against family caregivers and physicians who had helped terminally ill individuals to die. Some cases were eventually dropped after appeals (e.g., Dr. Morrison, in Nova Scotia); others led to convictions (e.g., Dr. Généreux in Quebec). Other cases in Manitoba, British Columbia, Quebec, and Ontario added to the sense that the law needed to be clarified (Butler et al., 2013).

On June 15, 2005, Francine Lalonde, a Bloc Québécois member of the Canadian parliament, had introduced a private member's bill that would have permitted a medical practitioner or someone assisted by a medical practitioner to aid another person to die if that person has a terminal illness or is experiencing severe physical or mental pain and "appears to be lucid" when he or she requests death. The measure failed to gain support from the federal government, and was not passed. Neither was a similar 2008 bill. Lalonde reintroduced her bill in the next session; it was defeated 228 to 59 in May 2010. (Sadly,

Ms. Lalonde announced in 2010 that she would not stand for re-election, because she had bone cancer.)

## Differing Views

Proponents of euthanasia and (physician-) assisted suicide stress the freedom of individuals to control the time and circumstances of their own death and sometimes view euthanasia as no different than refusing life-sustaining treatment. Opponents fear that vulnerable individuals could be coerced into euthanasia and (physician-) assisted suicide to ease the emotional and financial burden of caring for them. They also often point to the danger of easing the pressure on the medical community/system to provide optimum care and to find new cures and therapies. What is sometimes called the "slippery slope argument" suggests that allowing physician-assisted suicide can lead to encouraging those with disabilities to kill themselves, and eventually to the genocidal policies of Nazi Germany (Stingl, 2010).

Ethical frameworks can be used to support different positions (see Chapter 1, section 3.6, Ethical Frameworks). One key professional value for health care providers is to do no harm. Some argue that this means it would never be permissible to even assist in the killing of a patient; others interpret it as meaning that it is unethical to prolong a patient's life or provide lifesaving care when it is thought this will offer no benefit and may even cause unnecessary pain and suffering. Clinicians face a difficult challenge, as they must consider what is best for the patient, the views of the patient and his or her family, and their own beliefs.

Many religious groups argue that divine intervention and not human action should decide on time and context of death. While some groups allow for withholding and/or withdrawing of futile therapy and others believe in providing care at any cost, most of the world's major religions are against euthanasia. One author attempted to clarify the views of many religions on a series of related questions (Bülow et al., 2008). He divided his analysis into the following questions:

- Whether it was appropriate to withhold treatment. This could be subdivided into whether the treatment could be deemed "futile." He concluded that virtually all religions (other than the Greek Orthodox Church) would accept the decision to withhold treatment that was unlikely to be successful.

- Whether treatment, once started, could be withdrawn. Most (but not all) religions would also allow this, if the treatment was futile and also burdensome, dangerous, and/or extraordinary.
- Whether artificial nutrition, once started, could be withdrawn. Most, but not all, religions did not consider this to be appropriate.
- Whether the "double effect" could be employed. This term refers to administration of medications with the goal of alleviating pain, but which might also, unintentionally, hasten death. Most allow this, albeit not explicitly.
- Whether euthanasia was accepted. Most (but again not all) religions appeared to draw the line at intentional killing.

The author accordingly encouraged physicians to be culturally sensitive and learn about their patients' religious/spiritual beliefs and their views on the end of life. This assumes a unanimity that may not always be the case (including the potential for disagreements within families, but also between families and health care professionals).

## Active and Passive Euthanasia

One frequent distinction in the discussion of euthanasia is between active and passive mercy killing. Passive euthanasia is often associated with withholding treatment and allowing a person to die; this can be seen as "allowing nature to take its course." In contrast, active euthanasia involves taking direct action designed to help a patient to die. The line is not always clear; as noted above, the concept of "double effect" may involve giving a high (and potentially fatal) dose of painkillers, justified on the grounds that the intent was the relief of pain and that the death was somehow incidental. However, not all accept this distinction.

Another issue relates to who is involved in implementing euthanasia. For example, should the patient request that his or her life be ended, the actions needed to implement that request could be carried out by the physician (e.g., through a lethal injection), or by the patient and/or others who may assist them. The term physician-assisted suicide is often used to refer to situations where the physician makes available the means necessary for an individual to end his or her life when that individual chooses, but leaves administration to the patient, with or without help. A related distinction is whether patient wishes should be heeded, regardless of clinical outlook. This has two dimensions. Should physicians give whatever potentially painful and expensive treatment patients wish, even if these are unlikely to be helpful? (Ethicists often refer to this as the issue of futility.) Conversely, should patient wishes be followed with respect to his or her death? Does this depend on his or her medical condition? How much attention should be paid to the anticipated life expectancy? The extent of physical suffering? Mental suffering? The mental competency of the patient? Should those who are depressed be able to end their lives, even if their views were likely to change once they received appropriate mental health treatment?

A related question involves autonomy. Patients may request limitations on their treatment. The concept of avoiding "heroic measures" can be seen as requesting passive euthanasia should a certain stage in one's disease be reached. Advance directives are one approach to specifying, in advance, which treatments are desired; the term refers to written instructions regarding an individual's medical treatment preferences in case of illness/incapacity. Various forms of advance directives may include a living will (a legal document that specifies treatment preferences), a medical power of attorney (a legal document designating an individual to make medical decisions on behalf of a person in case of incapacity), and/or a do not resuscitate (DNR) order, which requests that the health care setting (which may include hospitals, but also long-term care, etc.) and those practicing in it should not use cardiopulmonary resuscitation (CPR) to revive that patient. In 2009, the Canadian Hospice Palliative Care Association (CHPCA) began a five-year national framework and implementation project to enhance advance care planning in Canada.

Another set of policies seeks to make euthanasia unnecessary. The advocates of hospice and palliative care argue that provision of holistic, integrated end-of-life care services, aimed at alleviating pain and suffering, will help ensure a "good death." Brought to North America in 1971, this holistic, multidisciplinary approach has spread to more than 600 programs in Canada to date. However, such programs are unevenly distributed across the country, are small with regard to service capacity, vary considerably in service provision and quality, and often rely entirely on volunteers (Wilson, 2003). In 2005, the Canadian Hospice Palliative Care Association estimated that only about 15% of patients in Canada had access to hospice/palliative care services. Both the Senate of Canada and the Parliamentary Committee on Palliative and Compassionate Care have issued reports urging greater expansion of best practices for end-of-life care (Albrecht et al., 2011). This movement does not directly address how such services should respond to individuals who wish to have their life ended; instead, it encourages the use of hospice and palliative care as an alternative to euthanasia.

### Role of Interest Groups and the Media

Several interest groups have become involved in this issue. In addition to providers, they include several groups representing patient/consumer interests. Dying with Dignity (DWD) seeks to allow assisted suicide; the Euthanasia Prevention Coalition (EPCC) seeks to prevent it. (See Appendix E for links to their respective websites.) The media have also devoted considerable attention to this question.

### Back to the Courts

In 2011, the BC Civil Liberties Association launched a new court challenge to overturn the prohibition of assisted suicide. The initial plaintiffs were the daughter and son-in-law of Kay Carter; they had taken their elderly mother to help her receive assisted suicide in a Switzerland clinic, and argued both that her right to assisted death in Canada had been denied, and that they had technically broken Canadian law by assisting her. However, Mrs. Carter had been reported as writing to her family that she alone had made that choice. The lawsuit was subsequently amended by adding Gloria Taylor, a 63-year-old resident of British Columbia who had ALS, to the lawsuit. Her lawsuit sought the right to commit suicide. Her affidavit indicated that she had been told in January 2010 that she would likely die within a year, and that she "want[ed] the legal right to die peacefully, at the time of her own choosing, in the embrace of her family and friends." In August, the BC Supreme Court agreed to expedite her case, over the objections of the federal and provincial governments. However, the courts rejected another challenge, by the Farewell Foundation, arguing that this group did not have standing because their lawsuit was filed on behalf of anonymous members. Instead, the Farewell Foundation was granted intervener status in the Carter/Taylor case. The Euthanasia Prevention Coalition has also applied for intervener status; at the time of writing, no decision had been made. Both groups have used this case as the basis of an appeal for donations.

In reaction to this court care, the federal justice minister, Conservative Rob Nicholson, told reporters that Parliament would not revisit the question of assisted suicide. He noted that the rejection of the Lalonde bill (C-384) clearly indicated that the question of euthanasia had been dealt with, and rejected. Ms. Taylor's lawyer, Joe Arvay, was quoted as saying, "Parliament obviously has an important role to play in the political process, but when it comes to determining what our fundamental rights and freedoms are, the court has the last word because the constitution is the supreme law of the land and not Parliament. ... Obviously [Mr. Nicholson] knows Parliament does not have the last word."

DECISION POINT

You are a policy analyst for the joint Department of Justice/Health Canada Task Force. You have carefully studied earlier attempts to amend the law in this regard (see Appendix C) and are familiar with how the issue is handled in other jurisdictions (Appendix D). In light of the current court case, but bearing in mind various reports on hospice/palliative care in Canada, what is your advice to the task force and why? Should Canadians be allowed to terminate their lives, and if so, should they be able to do this with assistance, including under the supervision of a qualified physician?

SUGGESTED QUESTIONS FOR DISCUSSION

1. Should euthanasia and physician-assisted suicide be permitted? If yes, what restrictions/limitations, if any, should be imposed? How, if at all, should vulnerable populations be protected (e.g., against pressure to end "unproductive lives")?
2. Discuss: the principle of autonomy; the role of religious beliefs; and the slippery slope argument.
3. Are withholding/withdrawing of treatment similar or different from (physician-) assisted suicide and euthanasia?
4. What is the role of interest groups in the public policy process? Of the media? Who are the key players concerned with this issue?
5. What difference would it make if these decisions were made by: Legislatures? Courts? Providers? Patients and their families?

## APPENDIX A: AMYOTROPHIC LATERAL SCLEROSIS (ALS)

Amyotrophic lateral sclerosis (ALS), also known as Lou Gehrig disease, is a devastating neurodegenerative illness. Degeneration of the upper and lower motor neurons in the brain and spinal cord hampers motoric/movement control, eventually leading to paralysis. Walking, speaking, eating, swallowing, breathing, and other basic functions become more difficult with time. According to the ALS Society of Canada, neurodegenerative diseases such as ALS, Alzheimer disease, Huntington disease, and Parkinson disease are predicted to surpass cancer as the second leading cause of death in Canada by 2040.

Approximately 2,500–3,000 Canadians currently live with ALS. The illness has no known cure or effective treatment, although physical therapy and occupational therapy can help to maintain strength and function, and speech therapy can assist with preserving an ability to communicate as speaking problems develop. In end-stage disease, the ability to breathe and, to a lesser extent, the ability to swallow seem to determine prognosis. The former can be managed by artificial ventilation, and the latter by gastrostomy or other artificial feeding, unless the patient has recurrent aspiration pneumonia. Eighty per cent of people with ALS die within two to five years of diagnosis (ALS Society of Canada, 2012).

## APPENDIX B: EXCERPTS FROM RELEVANT LAWS AND BILLS

The Canadian *Charter of Rights and Freedoms* (see Chapter 1, section 2.2.2)
   includes among the *Legal Rights* clauses related to the following:
   *Life, liberty, and security of person*: "7. Everyone has the right to life,
   liberty and security of the person and the right not to be deprived
   thereof except in accordance with the principles of fundamental
   justice."
   *Treatment or punishment*: "1. Everyone has the right not to be subjected to any cruel and unusual treatment or punishment."
Among the *Equality Rights* are:
   *Equality before and under law and equal protection and benefit of law*:
   "15. (1) Every individual is equal before and under the law and has
   the right to the equal protection and equal benefit of the law without discrimination and, in particular, without discrimination based
   on race, national or ethnic origin, colour, religion, sex, age or mental
   or physical disability" (Department of Justice Canada, 1982).

The *Criminal Code* includes this provision: "241. Every one who a) counsels a person to commit suicide, or b) aids or abets a person to commit suicide, whether suicide ensues or not, is guilty of an indictable offence and liable to imprisonment for a term not exceeding fourteen years" (Department of Justice Canada, 1985).

APPENDIX C: PREVIOUS ATTEMPTS TO CHANGE EUTHANASIA LAW IN THE CANADIAN PARLIAMENT

A number of attempts have been made to change the *Criminal Code* to permit euthanasia; at the time of writing, none had passed. Among them were the following:

*Bill C-203* was introduced by Robert Wenpan, Progressive Conservative, on May 16, 1991 in an attempt to amend the Criminal Code to protect a physician from criminal liability when administering pain-relieving treatment to a patient, even if the effect of that treatment might hasten death. Passing second reading on September 24, 1991, the bill was sent to legislative committee and 25 witnesses were heard until February 18, 1992, when hearings were adjourned with no date for resumption.

*Bill C-261* was introduced by Chris Axworthy, New Democratic Party, on June 19, 1991 as an Act to Legalize Euthanasia for persons suffering from an irremediable condition. A request for euthanasia would have to be reviewed by a referee appointed by the attorney general, leading to a euthanasia certificate to be executed by a qualified medical practitioner. The bill was dropped from the order paper upon second reading on October 24, 1991.

*Bill C-385* was introduced by Svend Robinson, New Democratic Party, on December 9, 1992 as an Act to Allow Physician-Assisted Suicide upon request of a terminally ill person based on the principle of autonomy. With the closing of the 34th Session of Parliament, the attempt died on the order paper.

*Bill C-215* was another attempt to pass the previous bill by Svend Robinson of the New Democratic Party to allow physician-assisted suicide upon the request of a terminally ill patient. It was introduced again on February 16, 1994, debated at second reading on February 22, 1994, and then dropped from the order paper.

*Bill C-407* was introduced by Francine Lalonde, Bloc Québécois, on June 15, 2005; the bill would allow any person, under certain conditions, to aid a person close to death or suffering from a debilitating illness to die with dignity if the person has expressed the free and informed wish to die. The bill was debated at second reading on October 31, 2005 but died on the order paper with the closing of the 38th Parliament.

*Bill C-562* was the second bill by Francine Lalonde of the Bloc Québécois to allow what it called a right to die with dignity; it was introduced on June 12, 2008, and would allow a medical practitioner, subject to certain conditions, to aid a person who is experiencing severe physical or mental pain without any prospect of relief or who is suffering from a terminal illness to die once the person had expressed his or her free and informed consent to do so. The bill died on the order paper with the closing of the 39th Parliament. In addition, Senator Sharon Carstairs introduced two Senate bills towards advance directives and medical decision making in 1996 (S-13) and 1999 (S-2); Senator Lavoie-Roux proposed a Senate bill on patient protection (S-29) in 1999. All bills died without being voted on.

*Bill C-384*, as noted in the case, was also defeated. Titled "An Act to Amend the Criminal Code (Right to Die with Dignity)," it received first reading on May 13, 2009. The proposed bill included the following provisions:

Summary: This enactment amends the Criminal Code to allow a medical practitioner, subject to certain conditions, to aid a person who is experiencing severe physical or mental pain without any prospect of relief or is suffering from a terminal illness to die with dignity once the person has expressed his or her free and informed consent to die.

Her Majesty, by and with the advice and consent of the Senate and House of Commons of Canada enacts as follows:

1. Section 14 of the Criminal Code is replaced by the following:
14. Subject to subsections 222(7) and 241(2), no person is entitled to consent to have death inflicted on him or her, and such consent does not affect the criminal

responsibility of any person by whom death may be inflicted on the person by whom consent is given.

2. Section 222 of the Act is amended by adding the following after subsection (6):

(7) Despite anything in this section, a medical practitioner does not commit homicide within the meaning of this Act by reason only that he or she aids a person to die with dignity, if

(*a*) the person

    (i)   is at least 18 years of age,

    (ii)  either: A) continues, after trying or expressly refusing the appropriate treatments available, to experience severe physical or mental pain without any prospect of relief, or B) suffers from a terminal illness,

    (iii)  has provided a medical practitioner, while appearing to be lucid, with two written requests more than 10 days apart expressly stating the person's free and informed consent to opt to die, and

    (iv)  has designated in writing, with free and informed consent, before two witnesses with no personal interest in the death of the person, another person to act on his or her behalf with any medical practitioner when the person does not appear to be lucid; and

(*b*) the medical practitioner

    (i)   has requested and received written confirmation of the diagnosis from another medical practitioner with no personal interest in the death of the person,

    (ii)  has no reasonable grounds to believe that the written requests referred to in subparagraph (*a*)(iii) were made under duress or while the person was not lucid,

    (iii)  has informed the person of the consequences of his or her requests and of the alternatives available to him or her,

    (iv)  acts in the manner indicated by the person, it being understood that the person may, at any time, revoke the requests made under subparagraph (*a*)(iii), and

(v)   provides the coroner with a copy of the confirmation referred to in subparagraph (i).

(8)  For the purposes of subsection (7), "medical practitioner" means a person duly qualified by provincial law to practice medicine.

3. Section 241 of the Act is renumbered as subsection 241(1) and is amended by adding the following:

(2)  A medical practitioner is not guilty of an offence under this Act by reason only that he or she aids a person to commit suicide with dignity, if

(*a*)  the person who commits suicide meets the conditions set out in paragraph 222(7)(*a*); and

(*b*)  the medical practitioner meets the conditions set out in paragraph 222(7)(*b*).

(3)  For the purposes of paragraph (2), "medical practitioner" means a person duly qualified by provincial law to practice medicine. (Government of Canada, 2009)

## APPENDIX D: EUTHANASIA AND ASSISTED SUICIDE IN OTHER JURISDICTIONS

### United States

A key US legal case regarding the cessation of treatment was Karen Ann Quinlan. At the age of 21, she suffered permanent brain damage and went into a coma as a result of alcohol and drug consumption. When the hospital refused to remove the respirator, her parents battled in the courts. In 1976, the New Jersey Supreme Court ruled in favour of the parents and the respirator was removed. However, she continued to be fed through tubes, and remained alive, still in a coma, in a nursing home until she died in 1985. Another case, that of Terri Schiavo, pitted the views of her husband, who wished to have treatment discontinued, and her parents, who did not. This case was fought at many levels between 1998 and 2005, even involving the US Supreme Court and the US government; she died in 2005, soon after her feeding tube was finally disconnected.

At the time of writing, the states of Oregon and Washington had enacted legislation that allowed physician-assisted suicide within certain restrictions.

Under the Oregon law (*Death with Dignity Act*, 1997), a capable Oregon resident diagnosed with a terminal illness can request in writing a lethal dose of medication from his or her physician for the purpose of ending one's life. The terminal diagnosis needs to be confirmed by a second physician after the request has been made, and the prescription can be written only upon a second (verbal) request at least 15 days after the initial request. The full text of the legislative statute is available online. The website also gives an annual report on key facts and figures (Oregon Government, 2014).

The Washington State *Death with Dignity Act* went into effect in 2008. The full text and data on uptake was posted on its website (Washington State Department of Health, 2014).

Following a 2009 Montana Supreme Court ruling (Baxter decision) that there was nothing in state law to prevent physicians from prescribing lethal drugs to mentally competent, terminally ill patients, Montana became the third US state to allow physician-assisted suicide. This has been controversial; in 2011, a bill was submitted in the state legislature to overrule this decision; it was defeated by the Montana Senate Judiciary Committee, but the debate continues.

### Europe

At the time of writing, Belgium, Luxembourg, the Netherlands, and Switzerland had legalized physician-assisted suicide.

Belgium legalized euthanasia and physician-assisted suicide for adults in 2002. Two physicians need to conclude on a terminal diagnosis, and a psychologist needs to be consulted if the patient's competence is in any doubt. A provision is also made for honouring an advance directive that is not older than five years. The Federal Control and Evaluation Commission was established to provide reports to Parliament.

A similar law (Bill 4909) was passed in Luxembourg in 2008 and took effect in February 2009.

The Netherlands passed specific legislation allowing euthanasia and physician-assisted suicide in 2002. This codified existing practice, since the Dutch courts had stopped prosecuting this offence in 1984. Guidelines applied regarding consent (the law does not permit euthanasia on children under the age of 12), and at least two doctors had to confirm a terminal prognosis or unbearable suffering.

In Switzerland, physician- (and non-physician-) assisted suicide has been legal since 1941, but euthanasia was forbidden. Lethal drugs were available through right-to-die organizations that usually required medical certification of a hopeless or terminal condition. The law also did not restrict its provisions to Swiss residents; a number of foreigners (including some Canadians) have accordingly travelled to Switzerland for physician-assisted suicide. Some of these cases have received considerable media attention. Kay Carter, whose family members are plaintiffs in the legal case, obtained assisted suicide at the Dignitas suicide centre in Switzerland in January 2010.

APPENDIX E: REFERENCES CITED AND FURTHER READING

Albrecht, H., Comartin, J., Valeriote, F., Block, K., & Scarpaleggia, F. (2011). *Not to be forgotten: Care of vulnerable Canadians.* Parliamentary Committee on Palliative and Compassionate Care. http://pcpcc-cpspsc.com/wp-content/uploads/2011/11/ReportEN.pdf

ALS Society of Canada. (July 2012). *ALS Society of Canada.* http://www.als.ca/

Bülow, H.H., Sprung, C.L., Reinhart, K., Prayag, S., Du, B., Armaganidis, A., et al. (2008). The world's major religions' points of view on end-of-life decisions in the intensive care unit. *Intensive Care Medicine, 34*(3), 423–30. http://dx.doi.org/10.1007/s00134-007-0973-8

Butler, M. Tiedemann, M., Nicol, J., & Valiquet, D. (2013). *Euthanasia and assisted suicide in Canada* (Publication No. 2010–68E). Ottawa: Library of Parliament. http://www.parl.gc.ca/Content/LOP/ResearchPublications/2010-68-e.pdf

Carstairs, S. (2005). *Still not there: Quality end-of-life care: A progress report.* http://www.virtualhospice.ca/en_US/Main+Site+Navigation/Home/Support/Resources/Books_+Links_+and+More/Hospice+and+palliative+care/Online+Resources/Still+Not+There_+Quality+End_of_Life+Care_+A+Progress+Report.aspx

Department of Justice Canada. (1982). *Canadian Charter of Rights and Freedoms.* Government of Canada. http://laws.justice.gc.ca/eng/Const/page-15.html

Department of Justice Canada. (1985). *Criminal Code: R.S.C., 1985, c. C-46.* Government of Canada. http://laws-lois.justice.gc.ca/eng/acts/C-46/page-113.html

Government of Canada. (2009). *Bill C-384*. Government of Canada. http://
www.parl.gc.ca/HousePublications/Publication.aspx?Docid=3895681&file=4

Nicol, J., Tiedemann, M., & Valiquet, D. (2013). *Euthanasia and assisted suicide:
International experiences* (Publication No. 2011-67-E). Library of Parliament.
http://www.parl.gc.ca/content/lop/researchpublications/2011-67-e.pdf

Oregon Government. (2014). *Death with Dignity Act*. http://public.health
.oregon.gov/ProviderPartnerResources/EvaluationResearch/Deathwith
DignityAct/Pages/index.aspx

Special Senate Committee on Euthanasia and Assisted Suicide. (1995). *Of life
and death: Final report*. http://www.parl.gc.ca/Content/SEN/Committee/
351/euth/rep/lad-e.htm

Stingl, M. (2010). *The price of compassion: Assisted suicide and euthanasia*. Peter-
borough, ON: Broadview Press.

Washington State Department of Health. (2014). *Death with Dignity Act*.
http://www.doh.wa.gov/YouandYourFamily/IllnessandDisease/Death
withDignityAct.aspx

Wilson, D. (2003). *Integration of end of life care: A Health Canada synthesis research
project*. University of Alberta. http://books1.scholarsportal.info/viewdoc
.html?id=365464

The following websites may also be helpful:

Canadian Hospice Palliative Care Association (CHPCA), www
.chpca.net

Dying with Dignity (DWD), www.dyingwithdignity.ca

Euthanasia Prevention Coalition (EPCC), www.epcc.ca

Farewell Foundation, http://www.farewellfoundation.ca/

Network for End of Life Studies, http://www.dal.ca/content/
dalhousie/en/home/sites/nels.html

University of Toronto Joint Centre for Bioethics (JCB), http://www
.jointcentreforbioethics.ca

# 23 Screen Tests

## Genetic Testing in the Nursery and the Workplace

YVONNE BOMBARD, MARION BYCE, JOE T.R. CLARKE, CÉLINE
CRESSMAN, REA DEVAKOS, DANIEL FARRIS, DAUNE MACGREGOR,
ZAHAVA R.S. ROSENBERG-YUNGER, NATASHA SHARPE, AND
RAISA B. DEBER

Genetic testing is a powerful tool that can help identify individuals at high risk for disease and/or vulnerability to environmental chemical hazards. However, there are numerous individual and societal implications regarding when these tests should be required, who should have access to test results, and what can be done with the information. Two scenarios are presented: genetic screening in the context of reproductive decisions, and genetic testing for insurance and employment purposes.

This case addresses several policy issues, including: screening; insurance; and the ethical issues relating to individual vs. societal rights, including issues of autonomy, privacy, and the risk of discrimination on the basis of genetic test results.

### Appendices

Appendix A: A Primer on Human Genetics
Appendix B: Genetic Diagnostic Technology
Appendix C: Types of Genetic Screening Programs
Appendix D: Tests Being Considered for Employment Example
Appendix E: References Cited and Further Reading

### The Case

Many forms of disease have genetic components. Ideally, if these are detected early enough, they can be treated, and their adverse effects controlled or eliminated. (See Appendix A for a primer on genetics.)

With the development of genetic diagnostic technology (see Appendix B), it is increasingly feasible to test for particular conditions among those who do not show any symptoms of disease.

As noted in Chapter 1, section 8.2 (Screening), screening is defined as "the presumptive identification of unrecognized disease or defect by the application of tests, examinations, or other procedures which can be applied rapidly. Screening tests sort out apparently well persons who probably have a disease from those who probably do not" (Wilson & Jungner, 1968, p. 11). Most countries accept the World Health Organization's list of factors that epidemiologists believe should be taken into account in evaluating screening programs; these focus on questions related to sensitivity (defined as the ability to correctly pick up positive cases), specificity (defined as the ability to correctly rule out disease), and prevalence (defined as the proportion of people in a given population who have the condition being screened for), as well as the costs and consequences of false positive and false negative results (see also Chapter 1, sections 8.2.1, 8.2.2, and 8.2.3).

Note that there is a fine line between screening and testing; the term *testing* usually applies to individuals who are seen as having a higher probability of having a particular condition, and the term *screening* to tests performed in the general population. Note also that evaluation of screening programs may seek to weigh the costs vs. the benefits.

Screening programs can vary in their timing and purpose (see Appendix C for types of genetic screening programs). In terms of timing, one can screen before birth (*prenatal*), shortly after birth (*newborn*), or among various members of the population. The purposes may be various combinations of: preventing the birth of individuals who would have had a particular condition, identifying affected individuals to allow early detection and treatment, and/or identifying those who are carriers of the condition. (By definition, once symptoms are evident, one would no longer refer to such tests as screening, since they would now be used to confirm or rule out a diagnosis.) The value of screening programs thus depends on such factors as whether there is clinical benefit to the affected individuals, the likelihood and implications of false positive tests, and the costs of the tests and associated diagnostic workups.

One of the earliest screening success stories was phenylketonuria (PKU). This relatively rare condition was found to be caused by a deficiency of an enzyme needed to metabolize phenylalanine (Phe), one of the naturally occurring amino acids needed by the human body to synthesize proteins. Phe, like the other so-called "essential amino acids," cannot be directly produced by the body, but must be obtained from food. In most people, the body will then metabolize Phe into tyrosine (another naturally occurring amino acid). For those with PKU, however, this reaction does not occur, and the build-up of Phe and its by-products can lead to irreversible brain damage (mental retardation, seizures, etc.). There is no cure. However, ensuring that the affected individual has a diet low in Phe and high in tyrosine can prevent the damage.

The success of this dietary therapy for children with PKU prompted the search for a reliable test to identify affected babies before they developed irreversible brain damage. The Guthrie test was simple to perform, inexpensive, and extremely sensitive; the test was conducted on a few drops of blood obtained by pinprick from the heel of newborn babies. Since the mid-1960s, almost every infant born in the Western world has been tested, within a few days of birth, for PKU. As a result of early detection and early (dietary) treatment, thousands of children and young adults born with this condition have averted the symptoms of severe mental retardation.

The successful application of genetic testing for PKU in newborns spawned an interest in the potential prevention of other genetic disorders through screening. Enormous advances in genetic technology, particularly genetic testing by DNA analysis, have made tests available for the early detection of a wide range of genetic disorders. There is considerable variation across jurisdictions in which of these tests are used (Green et al., 2006; Khoury et al., 2003). For example, in the United States, although newborn screening protocols vary from state to state, as of 2011, all states were required to screen for at least 21 specific conditions, with some states screening for 30 or more.

What can be done with the screening results depends on what is known about each condition, and when the tests are performed. In some cases, where treatments are available, disability or death can be prevented. In others, tests might give information about conditions for which no treatment yet exists. Parents may be offered selective termination of the affected pregnancy (if the test was performed prenatally), and/or given information to develop strategies to help them prepare to care for a child who will have that condition. Testing might also give information about late-onset diseases (e.g., Huntington disease); this information may eventually be valuable, but would not lead to immediate action. Other genetic tests exist for conditions where no causal linkage between the test result and the health risks has yet been established, and the test results are said to indicate a "propensity" (elevated risk) of particular conditions, as opposed to providing a diagnosis.

The rapid advancement of genetic technology has thus generated concerns about the potential for abuse of this technology. As noted, analysis of genetic information has the potential to detect a vast number of risks for which no preventive or therapeutic intervention is yet feasible. Any tests may also yield false positive or false negative results (see Chapter 1, section 8.2.2, Assessing Screening Tests). Concerns have accordingly been expressed as to what, if anything, should be done to protect individual rights to privacy, confidentiality, and self-determination. Another consideration is financial interests, both of those who develop and market the genetic tests and of companies who might be able to avoid expensive health problems among their employees. Genetic information can lead to discrimination against some individuals with respect to employment or insurability. (Arguably, this does not differ much from the previous practice of using family history of certain conditions as a proxy for risk.) As noted in Chapter 1, section 5.9 (Insurance, Elasticity, and Moral Hazard), premiums charged by insurance companies are based on calculations of risk. Should insurance companies have the right to require prospective clients to undergo genetic testing for disease susceptibility? Similarly, should employers have the right to test prospective employees for vulnerability to environmental chemical hazards that they may be exposed to on the job? A related issue is that of confidentiality. How secure are the results of genetic testing? Where, and for how long, are the samples and test results stored? Who should have access to the test results? Should they be shared with other health providers, employers, insurance companies, and/or family members?

You have been asked to help clarify how genetic testing should be implemented, including attention to developing guidelines as to which genetic testing is appropriate, how the information could be used, and who should have access to the resulting information. You have been asked to discuss two specific examples – newborn screening and screening in the workplace.

### Newborn Genetic Screening Example

In 2000, the Ontario Ministry of Health and Long-Term Care (MOHLC) instituted the Provincial Advisory Committee on New Predictive Genetic Technologies to assist Ontario in developing a policy framework for the introduction of these services. This committee was also asked to create guidelines, principles, broad criteria, and advice to direct decisions on how new genetic services should be incorporated into the system, including the likely impact on patients, the physician-patient relationship, the health care system, and society. This multidisciplinary committee had a varied membership who brought expertise in genetics and genetic counselling, laboratory medicine, clinical epidemiology, family medicine, law, ethics, and psychosocial issues; it included representatives from the Canadian Cancer Society, the Heart and Stroke Foundation, the Huntington Society of Canada, the Ontario Association of Medical Laboratories, the Ontario College of Family Physicians, the Ontario Hospital Association, and the Ministry of Health and Long-Term Care.

Your province has now followed suit. As a member of the Provincial Advisory Committee you have been asked by your ministry of health to review the current state of genetic technology and to advise the government on policies regarding screening for genetic susceptibility to disease. You are asked to begin by making recommendations about five potential tests for newborn children, as described below.

## Test 1. Screening Newborn Infants for Congenital Hypothyroidism

Congenital hypothyroidism is a condition in which the thyroid gland is absent, or does not produce enough of the hormone thyroxine. Sometimes it is caused by an inherited defect in the synthesis of thyroxine. It affects about 1 in every 3,000 to 4,000 infants born in Ontario. Those affected with the disease invariably become mentally retarded unless treated from early infancy with replacement doses of thyroxine. Infants with the disease can be detected by measuring the levels of thyroxine or a related compound, thyrotropin (TSH). An inexpensive screening test is available that uses a small blood sample obtained from the newborn child; the test is highly sensitive, with acceptable specificity.

## Test 2. Screening Newborn Infants for Sickle Cell Anemia

Sickle cell anemia is a severe type of anemia. It is an autosomal recessive disorder, meaning that it occurs primarily if both parents carry the sickle cell trait. This trait is most common in people whose families come from Africa, certain South or Central American countries (especially Panama), the Caribbean islands, Mediterranean countries (such as Turkey, Greece, and Italy), India, or Saudi Arabia. It is much rarer among Caucasians (with estimates ranging from 1 in 2,000 to 1 in 10,000). In the United States, where 2 million have the trait, it is present in about 1 in 12 African Americans, resulting in sickle cell anemia in approximately 1 in 500 African American births, and in 1 of every 36,000 Hispanic American births. The signs and symptoms vary, but are often associated with anemia and pain and decreased ability to fight infections. The goal of screening newborns is to identify affected infants and treat them with prophylactic antibiotics, before they develop life-threatening infections. However, the treatment of other complications resulting from the disease, which may include severe anemia, growth failure, heart disease, kidney failure, strokes, and episodes of excruciating abdominal and bone pain, is less successful. Parents who might not have known their carrier state can also be made aware whether future births may be at risk, although typically that is not the purpose of screening infants.

## Test 3.  Screening Newborn Infants for Krabbe Disease

Krabbe disease is a very rare neurodegenerative disorder resulting from a gene defect (prevalence is about 1 in 100,000). People with that defect do not make enough galactocerebroside beta-galactosidase (galactosylceramidase), a substance that the body requires to make myelin, the material that surrounds and protects nerve fibres, and is necessary to allow the nervous system to work properly. Krabbe disease is most common among people of Scandinavian descent.

There are two forms of Krabbe disease. Early-onset Krabbe disease appears in the first months of life. Most children with this form of the disease die before they reach age two from complications arising from feeding difficulties and failure to thrive. The only treatment at the time of writing was bone marrow transplant, which is both expensive and potentially dangerous, and whose potential benefits were still being investigated (Burke et al., 2011). In contrast, late-onset Krabbe disease begins in late childhood or early adolescence, and is characterized by vision and muscular problems. The course of the disease is highly variable, with more than half of the cases detected remaining asymptomatic. The objective of screening infants for Krabbe disease is to identify the early-onset form to enable early treatment; however, the screening tests identify both early- and late-onset disease. Identifying late-onset disease creates potential issues concerning overdiagnosis of a condition that may not ever cause symptoms or health problems.

### Test 4.  Screening Newborn Infants for Duchenne Muscular Dystrophy (DMD)

DMD is a slowly progressive X-linked recessive muscle disease, which means that it primarily affects boys. It usually presents when the child is between 6 and 10 years old, resulting in muscle weakness progressing over the years to complete paralysis by the mid-teens. At the time of writing, there was no cure for the disease; treatment was primarily supportive, including ventilatory support for the last several years of life. Those affected generally died of complications of prolonged paralysis in their twenties. DMD is identifiable in the newborn period by a blood test that measures creatine kinase. Screening can be newborn, prenatal, and/or carrier. Newborn screening uses mutation analysis to identify infants with the disease; however, since there was no treatment for DMD, very few jurisdictions did this (Bombard et al., 2009, 2010). Prenatal screening of fetuses would allow couples the option of terminating the pregnancy should the disease be present. These tests examine DNA from fetal tissue or cells obtained by chorionic villus sampling (CVS) or amniocentesis (see Appendix B); the tests are highly sensitive and specific as long as the mutations causing the disease are known, but are expensive. Pregnancy termination also presents ethical issues. Carrier screening permits the early detection of female carriers of the gene; genetic counselling (including prenatal diagnosis) may then prevent recurrence of the disease in subsequent children. Identification of these carriers of DMD mutations requires molecular genetic testing by a laboratory specializing in the procedure. However, if there is no history of DMD in any other member of the family, there is a 30%–35% probability that the affected child has the disease as a result of a new mutation; when that happens, the mother is not a carrier of a mutant DMD gene mutation and the risk of the disease occurring in subsequent offspring is negligible.

### Test 5.  Screening Newborn Infants for Cystic Fibrosis (CF)

Cystic fibrosis is an autosomal recessive disorder characterized by chronic progressive lung disease and intestinal malabsorption. Infants with CF require long-term treatment with antibiotics, respiratory therapy, and nutritional supplements, but at the time of writing, almost all would die from respiratory failure in early adulthood. It affects about 1 of every 2,500 infants born, and 1 in 25 Caucasians is a carrier of the CF gene.

Screening for CF, like screening for DMD, can be newborn, prenatal, and/or carrier. Newborn screening identifies infants with the disease by testing for deficiency of intestinal enzymes in the blood. Diagnosis requires a sweat chloride test. Infants detected early and started on treatment before they develop permanent lung damage do better in the long term, though the overall effect on longevity is still controversial. The newborn screening test is expensive and not highly sensitive, and false positives are common. Prenatal screening of fetuses affected with CF is possible by analysis of tissue obtained by CVS or by analysis of cultured cells obtained by amniocentesis. The prenatal screening test is based on identification of the specific CF mutation in DNA from fetal tissue or cells; it is highly sensitive and specific, so long as the mutations causing the disease are known, but it is expensive. Carriers of the CF gene are identifiable by a blood test, based on analysis of specific mutations. Carrier couples, who would be at high risk for having affected offspring, can be offered prenatal diagnosis. However, the only current way of preventing a child from being born with CF is selective termination of pregnancy to prevent the disease. The DNA screening test for carriers is only 85% sensitive, depending on the number of different CF mutations tested for, but it is 100% specific (which means that false positives are exceedingly rare). The test is expensive.

### Genetic Testing For Employment and Insurance Purposes Example

Your second example concerns genetic testing in the workplace. An auto parts company is planning to open a branch plant in your province. The senior management has met several times during the planning process and has prepared submissions for the chief executive officer and the board of directors of the company, providing information on costing and potential timelines to establish the new plant.

The vice-president of human resources has requested a special combined meeting of the senior management team and the board of directors to review plans for recruitment of workers for the new plant. Owing to the high unemployment rate in the region where the plant is to be established, the company anticipated that it will receive many applications. At the meeting, presentations were made by an expert consultant who is a specialist on genetic screening, and from Dr. A.T., the physician employed by the company as director of occupational health and safety. Prior discussion with Dr. A.T. had led Human Resources to consider a policy for new employees that would involve genetic screening as a pre-employment condition. The matter was recognized to be potentially controversial, prompting this special meeting with the board. Also present at the meeting, at the request of the Canadian Auto Workers Union (CAW), was the president of the union local and the in-house legal counsel for the company. At the meeting, the union president argued against using genetic testing to screen out high-risk individuals. She expressed some concern that one consequence would be relaxing environmental safety standards, which in turn would place even the genetically low-risk workers at higher risk as a result of exposure to increased levels of toxic pollutants.

In a report circulated prior to the meeting, the expert consultant, who was also a university-based medical geneticist, provided the company with an outline of the current status of genetic testing in Canada. The report included a detailed list of all genetic tests currently available (both on a research as well as a commercial or service basis). The consultant recommended using genetic screening for prospective employees, focusing on: conditions likely to increase susceptibility to work place hazards and exposures, conditions with a high rate of employee absenteeism, and several rare neurodegenerative disorders with onset in midlife. All the conditions were deemed to have implications for individual functioning and colleague safety in the plant, as well as for the potential costs of disability and life insurance. Specifically, the consultant recommended screening for the following conditions (see Appendix D for more information about them): hemoglobinopathies (including sickle cell disease and thalassemia), lipid disorders, alpha1 antitrypsin deficiency, adult-onset Gaucher disease, and Huntington disease.

Dr. A.T., the medical director, indicated that he had reviewed the recommendations and had a number of concerns regarding the potential for discrimination. However, he pointed out that the province's Occupational Health and Safety Act does allow for exclusion of prospective employees, based on job description. He recommended introduction of testing for alpha1 antitrypsin deficiency, because of the high workplace exposure to dust from the finishing of various auto parts produced in the plant. Unless workers who were at high risk for emphysema were excluded, costly airflow modifications to the plant would be necessary.

The pension and benefits analyst for the company expressed concerns that the company currently faced the potential of having to insure applicants who knew they were at high risk, but did not pass that information on to the employer or the insurance company. She also noted the potential for bad publicity if the company (or the insurance companies it dealt with) were seen as discriminatory (see Chapter 1, section 5.8, Role of Media). Indeed, if there was enough adverse public reaction, there was some concern that the government could react with legislation.

A university-based bioethicist, retained by the company, commented that employers are generally accepted to have the right to perform pre-employment physical and mental examinations on prospective employees, to the extent that they are critical to the prevention of work-related injury and disease. The preventive value of employment medical examinations must be weighed against the adverse effects on privacy and the potential for discrimination and against the alternative of making the workplace safer for all employees. He was not convinced that the company should introduce any of these genetic screening tests.

DECISION POINTS

As a member of the provincial advisory committee, what do you recommend should be done about these five tests for newborn children?

As a member of the board of directors, what policy do you recommend that the company adopt with respect to genetic testing of your employees for the new plant?

SUGGESTED QUESTIONS FOR DISCUSSION

1. What criteria would you use to evaluate the merits of genetic screening programs? What should (or should not) be screened for?
2. What should the requirements be for consent to testing in a genetic screening program? Should individuals have the right not to know their status with regard to genetic risk? Should they have the right not to be tested? Should they be encouraged/obligated to share the test results with other family members? Would this differ

depending on what treatments are available? Who should have access to the results of genetic screening tests, and under what circumstances? What, if any, provisions should be made for follow-up care and counselling?

3. How would your recommendations differ when considering screening for newborns or children? Under what circumstances might the government endorse screening infants for a genetic condition for which there is currently no effective treatment?

4. How important is it for jurisdictions to have uniform policies about screening?

5. What should the company's policy be? Should insurance companies have the right to require individuals to undergo genetic testing before issuing disability or life insurance? Should they have the right to request the results of previous genetic tests? Should they be able to use information about family history of various diseases? What safeguards may be needed to protect insurance companies from adverse selection? Discuss the similarities and differences between information from family history and information from genetic tests.

6. Should workers be required to undergo screening for genetic sensitivity to environmental exposures in the workplace? What is the responsibility of the employer with regard to protection of the health of workers who test negative in such a screening program?

## APPENDIX A: A PRIMER ON HUMAN GENETICS

In humans the genetic material (genes) are arranged on 46 chromosomes; they form 23 pairs. One chromosome in each of these pairs is inherited from each parent. Twenty-two of these homologous pairs are known as the autosomes. The remaining pair is known as the sex chromosomes; they are denoted X and Y. Females have two X chromosomes, whereas males have one X and one Y.

Each gene is found at a specific locus, or position on a particular chromosome. Each pair of chromosomes is supposed to have (roughly) the same genes. However, not all genes are identical; variations ("mutations") may occur over time, leading to alternative forms of a particular gene. These alternative forms are called alleles. Depending on how many mutations have occurred, there may be many different alleles for a given locus in a population of individuals. Alleles occurring at a frequency of greater than 1% in the population are called polymorphisms.

One member of each chromosome pair is inherited from each parent. If a person inherits the same allele from both parents, they are homozygous for that locus; if they inherit different alleles, they are heterozygous.

Genetic disorders may be caused by a single deleterious gene, or be multifactorial. Mutations may be inherited from an affected parent, or occur as a result of a new genetic mutation (which may also be caused by environmental exposure).

Single gene disorders, which are called Mendelian conditions, are the most straightforward. In turn, they can be divided into two categories.

For dominant mutations, the defect causes disease even when it affects only one of the pair of alleles at a particular locus. Note that most individuals affected with dominant disorders are heterozygous at the crucial locus, since the disease will occur in spite of the presence of a normal allele at the same locus on the other member of a chromosome pair. About 1,000 dominant disorders have been described. They range in severity from trivial conditions (e.g., brachydactyly, which gives the individual abnormally short fingers) to severely disabling conditions (e.g., achondroplastic dwarfism), to fatal conditions (e.g., Huntington disease).

Recessive mutations produce disease only if both alleles of a particular gene are defective. Recessive diseases thus occur only when the same two deleterious alleles are found at the same loci of a chromosome pair. Someone with one abnormal and one normal allele is called a carrier; although they do not have the disease, they may transmit it to their children, particularly if both parents are carriers. For example, if both parents are heterozygous for a mutant allele (which we will denote as $A_M$), but also have the normal allele (which we will denote as A), then each child the parents conceive has a 25% chance of getting the disease by inheriting the mutant allele from both parents (homozygous $A_M A_M$), a 50% chance of being a carrier by inheriting a mutant allele from one parent and a normal allele from the other (heterozygous $AA_M$), and a 25% chance of inheriting a normal allele from both parents (homozygous AA).

However, if the defect is on the sex chromosomes, males will be more susceptible, because they have one X and one Y chromosome, which means that there is less possibility of having a normal allele to offset the defective one. For reasons not well understood, the Y chromosome appears to carry only a few genes, which means that most of the sex-linked diseases are caused by genes carried on the X chromosome. Consider a woman who is a carrier of the X-linked trait for hemophilia; we will denote the normal allele by X and the hemophilia allele by $X_h$. This woman would be designated as $XX_h$ (female carrier). She is married to a man who has a normal X allele; he would be designated as XY. Since their children will inherit one sex chromosome from each parent, they could be XX (normal female), $XX_h$ (female carrier), XY (normal male), or $X_hY$ (male with hemophilia). No daughters will express the disorder, but each (on average) will have a 50% chance of being a carrier of the mutant gene and therefore being at risk for bearing affected sons. Each of the sons of a carrier female will have a 50% chance of being affected with hemophilia, and an equal chance (50%) of being normal. More than 100 X-linked disorders are known in humans, including hemophilia and Duchenne muscular dystrophy.

However, most genetic conditions are not inherited according to the patterns of inheritance of single gene disorders. They are called multifactorial, or polygenic, to indicate that many factors, besides single mutations, will affect the occurrence of disease in any particular individual. These disorders, which are more common than single gene disorders, may run in families, but the risk that other family members will inherit them is generally much lower than for single gene disorders. The risk that any particular relative of a person affected with a multifactorial or polygenic disorder will also have that condition is accordingly estimated empirically, on the basis of experience with the population as a whole. The neural tube defects represent an important class of multifactorial or polygenic disorders. These include anencephaly (the failure of the cranial cavity to close properly during fetal development) and spina bifida (the failure of the fetal spinal column to close properly). Anencephaly is estimated to occur in 1 of 10,000 births; it is incompatible with life. Spina bifida, although still rare (estimated at 1–2 per 1,000 live births), is also among the more common serious disorders, but it varies considerably in severity. Infants with spina bifida may be paralyzed from the waist down and often have a build-up of fluid inside the skull (hydrocephalus); such children often require lifelong medical treatment and care.

Interest has also been growing rapidly in a large group of common disorders arising in adults that appear to occur as a result of interaction between genetic factors, sometimes called "genetic susceptibility genes," and environmental factors, such as diet. They include such disorders as diabetes mellitus, coronary artery disease, lipid disorders, cancer, and some forms of mental disease. The conditions definitely tend to run in families, and they have many of the characteristics of multifactorial or polygenic disorders. However, the effect of environmental factors on the development of overt disease appears to be much greater than for other genetic conditions. Much of the molecular genetic research undertaken in recent years is directed at identifying genes responsible for the increased susceptibility to these disorders in particular individuals and their families.

Another type of genetic disease, the chromosomal disorders, is caused by structural rearrangements or changes in the number of chromosomes per nucleus. Large amounts of genetic material are involved in these rearrangements, and there is little hope for treatment of affected persons. Most commonly occurring chromosomal abnormalities are abnormalities of chromosome number, called aneuploidy, either trisomies (the presence of an additional chromosome) or monosomies (the absence of one chromosome of a pair).

Trisomies are relatively common; they include Down syndrome (an extra chromosome 21), Patau syndrome (an extra chromosome 13), and Edwards syndrome (an extra chromosome 18). Children with the trisomies involving the autosomes usually have multiple congenital abnormalities, while sex chromosome trisomies are far less debilitating. Individuals with an XXY chromosome complement (Klinefelter syndrome) look like normal males. They may experience some difficulties with normal sexual development and sterility, but are able to lead fairly normal lives. Individuals with an XXX chromosome complement are almost indistinguishable from normal females. In contrast, the only known sex chromosome monosomy that is compatible with life is Turner syndrome (XO), which is relatively common. Individuals with Turner syndrome look like girls, though they have no real ovaries and are generally very short in stature.

Abnormalities of the number of chromosomes are almost always sporadic; the parents of affected children are generally normal. The defects are caused by errors in the separation of the chromosomes when the sperm and eggs are produced (meiosis); the risk of abnormalities of chromosome number is known to increase with the age of the mother.


APPENDIX B: GENETIC DIAGNOSTIC TECHNOLOGY

There are a number of technologies that can be used to test for genetic disease. These include biochemical testing, DNA testing, and chromosome analysis.

Biochemical testing relies on showing accumulation of a compound as a result of a genetic defect in its elimination (e.g., phenylalanine in PKU), demonstrating deficiency of a compound as a result of a defect in its production (e.g., thyroid hormone in congenital hypothyroidism), or demonstrating deficiency of a specific enzyme associated with a particular genetic disease (e.g., hexosaminidase A in Tay-Sachs disease). The advantages of biochemical genetic testing are technical simplicity, relatively low cost, and the potential for rapid analysis through automation.

Molecular genetic (DNA) testing requires knowledge of the exact nature and prevalence of specific nucleotide sequence changes associated with particular diseases. Two ways DNA sequence information can be used diagnostically are specific mutation analysis and genetic linkage analysis. Specific mutation analysis can be performed when the specific mutations causing disease are known. For example, the mutation ΔF508 is a common mutation in the CFTR gene; this mutation is one of many that can cause cystic fibrosis. Demonstrating the presence of the mutation is relatively easy. In the case of cystic fibrosis, and many other conditions, direct mutation analysis is the only reliable way to identify carriers of disease-causing mutations because biochemical genetic testing is not practical. In other situations, the gene causing a particular disease may not be known, but it is known to be located very close to another gene that is well characterized and exists in several polymorphic forms. By tracking the association of disease with a specific linked polymorphism in a family, the risk of disease in any particular individual can be calculated. This type of genetic linkage analysis requires DNA samples from affected and healthy relatives, as well as from the person who is seeking the genetic testing. For many years, genetic linkage analysis was the most reliable way to determine the risk of Huntington disease in blood relatives of an affected individual. However, it was not always fully accurate, or always practical. One problem was the need to obtain blood or tissue samples from relatives, some of whom might be dead, and others of whom might not want to know if they were affected.

Chromosome analysis requires fresh samples of tissues, such as blood or amniotic fluid cells, containing cells capable of mitosis. Cells are stimulated to divide and fixed at a stage of cell division (metaphase) when the chromosomes are compacted and easy to see by light microscope. Photographs of the cells are taken, and the chromosomes are sorted according to size and shape to produce a karyotype. The patient's karyotype can then be compared with the normal karyotype to identify abnormalities of number, size, or structure. Abnormalities in chromosome number or major structural abnormalities can be detected by an automated, computed-assisted technique. Smaller, submicroscopic abnormalities in chromosome structure are detectable by a technique called fluorescence in situ hybridization (FISH) analysis. The chromosomal abnormalities causing conditions like Down syndrome, Turner syndrome, or Klinefelter syndrome can all be diagnosed using this approach. The interpretation of more subtle chromosomal abnormalities requires considerable skill and experience.

Biochemical genetic testing is inherently more sensitive than direct mutation analysis. For example, there are many dozens of mutations in the gene for phenylalanine hydroxylase causing PKU. To test for each mutation by molecular genetic (DNA) testing is impractical; however, all are associated with increased phenylalanine concentrations in the blood. Similarly, there are over 50 mutations of a particular gene (HEXA) that have been found to be associated with Tay-Sachs disease; all cause a deficiency in the same compound (hexosaminidase A). In both cases, a single biochemical assay tests for the presence of dozens of different mutations, all of which affect enzyme activity and produce disease.

It is now possible to detect the presence of many genetic disorders in embryos and fetuses, and the number that can be detected is increasing rapidly. Development of many new techniques for prenatal diagnosis of genetic diseases has coincided with an increased, although not universal, acceptance of the termination of undesired pregnancies. However, in contrast with tests performed on adults or newborns (which may require a blood sample), prenatal screening usually requires that samples be collected by one of two relatively expensive surgical procedures – amniocentesis or chorionic villus biopsy. Amniocentesis is generally done at 15–20 weeks of gestation. It involves the introduction of a fine needle through the abdominal wall and uterus, into the amniotic sac surrounding the fetus, in order to obtain a sample of amniotic fluid. Fetal cells suspended in the fluid are harvested and cultured for biochemical, molecular, or chromosome analysis. The risk to the pregnancy is small but not zero (approximately 0.5% risk of miscarriage). Because of the need to culture the cells for analysis, genetic testing takes 2–4 weeks. Chorionic villus sampling (CVS) involves the introduction of a fine catheter through the cervix or abdominal wall to obtain a small (25 mg) sample of the embryonic placenta, and is done at 10–12 weeks of gestation. Biochemical, molecular, or chromosomal genetic testing of samples obtained through CVS generally takes only a few days because the amount of tissue obtained is much greater than that obtainable by amniocentesis. Again, risk to the pregnancy is small but not zero (approximately 2% risk of miscarriage). The main advantage of CVS, as compared with amniocentesis, is the speed with which a fetal diagnosis can be made. These prenatal diagnostic procedures are done only in the case of pregnancies at high risk for fetal abnormalities; the risk may be determined by the presence of a family history of a specific heritable genetic disorder and/or by maternal screening.

Maternal screening can take three forms: maternal age, maternal serum screening, and midtrimester ultrasound examination. The incidence of chromosomal abnormalities, such as trisomy 21, rises rapidly with maternal age beyond age 35. When the mother is 35, the risk of the fetus having a major chromosomal abnormality is about the same as the risk of miscarriage following amniocentesis. Accordingly, women scheduled to deliver beyond their 35th birthday are often offered amniocentesis to allow chromosome studies to be performed. Maternal serum screening (MSS) can be used to detect biochemical compounds suggesting disease. For example, the presence of open neural tube defects (spina bifida) in the fetus is associated with an increase in the level of alpha-fetoprotein (AFP) in maternal serum. Other fetal chromosomal defects are associated with abnormally low levels of estriol and human chorionic gonadotropin (HCG) in maternal serum. Testing maternal serum AFP, estriol, and HCG levels during pregnancy has thus become routine in many places in Canada; any abnormalities can then be followed up by ultrasound examination and amniocentesis. Midtrimester ultrasound examination can be used to identify many birth defects, such as major structural abnormalities of the brain, heart, and limbs; this requires skilled ultrasound examination at 16–20 weeks of gestation. Some of the defects detected are trivial, or may even disappear before the birth of the infant. Progress in imaging technology has placed increased pressure on geneticists and perinatologists to interpret ultrasound examination findings showing novel variations in structure. Identification of abnormalities by ultrasound examination is often followed by amniocentesis and chromosome analysis of amniotic fluid cells.

APPENDIX C: TYPES OF GENETIC SCREENING PROGRAMS

The goal of screening for the purposes of reproductive planning is to identify individuals or couples at high risk for having children affected with specific genetic disorders prior to pregnancy, to allow them the opportunity to consider different reproductive strategies to decrease the risk of disease in their offspring. If that risk is high enough, however, the program would probably be considered genetic testing rather than genetic screening (see Chapter 1, section 8.2, Screening). Some programs are often concentrated among members of communities/ ethnic groups known to have a relatively high proportion of carriers of a particular disease, such as Ashkenazi Jews (Tay-Sachs disease) or African Americans (sickle cell disease). For example, as noted in the case, about 15%–20% of African Americans are carriers of the sickle cell anemia gene mutation. Carriers are identifiable by a simple blood test. Although carriers are completely asymptomatic, if both parents are carriers, each child has a 25% chance of inheriting the gene mutation from both parents and thus having sickle cell anemia. The objective of screening for carriers of the sickle cell gene mutation might be to identify couples at risk of having offspring affected with the disease. Strategies might include screening pregnant women and their partners, screening all people of childbearing age in high-risk populations, or screening all people of childbearing age regardless of estimation of prior risk. Should both partners screen positive, their options might include various combinations of genetic counselling to prevent disease occurrence in potential offspring, or even prenatal testing of the fetus at 15–16 weeks of gestation, and potential termination of the pregnancy if the fetus is found to be affected. What to do with screening results can thus present ethical dilemmas.

Many women undergo prenatal screening blood tests or midtrimester ultrasound examination of the fetus to identify fetuses at high risk for severe birth defects, such as chromosomal abnormalities (e.g., Down syndrome) or neural tube defects. High-risk women (which may include couples already identified as being carriers of specific disorders) are generally offered definitive diagnostic testing, usually by amniocentesis, and given the option to terminate the pregnancy by abortion if the fetus is confirmed to have a major birth defect. Although many genetic disorders can now be detected prenatally, it should be noted that no universal prenatal screening programs have been set up; only pregnancies known to be at an increased risk for a genetic defect (often determined through family history) are tested. One rationale was that the high cost of the invasive procedures and the risk attached to them (although very small) did not warrant their use on a universal basis. In contrast, alphafetoprotein (AFP) testing and ultrasonography were seen as sufficiently safe, non-invasive, and inexpensive to be applied even to low-risk pregnancies.

The goal of screening newborns for genetic diseases is to allow early detection, followed by early therapeutic intervention to prevent the onset or minimize the severity of resulting defects. Usually therapy must be instituted before irreversible physiological changes have occurred. Neonatal screening programs generally target disorders for which there is a treatment (i.e., phenylketonuria and congenital hypothyroidism). An important justification for mass screening exists for those conditions where waiting for a diagnosis until after clinical symptoms appear may mean that it is too late for the maximum benefit of therapy.

Genetic screening may also be undertaken simply to determine the prevalence of a specific genetic variation in a certain population, by testing large numbers of the group, without linking the test results with specific individuals. Here the goal is simply to collect information; it does not include measures to detect specific high-risk individuals or couples or to act on the results.

Mass screening programs test the population at large for the presence of disease. In the case of genetic screening, mass screening would identify both carriers and affected individuals. The cost-effectiveness of this sort of population screening is dependent upon the prevalence of a disorder among a particular population, as well as the cost and availability of treatment (see Chapter 1, section 8.1, Economic Analysis: Cost-effectiveness, and section 8.2.3, The Role of Prevalence).

Some disorders are more prevalent among some populations than others, and it may be more cost-effective to do target group screening only in those populations where the prevalence is high enough to warrant it. However, this strategy may miss cases among the lower-risk populations. Those responsible for screening programs have argued that, when instituting target group screening programs, it is important to word policies and legislation carefully in order to avoid stigmatizing and discriminating against a particular group. They use as an example the experiences in the United States, where legislated sickle cell anemia screening programs instituted in the 1960s and 1970s were seen to have stigmatized those with the sickle cell trait; references to using the results to "avoid breeding" also led to fears that the program had eugenic aims.

APPENDIX D: TESTS BEING CONSIDERED
FOR EMPLOYMENT EXAMPLE

The following information was provided to the board of the auto parts company about the conditions being considered for screening.

*Hemoglobinopathies.* The information focused on sickle cell disease and beta-thalassemia, two particularly common hereditary disorders of hemoglobin synthesis that could cause severe, debilitating disease. Both are autosomal recessive disorders, causing no significant abnormalities in carriers of the respective genes.

*Sickle cell disease* is caused by a mutation resulting in the substitution of normal hemoglobin by hemoglobin S (HbS). Individuals who are homozygous for HbS develop chronic anemia, recurrent attacks of severe abdominal and bone pain, recurrent attacks of severe hemolytic anemia, organ infarction, and enlargement of the spleen. Early death is common, often from overwhelming bacterial infections. Treatment of the disease is primarily symptomatic. Carriers of HbS may experience painful crises on exposure to low oxygen levels, such as experienced during high-altitude flying or mountaineering without oxygen. Sickle cell disease is particularly common in black Africans and African Americans, affecting up to 1 in 650 American black children; about 8% are heterozygous carriers of the HbS gene. In west-central Africa, up to 30% of the population are carriers. Affected infants are detectable early in infancy by a simple blood test, based on measurement of HbS. Prophylactic treatment with antibiotics has been shown to prevent life-threatening infections, which are particularly common in the first few years of life. The screening test is inexpensive, sensitive, and specific, but the cost-effectiveness of population screening is still considered by some to be unproven. One issue is whether screening should be focused on infants of black American parents, or applied to the entire population of newborn infants. Carriers of HbS are also identifiable by a simple blood test, and carrier couples can then be offered the option of prenatal diagnosis and selective termination of pregnancy. Prenatal testing involves HbS mutation analysis in fetal tissue obtained by CVS or in cultured cells obtained by amniocentesis.

*Beta-thalassemia* is another common, hereditary defect of hemoglobin synthesis. It is caused by a defect in hemoglobin production. Affected infants develop severe, transfusion-dependent anemia in the second half of the first year of life. Treatment with repeated blood transfusions corrects the anemia, but it also causes iron overload, which causes early death, usually from the effects on the heart and liver. Iron overload is preventable by treatment with desferroxamine injections, but this is inconvenient and extremely expensive. Beta-thalassemia is particularly common in individuals originating from the Mediterranean Basin and Asia. Carrier detection is possible with a simple, inexpensive blood test. Confirmation of carrier status is somewhat more complex and expensive. Carrier couples can be offered prenatal diagnosis, by mutation analysis of fetal tissues or cells, and selective abortion if the fetus is found to be affected. In certain areas, like Cyprus and Sardinia, carrier detection screening programs have drastically decreased the incidence of the disease.

*Lipid disorders* are a mixed group of disorders characterized by high levels of cholesterol in plasma, sometimes associated with increased concentrations of triglycerides. In most cases, the condition is acquired as the secondary result of some other problem, such as diabetes or alcoholism. In some, it is the result of a familial abnormality of plasma lipid metabolism. The most serious of the primary, hereditary disorders of lipid metabolism is familial hypercholesterolemia (FH). FH is an autosomal dominant condition caused by a defect in the transport of cholesterol into cells. It is characterized by a high risk of early-onset coronary artery and cerebrovascular disease, including myocardial infarction and stroke caused by accelerated atherosclerosis. The disease affects about 200 individuals per 100,000 population. Testing for hypercholesterolemia is simple and inexpensive, but accurate interpretation of the results of testing is more difficult. Treatment with a low-fat diet and drugs can be effective in decreasing plasma cholesterol levels and the risk of premature arterial disease, but rarely to normal levels.

About 1 in 3,500 individuals in the population are homozygous for *alpha-1-antitrypsin deficiency*, an autosomal recessive condition predisposing to chronic obstructive lung disease and emphysema, particularly on exposure to irritants, including many industrial chemicals or tobacco smoke. Avoidance of exposure to airway irritants significantly decreases the risk of lung disease. Testing for the condition is relatively simple and inexpensive, and the sensitivity and specificity of the tests are high.

*Adult-onset Gaucher disease* is an autosomal recessive disorder of glycolipid metabolism caused by deficiency of a lysosomal enzyme, beta-glucosidase. It is characterized by enlargement of the liver and spleen, with progressive thrombocytopenia (deficiency of blood platelets), sometimes causing a life-threatening bleeding tendency. Affected individuals also suffer acute episodes of severe bone pain, similar to those occurring in people with sickle cell disease. The disease is particularly common among Ashkenazi Jews, affecting up to 1 in 500 individuals; as many as 1 in 12 are carriers of the Gaucher disease gene. In the Jewish population, affected individuals and carriers are easily identified by DNA testing. The condition is so mild that most affected individuals never know they have the disease. However, in some, the disease is severely debilitating. Effective treatment by enzyme replacement therapy is possible, but it is extremely expensive, at the time of writing costing $200,000 to $300,000 per year for an affected adult.

*Huntington disease* is an autosomal dominant, adult-onset, neurodegenerative disease characterized by uncontrollable, abnormal movements of the extremities, depression, emotional lability, and progressive dementia. The movement disorder generally begins at 35–40 years of age. However, affected individuals are identifiable at any age, even prenatally, by analysis of DNA, extracted from small blood samples, for the typical trinucleotide repeat mutation characteristic of the disease. There is no effective treatment for the condition; it generally culminates in death from the complications of severe neurological impairment 15–20 years after the onset of symptoms.

## APPENDIX E: REFERENCES CITED AND FURTHER READING

Bombard, Y., & Lemmens, T. (April 2010). Insurance and Genetic Information. In: *Encyclopedia of Life Sciences (ELS)*. Chichester: John Wiley & Sons, Ltd. DOI: 10.1002/9780470015902.a0005203.pub2.

Bombard, Y., Miller, F.A., Hayeems, R.Z., Avard, D., & Knoppers, B.M. (2010). Reconsidering reproductive benefit through newborn screening: A systematic review of guidelines on preconception, prenatal, and newborn screening. *European Journal of Human Genetics, 18*(7), 751–60. http://dx.doi.org/10.1038/ejhg.2010.13

Bombard, Y., Miller, F.A., Hayeems, R.Z., Avard, D., Knoppers, B.M., Cornel, M.C., et al. (2009). The expansion of newborn screening: Is reproductive benefit an appropriate pursuit? *Nature Reviews: Genetics, 10*(10), 666–7. http://dx.doi.org/10.1038/nrg2666

Burke, W., Tarini, B., Press, N.A., & Evans, J.P. (2011). Genetic screening. *Epidemiologic Reviews, 33*(1), 148–64. http://dx.doi.org/10.1093/epirev/mxr008

Green, N.S., Dolan, S.M., & Murray, T.H. (2006). Newborn screening: Complexities in universal genetic testing. *American Journal of Public Health, 96*(11), 1955–9. http://dx.doi.org/10.2105/AJPH.2005.070300

Hanley, W.B. (2005). Newborn screening in Canada – Are we out of step? *Paediatrics and Child Health (Oxford)*, *10*(4), 203–7.

Khoury, M.J., McCabe, L.L., & McCabe, E.R.B. (2003). Population screening in the age of genomic medicine. *New England Journal of Medicine*, *348*(1), 50–8. http://dx.doi.org/10.1056/NEJMra013182

Pollitt, R.J. (2007). Introducing new screens: Why are we all doing different things? *Journal of Inherited Metabolic Disease*, *30*(4), 423–9. http://dx.doi.org/10.1007/s10545-007-0647-2

Wilson, J.M.G., & Jungner, G. (1968). *Principles and practice of screening for disease* (Public Health Paper No. 34). World Health Organization. http://whqlibdoc.who.int/php/WHO_PHP_34.pdf

Wilson, K., Kennedy, S.J., Potter, B.K., Geraghty, M.T., & Chakraborty, P. (2010). Developing a national newborn screening strategy for Canada. *Health Law Review*, *18*(2), 31–9.

The following websites may also be helpful:

Canadian Agency for Drugs and Technology in Health (CADTH) Environmental Scan Summarizing Newborn Screening in Canada, http://www.cadth.ca/en/products/environmental-scanning/environmental-scans/newborn-screening

National Heart, Lung and Blood Institute of the US National Institutes of Health, Sickle Cell Anemia, http://www.nhlbi.nih.gov/health/health-topics/topics/sca/

Newborn Screening Ontario Fact Sheets, http://www.newbornscreening.on.ca/bins/content_page.asp?cid=7-21

Ontario Ministry of Health and Long-Term Care, Executive Summary and Full Report of the Provincial Advisory Committee on New Predictive Technologies, http://www.health.gov.on.ca/english/public/pub/ministry_reports/geneticsrep01/genetic_report.html

US National Library of Medicine, Genetics Home Reference, http://ghr.nlm.nih.gov/nbs

# About the Contributors

**Raisa B. Deber**, PhD, is a Professor at the Institute of Health Policy, Management and Evaluation (HPME), Faculty of Medicine, University of Toronto. She has lectured, mentored, published, and consulted on health policy at local, provincial, national, and international levels. Her current research, conducted with colleagues and students, includes examination of the public-private mix in health care financing and delivery (including the implications of the distribution of health expenditures), health human resources, primary health care, issues associated with the movement of care from hospitals to home and community, patient engagement, and approaches to accountability. In 2009 Professor Deber received one of Canada's most prestigious lectureships, the Emmett Hall Memorial Lectureship; it recognizes outstanding contributions to the health ideals articulated by Justice Hall: equity, fairness, justice, and efficiency. In 2012, she was elected a fellow of the Canadian Academy of Health Sciences.

**Catherine L. Mah**, MD, FRCPC, PhD, is a paediatrician, Scientist at the Centre for Addiction and Mental Health, and Assistant Professor at the Dalla Lana School of Public Health, University of Toronto in the Divisions of Public Health Policy and Clinical Public Health. Dr. Mah leads a multidisciplinary program of research at the intersection of food policy, social policy, and population health. She has received funding from the Canadian Institutes of Health Research, the Public Health Agency of Canada, and the Japan Foundation. Dr. Mah has worked with stakeholders in Ontario and internationally on policy framing, policy in practice, and ethics of policy, for issues including household food insecurity, food advertising, menu labelling, and healthy food environments.

These case studies arose from Raisa B. Deber's graduate course, Case Studies in Canadian Health Policy, in HPME at the University of Toronto. As can be seen, these cases tap a wealth of knowledge and expertise. Most of the students taking the course are midcareer professionals, enrolled in a variety of programs and departments, including MSc/PhD programs, and Master of Health Science (MHSc) professional programs. Most of these cases arose from real-life situations the initial case author(s) had encountered that offered generalizable insights, and were further developed in subsequent years in active collaboration with other students who had chosen to present and develop that case. Note that their initial contributions to the cases were in their role as student, although they were kind enough to read and comment on the revised versions.

Here, briefly, is some information about the co-authors and what they told us that they were doing when they signed off on the revised case, recognizing that in this rapidly changing environment, "currently" may no longer reflect what they are doing today. Any views expressed do not necessary reflect the views of their current employers, although (as noted in the acknowledgments) we are gratified by the positive reactions we have received.

**Monica Aggarwal**, PhD, is a health care consultant with extensive experience in: primary care; eHealth; policy development and service design; program and project design, planning and implementation; health services research, analysis and evaluation; and change management. She has a special interest in improving primary and mental health care services for patients through health services research, policy development, and management.

**Mohamad Alameddine**, PhD, is currently Assistant Professor at the Department of Health Management and Policy at the Faculty of Health Sciences, American University of Beirut (AUB). He joined AUB in 2008, coming from the University of Toronto where he worked as a senior research associate and prior to that as Director of International Development at the Faculty of Medicine. He holds a PhD in health management and Policy from the University of Toronto and a Master's degree in public health from AUB. His main research interests are health human resources labour force dynamics, recruitment and retention practices, and the quality of work environments. He has a number of publications in the field and is regarded as a regional health systems consultant.

**Nurlan Algashov**, MD, MHSc, was born in Almaty, Kazakhstan, and completed his MD at the Kazakh National Medical University in 2005. He received the International Presidential Scholarship "Bolashak," and obtained his MHSc from the University of Toronto in 2008. He worked as an expert-analyst in the health sector in the JSC National Analytical Center under the Government and the National Bank of the Republic of Kazakhstan. After that he worked as a Senior Manager, then as a Director of the Department of Strategy and Analysis at Nazarbayev University in Astana. In 2012 he worked as a Deputy Chairman and then as an Acting Chairman at the Republican Research Center for Emergency Care. Currently he works as a Deputy Chairman at the National Medical Holding.

**Karen Arthurs**, RN, MHSc, has held a variety of management positions in acute care, government, private consulting, and community/public health. Currently she is Manager of Infant, Children, and Youth Services at Vancouver Coastal Health and oversees public health programs for high-risk maternity clients and young children in the Vancouver community.

**Marie Balitbit**, MHSc, CHE, DC, is currently responsible for regional site operations and business development at one of UHN Altum Health's outpatient rehabilitation facilities. She is also an Administrative Surveyor, traveling frequently to conduct accreditation surveys on rehabilitation organizations in the United States on behalf of the Commission on Accreditation of Rehabilitation Facilities (CARF). Previous roles held by Dr. Balitbit include: Director of Quality Management and Evaluation at Centric Health, National Healthcare Program Specialist for the Healthcare Services and Corporate Procurement Departments at Aviva Canada Insurance, and independently owned and operated a chiropractic clinic. She is a registered chiropractor, has an MHScs degree from the University of Toronto, and holds a Certified Health Executive designation from the Canadian College of Health Leaders.

**Patricia Baranek**, PhD, is currently a health services and policy research consultant in Toronto and has an adjunct appointment as Assistant Professor in the Institute of Health Policy, Management and Evaluation at the University of Toronto. She has co-authored *First Do No Harm, Evaluating Reform Remedies for Canadian Health Care* (UBC Press, 2002) and *Almost Home: Reforming Home and Community Care in Ontario* (University of Toronto Press, 2004).

**Charles Battershill**, PhD (York University), continues as York University contract faculty in social science and sociology. He specializes in sociology of work, industry, occupations, and professions and teaches about economic globalization. He does this while operating a modest financial planning business as a representative of Primerica Financial Services, Inc.

**Andrea Baumann**, RN, PhD, is Associate Vice-President of Global Health at McMaster University and the scientific director of the Nursing Health Services Research Unit, funded by the Ontario Ministry of Health and Long-Term Care. She is also a Professor in the School of Nursing and Director of the World Health Organization Collaborating Centre in Primary Care Nursing and Health Human Resources. Her many publications focus on decision-making and health human resource issues. In addition to her research, she has directed several international projects in relation to capacity building and higher education.

**Sherry Biscope**, MHSc, is currently working as a research consultant with Toronto Public Health.

**John Blake**, PhD, is an Associate Professor in the Department of Industrial Engineering at Dalhousie University in Halifax, Nova Scotia. He received a bachelor's degree in industrial engineering from the University of Toronto in 1988 and a doctorate in IE from the University of Toronto in 1997. He also holds an appointment with Canadian Blood Services' Research and Development Group. He is interested in the application of operational research techniques to problems in health care. These include wait times for medical care, operating room scheduling and operating room time allocation, case mix planning, platelet ordering and inventory analysis, blood product production and distribution, and multi-echelon supply chain management.

**Daniel Bolland**, MHSc, moved from health administration to work for Baxter pharmaceutical company, and then became interested in the software that it used to make, sell, ship, and run their books. After working as a consultant with Deloitte, he started his own consulting company, designing and implementing that same software, which is now owned by Oracle. He is now an independent Oracle consultant, working internationally.

**Yvonne Bombard**, PhD, received her Interdisciplinary doctorate in Medical Genetics at the University of British Columbia. She completed postdoctoral fellowships at the University of Toronto, Yale University, and Memorial Sloan-Kettering Cancer Center. Now a scientist at Li Ka Shing Knowledge Institute and Assistant Professor at IHPME at the University of Toronto, she conducts policy and health outcomes research in genomics, personalized medicine, and health technology assessment.

**Chris Bonnett**, MHSc, is President of H3 Consulting. His expertise is in workplace health strategy and health policy research, specializing in pharmaceuticals and the private sector. He has served as a volunteer board member for three health service organizations in the community and hospital sectors, and is a member and past Chair of the Canadian Council on Integrated Healthcare. He holds an MHSc from the University of Toronto, and is a PhD candidate in the School of Public Health and Health Systems at the University of Waterloo.

**Maureen Boon**, MHSc, is the Senior Advisor, Executive Office at the College of Physicians and Surgeons of Ontario. Maureen obtained her BSc from Queen's University and MHSc from the University of Toronto. She was responsible for developing and managing all college policies for nine years, most recently as Associate Director, Policy. Her current portfolio includes strategic planning, stakeholder relationship management, and eHealth project leadership.

**Karen Born** is a PhD candidate in health services research at the Institute of Health Policy, Management and Evaluation at the University of Toronto. She holds an MSc in international health policy from the London School of Economics and an honours BA in political science from McGill University.

**Laurie Bourne**, MHSc, is currently the Senior Manager of Access to Care Informatics at Cancer Care Ontario (CCO). Before joining CCO in 2010, Laurie was a consultant at the Courtyard Group healthcare consulting firm in Toronto, from 2007 to 2010. Previously she also was a health analyst for the Chief Medical Officer of Health (CMOH) at the Ontario Ministry of Health and Long-Term Care. Laurie holds an MHSc in Community Health and Epidemiology and an MHSc in Health Administration from the University of Toronto.

**Talar Boyajian** is a medical student at the University of Toronto, class of 2014. She has an MSc in Health Policy, Management and Evaluation from the University of Toronto and a Bachelor of Science in cell biology from McGill University. She has published research and worked in knowledge translation in the field of high-risk obstetrics.

**Susan Bronskill** is a scientist at the Institute for Clinical Evaluative Sciences and an Assistant Professor in the Institute of Health Policy, Management and Evaluation at the University of Toronto. She has a PhD in health policy from Harvard University and an MSc in Health Administration from the University of Toronto.

**Marion Byce** received her BSc in biology, University of Guelph, her MHSc in Health Administration, University of Toronto, and is a Registered Technologist (Cytogenetics). She presently owns and runs Spiritwood Farm in North Caledon with her husband and three daughters. Marion and her family train and sell show horses and teach horseback riding.

**Jane-Anne Campbell** worked for many years with incredible children and families, alongside dedicated colleagues, at Holland Bloorview Kids Rehabilitation Hospital in Toronto. She is currently a full-time mom with three amazing young daughters, whom she and her husband, Glen, adopted from China. She has a passion for the issues affecting children with special needs and their families, and is hoping to resume her PhD studies in this field.

**Heather Chappell,** MSc, CHE, is the National Director, Cancer Information and International Affairs at the Canadian Cancer Society. In this role, she oversees the development of cancer information and national/international cancer control strategic partnerships. She has a BSc in kinesiology from the University of Western Ontario, an MSc in health policy from the University of Toronto, and is a Certified Health Executive with the Canadian College of Health Leaders.

**Rachna Chaudhary** has practiced as an occupational therapist in Ontario for nine years, primarily working with children with varying special needs in the non-profit sector (e.g., children's treatment centres). She received her BSc (OT) from Queen's University in Kingston, ON, and her MHSc in Health Policy, Management and Evaluation (HPME) from the University of Toronto in 2011. Rachna has recently been appointed to the Board of Directors at the Scarborough Centre for Healthy Communities (SCHC), a not-for-profit community health centre (CHC) in the Greater Toronto Area, which services at-risk and marginalized populations. Rachna is passionate about evidence-based health care, the 12 determinants of health, children's health, positive organization culture, and using an ethical and systems-level approach to ameliorate the Canadian health care system.

**Munaza Chaudhry** is an independent health research consultant who has worked with federal and provincial governments, universities, and not-for-profit organizations in the areas of chronic disease management, primary health care, and quality improvement. She is currently completing her PhD in Health Policy, Management and Evaluation at the University of Toronto.

**Carole-Anne Chiasson**, MHSc, OT Reg. (Ont.), has worked at Holland Bloorview Kids Rehabilitation Hospital for nine years; her titles have included occupational therapist, manager, project support, and quality analyst. She is passionate about quality in health care, and about her family.

**Joe T.R. Clarke**, MD, PhD, MSc, FRCPC, FCCMG, is currently Professor Emeritus, University of Toronto (Department of Paediatrics), professeur d'enseignement clinique, University of Sherbrooke (Quebec), and past Chairman of the Provincial Advisory Committee on Maternal-Childhood Screening (Ontario). He is the sole author of three editions of *A Clinical Guide to Inherited Metabolic Diseases* (Cambridge University Press), first published in 1996, and of over 180 papers published in peer-reviewed medical scientific journals.

**Kathryn Clarke**, MHSc, RD, is currently working as a consulting dietician in long-term care.

**Andrea Cortinois**, PhD, has worked as a journalist, a researcher, a teacher, and a manager of health-related interventions on four continents, mainly in low-income countries. Born in Italy, he earned a Master of Public Health from the University of Wales College of Medicine, Cardiff, UK, and a PhD in Health Policy, Management and

Evaluation at the University of Toronto. Andrea works at the Centre for Global eHealth Innovation, Toronto General Hospital, where he leads the Multiculturalism and Health research stream within the People, Health Equity and Innovation (PHI) Research Group. He is an Assistant Professor at the Dalla Lana School of Public Health, University of Toronto, and teaches courses on migration and health and international health. His current research focuses on the application of new information and communication technologies to reach marginalized population groups.

**Maria Isabella (Marisa) Creatore**, PhD, is the manager of the Health Database Research Initiative and an epidemiologist at the Centre for Research on Inner City Health (CRICH) at St Michael's Hospital and the Institute for Clinical Evaluative Sciences (ICES). She has an MSc in epidemiology at Queen's University (2000) and a PhD from the University of Toronto (2013).

**Céline Cressman** is a PhD student in the Institute of Health Policy, Management and Evaluation at the University of Toronto. Her academic background includes an MSc in public health research from the University of Edinburgh, and a degree in social studies of medicine from McGill University. Her PhD thesis seeks to examine the structures of decision making and organization of service delivery in child health screening policy.

**Ian Dawe**, MD, MHSc, is the physician-in-chief at Ontario Shores Centre for Mental Health Sciences and an Associate Professor and head of the Division of General Psychiatry, Department of Psychiatry, University of Toronto.

**Doreen Day** is a senior project manager with the Ontario Provincial Council for Maternal and Child Health. She has completed an honours BSc from McMaster University and an MHSc in Health Administration from the University of Toronto and holds the qualification of certified health executive (CHE) from the Canadian College of Health Leaders.

**Rea Devakos** works in digital publishing and archiving and is the liaison librarian for the University of Toronto's Institute of Health Policy, Management and Evaluation. She holds an MLIS from UBC and an MHSc from the University of Toronto.

**Rinku Dhaliwal** graduated from McMaster University in 2002 with her BSc in nursing. Her interest in mental health led her to specialize in child and adolescent psychiatry as a registered nurse in an acute care hospital in the Waterloo Wellington LHIN. She obtained her MHSc from the University of Toronto in 2011, and is now focusing her career on developing strategies to support health system integration across the continuum of care.

**Sarah Dimmock** currently works at Women's College Hospital in Toronto where she directs strategic projects in areas of quality improvement and patient safety. As a clinical occupational therapist, Sarah specialized in neonatal intensive care and acute care pediatrics at the Hospital for Sick Children in Toronto. Sarah completed her MHSc in Health Administration at the University of Toronto, BHSc in occupational therapy at McMaster University, and a BA (Hons) in political science and history at McMaster University.

**Mark Dobrow**, PhD, is Director of Analysis and Reporting at the Health Council of Canada and Associate Professor in the Institute of Health Policy, Management and Evaluation at the University of Toronto. Previously, he was scientist and lead of the Cancer Services & Policy Research Unit at Cancer Care Ontario. His research interests include the optimization of the use of scientific and non-scientific evidence, performance management systems, and clinical/corporate accountability mechanisms to support/guide decision making by organizations that manage, organize, finance, and/or deliver health services.

**Adam M. Dukelow**, MD, MHSc, FRCP(C), CHE, is Associate Professor in the Division of Emergency Medicine at the University of Western Ontario. Dr. Dukelow's clinical practice is based at London Health Sciences Centre (University and Victoria Hospital Emergency Departments) and St. Joseph's Health Centre (London) Urgent Care Centre. Dr. Dukelow has a special interest in improving patient care through health administration.

**Laura Esmail**, PhD, is a Senior Manager at AcademyHealth (Washington, DC) where she helps lead projects on patient and stakeholder engagement, patient-centered outcomes research, and comparative effectiveness research. She obtained her doctorate in pharmaceutical policy from the University of Toronto and has over ten years of experience in the design, analysis, and dissemination of research that aims to improve patient outcomes and health policy.

**Sheryl Farrar**, BSc, MHSc, has worked in the fields of primary health care, hospital relationships with primary health care providers, and public health. She is currently a program manager in public health in Eastern Ontario.

**Daniel Farris** completed studies in biology and joined the Canadian Forces in 1985. He has a Certificate in Health Services Management from the Canadian Healthcare Association and an MHSc from the University of Toronto. He is a CHE and a graduate of the Canadian Forces Staff School and Land Forces Command and Staff School.

**David Ford** is a management consultant with health care consulting experience in London and Toronto. He previously worked with the Ontario Medical Association as a senior policy analyst and holds an MHSc from the University of Toronto.

**Brenda Gamble** received her PhD in Medical Sciences from the University of Toronto and is an Assistant Professor in the Faculty of Health Sciences at the University of Ontario Institute of Technology (UOIT). Her research areas include health human resources, accountability in health care, interprofessional practice, and the medical laboratory sector.

**Stephanie Gan**, following graduation from the University of Toronto, entered the ranks of the Canadian federal public service through the Accelerated Economist Training Program and is currently an analyst at the Privy Council Office.

**Katerina Gapanenko**, MD, PhD, received her MHSc in Health Administration from the University of Toronto, HPME, Faculty of Medicine.

**Michael Gardam**, MD, Director of Infection Prevention and Control at the University Health Network (since 2001), and former Director of Infectious Disease Prevention and Control at the Ontario Agency for Health Protection and Promotion (2008–10), is devoted to discovering new ways to prevent the spread of infectious diseases in health care settings and the community. He continues to champion the elimination of "superbugs" as Physician Director of the Community and Hospital

Infection Control Association Canada (CHICA) and the national lead of the "Stop Infections Now!" collaborative for Safer Healthcare Now!, and to run the tuberculosis (TB) clinic that he founded in 2000 at Toronto Western Hospital. He is an international expert consultant in patient and staff safety issues such as TB, SARS, pandemic influenza, medical device reprocessing, and hospital superbugs. He is also an Associate Professor of Medicine at the University of Toronto. He is a graduate of McGill University and the University of Toronto and is a fellow of the Royal College of Physicians and Surgeons of Canada in infectious diseases.

**Nada Victoria Ghandour** is the Statutory Specialist at the Region of Peel. She graduated with a Master's degree in Public Administration and Policy from Carleton University. She currently serves as the Vice Chair on the Municipal Education and Research Fund, and currently sits on the Access and Privacy Working group at the Association of Municipal Clerks and Treasurers of Ontario. She is working towards an Information Access and Privacy Protection certificate at the University of Alberta and continues to focus her research on access to information and privacy as it relates to municipal government administration.

**Erin Gilbart**, PhD, is an independent health care consultant with expertise in performance measurement, quality improvement, and the application of evidence-based clinical practice guidelines with an emphasis on the aging population. Recent work includes data analysis and report writing for a longitudinal study of assisted living and long-term care residents in Alberta. Her clients include academic institutions, government, and health care providers.

**Asmita Gillani** is the CEO of Aga Khan University Hospital, Nairobi, Kenya. Previously she served as chief operating officer for more than seven years and as CEO for six months at York Central Hospital in Richmond Hill, Ontario, before she was called upon to assume her current position. She holds an MHSc from the University of Toronto and a BSc (Hons) from the University of London. She is a Certified Health Care Executive with the Canadian College of Health Care Executives. She has received awards for her professionalism and volunteerism (including the Queens Golden Jubilee Award), published articles related to the health profession, and served on important Canadian health committees. Her contribution as a volunteer has been extensive, including as Chair of the Aga Khan Social Welfare Board for Canada and as

Vice President of the Aga Khan Council for Canada for two consecutive terms. Currently she serves on many public-private committees dedicated to furthering the quality and standards of care in the region.

**Carolyn Steele Gray**, MA, PhD, received her degree at the University of Toronto in Health Policy, Management and Evaluation in 2013. Her doctoral work focused on accountability in the home and community care sector in Ontario. She is working as a post-doctoral fellow at the Bridgepoint Collaboratory for Research and Innovation in Toronto. The post-doctoral work focuses on developing and implementing integrated care plans for complex continuing care patients and creating electronic patient reported outcomes tools. She holds an MA in Public Policy and Administration from Ryerson University where her work focused on performance measurement in supportive housing. In addition to her studies, Carolyn worked as a program evaluator for the York Institute for Health Research, Program Evaluation Unit, and has been involved in a number of health services research projects.

**Joanne Greco** is the Vice President, Infrastructure and Chief Nursing Officer at Closing the Gap Healthcare Group. As a passionate healthcare leader who has repeatedly demonstrated her ability to provide leadership excellence in community healthcare, Joanne has over 20 years of experience in various leadership roles at such organizations as the Toronto Central Community Care Access Centre (Director of Client Services) and the former North York Community Care Access Centre in Toronto. Some of Joanne's work experiences include leadership in various reviews and projects to improve health system processes and efficiencies, involving primary care, acute care, long-term care, and community care sectors. She holds a BSc in Nursing from the University of Windsor, and an MHSc in Health Administration, University of Toronto. Joanne also has certificates in Project Management, Lean Process Improvement, and is a Certified Health Services Executive.

**Shawna Gutfreund** holds an MA in philosophy with a specialization in bioethics from McGill University and an MHSc in Health Administration from the University of Toronto. She has worked as a research ethics coordinator, privacy officer, and policy analyst.

**Olivia Hagemeyer** completed an MHSc in Health Administration in 2009. She is a speech-language pathologist and manager of the

Augmentative Communication & Writing Aids Program at Surrey Place Centre in Toronto.

**Carrie-Lynn Haines** is a Registered Nurse who has had experience in a variety of roles over the past 30 years, including emergency department administrator, change agent, investigator, clinician, educator, consultant, and patient care advocate, and has worked in a variety of health care environments, including academic/tertiary and community hospitals, public health, the College of Physicians and Surgeons of Ontario, and the Ontario Hospital Association. She is currently Project Manager, Ontario at the Canadian Patient Safety Institute. She graduated with an MHSc degree in Health Administration from the University of Toronto in 2011.

**David Hoff** worked for 20 years for the Ontario Ministry of Health and Long-Term Care in a variety of director-level positions in policy and planning. He worked as a Public Member of the Consent and Capacity Board, and of the Ontario College of Pharmacists, and he works with the Canadian Coast Guard Auxiliary. He has master's degrees in philosophy (UWO) and public health (University of Michigan) and has also done graduate studies in health policy (University of Toronto) and epidemiology (UWO).

**Jeff Hohenkerk** is currently Vice President of Quinte Health Care in Ontario. Jeff has 28 years of experience, both in the public and private healthcare sectors. His experience includes medical diagnostic imaging, laboratory services, strategy, clinical informatics, capital redevelopment, performance management, and transformation. Jeff played a major role as a Provincial MRI Process Improvement Coach for the MOHLTC and Vice Chair of the Wait Times Strategy and Diagnostics Working Group to improve wait times for the province. He was also an active member of the CE LHIN Regional Rehab Working Group, the Clinical Education Leadership Council of the Michener Institute for Applied Sciences, the Breast Screening Program for Rouge Valley Hospital, and volunteers as a board member on several not-for-profit organizations. He holds a Master's degree in Health Administration, Lean Six Sigma Black Belt Certification, Bachelor of Applied Sciences, Diploma of Health Services Management, and a Medical Radiation Technology License. Jeff is a Certified Health Services Executive.

**Julie Holmes** is currently the Director of Ambulatory Services at St Joseph's Healthcare in Hamilton, Ontario. She has a BA degree from McMaster University and an MHSc degree from the University of Toronto.

**Paul Holyoke** has a PhD in Health Policy from the University of Toronto, an MSc (Econ) from the London School of Economics, and a law degree from the University of Toronto. He is Saint Elizabeth Health Care's director of research and program development, and he teaches at York University's School of Health Policy and Management. His current areas of research are personal support and rehabilitation services in home care and education programs and supports for unpaid family caregivers.

**Lisa Jackson**, MHSc, is a healthcare administrator with a broad range of skills in strategic planning, general management, and consulting. Lisa has varied career experience including working in three countries (Canada, United States, and Scotland). Lisa has particular expertise in implementing complex change-management initiatives that span the continuum of care.

**Carolina Jimenez**, MD, MSc, was born in Bogota, Colombia. She did an elective in the Department of General Surgery at the University of Toronto and a research elective at the Centre for Global eHealth Innovation as a medical student. After moving to Canada, she completed a Master's degree from the Institute of Health Policy, Management and Evaluation, under the supervision of Dr. Alex Jadad. Her thesis was a systematic review and content analysis of national information and communication technologies (ICT) and eHealth policies in Latin America and the Caribbean. She has continued doing research at the University of Toronto and the University Health Network.

**David Kirsch**, PhD, is a research fellow in the Global Health Diplomacy Program at the Munk School of Global Affairs. He has Master's-level degrees in computer science and health policy, and a PhD in medical science. He has a keen interest in healthcare and the public sector and is committed to improving program effectiveness through sensibly applied accountability and governance. His current research interests include accountability, governance, under-5 mortality, and innovation.

He advises governments and major businesses in the areas of strategic planning, business transformation, enterprise architecture, informatics, program evaluation, accountability, and governance.

**Joshua Kline**, MD, is a practicing family physician with Parkview Physicians Group and the Physician Leader of the Primary Care Service Line, Parkview Health, Fort Wayne, Indiana. He worked on this case while studying at the University of Toronto on a Fulbright scholarship.

**Christopher A. Klinger**, PhD, received his PhD in the Institute of Health Policy, Management and Evaluation (HPME) at the University of Toronto. After working as a long-term care nurse in Germany, he developed a passion for improving care for this population. He has also studied at the Research Summer School at Lancaster University's International Observatory on End of Life Care in the United Kingdom, worked for the National Hospice and Palliative Care Organization, Inc. (NHPCO) in Virginia, and taught health-systems courses at Fachhochschule Koblenz. He currently holds a research assistantship with the Bruyère Research Institute's (BRI) Palliative Care Education and Research Program in Ottawa, and co-chairs the National Initiative for the Care of the Elderly's (NICE) End-of-Life Issues Theme Team.

**Irene Koo**, MHSc, currently works as Quality Lead in Ambulatory Programs at SickKids Hospital. Prior to completing her MHSc, she worked as a physical therapist for over 10 years specializing in rehabilitation of children with neurological disorders. She has taught courses at George Brown College and the University of Toronto. Her interests are in looking at system efficiencies that allow a more seamless transition for families navigating the healthcare system.

**William Kou**, MHSc, is an epidemiologist at the York Region Community and Health Services Department in Ontario. He has worked on various projects, including population health assessment reports, the development of a balanced scorecard for public health, and an ongoing risk factor surveillance survey for adults.

**Nancy Kraetschmer**, MBA, PhD, is a senior health care leader with extensive experience in health policy, research and evaluation, and strategy. Her research interests include hospital accountability and performance measurement systems. In addition to her day job, she also holds an adjunct faculty position in the Institute of Health Policy, Management and Evaluation at the University of Toronto.

**Seija K. Kromm** holds an MA in economics from the University of Calgary and is currently a PhD candidate at the Institute of Health Policy, Management and Evaluation at the University of Toronto. Prior to her PhD studies, she worked as a laboratory technician in the area of fertility evaluation and treatment, and as a research associate in health economics.

**Kerry Kuluski** completed her PhD in health services research at the University of Toronto in 2010. Following this, she spent six months as a visiting scholar with the Health Experiences Research Group at the University of Oxford. Kerry is currently a research scientist at Bridgepoint Health in Toronto, where she is leading a program of research on complex chronic disease and patient experience.

**Lise Labrecque**, BSW, MHSc, Cert. Prog. Eval., is an evaluator and health promoter working in Ottawa, Ontario. She currently works in the public health sector, supporting management teams with strategy implementation and leadership development. Before going into public health, Lise spent 15 years developing, implementing, and evaluating community-based health promotion programs in Community Health Centres.

**Kenneth Cheak Kwan Lam**, PhD, is a Course Director in the School of Health Policy and Management and Adjunct Professor in the Graduate Program in Health at York University. Kenneth previously worked as a consultant with the OMHLTC and in various capacities with the Ontario Agency for Health Protection and Promotion (now renamed Public Health Ontario), The Change Foundation, and the Ontario Hospital Association. In addition to his doctorate in health policy from the University of Toronto, he also holds an Honours Bachelor of Arts with distinction in political science from the University of Toronto, a Master of Arts in political science from McMaster University, and a Master of Public Administration from the School of Policy Studies at Queen's University. Commencing in Fall 2013, Kenneth will be pursuing a Master of Studies in Law at the University of Toronto while continuing his teaching at York.

**Bev Lever**, BA, MSW, MHSc in bioethics, PhD candidate, has worked in executive positions in the public, private, and health research sectors. Her experience as the Vice-President of Provincial Government Relations/Stakeholder Partnerships with Canada's Research-Based Pharmaceutical Companies, as well as her position as Lead, Health Care Research for the Ontario Ministry of Health and Long-Term Care, positioned her well to address pharmaceutical/health care issues in a fair and ethical manner.

**Leah Levesque**, BScN, MHSc, CHE, is the Vice-President of Patient/Resident Services at the Arnprior and District Memorial Hospital and the Grove Nursing Home. She has worked in a variety of clinical settings, including critical care as a nurse, and later managed departments, including emergency, medicine/surgery, operating room, and PACU departments in both rural and urban settings. She completed her Master's degree in Health Administration at the University of Toronto in 2010.

**Esther Levy**, MHSc, has held a variety of management and policy positions in healthcare and with the Ontario government. Formerly a Speech-Language Pathologist in neuro-rehabilitation, she worked with the Ministry of the Attorney General's Office of the Public Guardian and Trustee on the operationalization of health consent and substitute decision making legislation. Within the Ministry of Children and Youth Services, she led a number of key policy and program initiatives in child welfare, and is currently the Director of the Child and Youth Development Branch.

**Judy Litwack-Goldman**, MHSc, President of Judy Litwack-Goldman Consulting, has extensive experience in strategic planning, capacity assessments, board development, fundraising, and communications for non-profit and charitable organizations. Since 1990, she has been helping non-profit organizations and charities adapt to change.

**Christopher J. Longo**, PhD, is Associate Professor, DeGroote School of Business, Health Policy and Management, and Member, Centre for Health Economics and Policy Analysis, McMaster University, and Associate Professor (status only), Dalla Lana School of Public Health, University of Toronto. He holds a BA in economics, York University; MSc, physiology, University of Western Ontario; and PhD, Health

Policy, Management and Evaluation, University of Toronto. Dr. Longo has over 20 years of industry and academic experience in clinical research, economic evaluation, and market access and policy strategies for pharmaceuticals. His research interests include: the economic and quality of life evaluation of health technologies (predominately pharmaceuticals) in the areas of cancer, diabetes, sepsis, and public health programs; the equity implications of efficiency initiatives on patients' financial burden for health care; global pharmaceutical pricing strategies; and behavioral factors that lead to higher individual consumption of healthcare resources. Although still involved in many research projects related to the healthcare system and its end users, he has refocused his research agenda. His latest research examines the costs and economic evaluation of interventions/programs throughout the cancer journey, with the intent of informing policy decision making.

**Helen Looker** has worked in several fields of research since graduating from the University of Toronto in 2005, including seeking best practices for injury prevention and as an interviewer for a McMaster University stroke rehabilitation study that compared costs of institutional vs. home delivery of services. Currently, with a MSc in Planning, Helen is acquiring technical skills for a career in the planning profession and looks forward to planning healthy communities.

**Nibal Lubbad**, MD, CCFP, MHSc, is currently working as a family doctor in Burlington, Ontario – a specialty she has much passion for. Born in Gaza, Palestine, she went to Russia for her MD, graduated from St Petersburg Academy of Medicine, and worked as a general practitioner in Palestine. In 2003, she completed her MHSc in Family and Community Medicine at the University of Toronto, and also received her academic fellowship in family medicine from that department. After working as a research officer in Health Policy, Management and Evaluation at the University of Toronto, including studies of the impact of primary health care on the acute care sector, she completed her Family Medicine Residency at McMaster University, Department of Family Medicine, Hamilton, Ontario.

**Daune MacGregor**, MD, is a Paediatric Neurologist and recently completed two terms as Associate Paediatrician-in-Chief, and Associate Chair, Clinical Services, in the Department of Paediatrics at the Hospital for Sick Children, University of Toronto. Her most recent appointment is as Associate Medical Director, SickKids International. She completed her medical training at the University of Saskatchewan, graduating cum laude in 1971. She then trained in Paediatrics and Neurology in Toronto at the Hospital for Sick Children and did postgraduate studies in Developmental Neurology at the Hospital for Sick Children, Great Ormond Street, London, England, and the Children's Hospital Medical Center at Harvard University in Boston, Massachusetts. She was appointed a Full Professor of Paediatrics and Neurology at the University of Toronto in 1995. Her research interests are in the study of cerebral vascular disorders including stroke and headache, and neurodevelopmental disorders including acquired brain injury in children. Dr. MacGregor is a past President of the Canadian Association of Child Neurologists. She is currently completing her MBA studies at Athabaska University.

**Leslie MacMillan**, MD, MHSc, is a hospital clinical associate in Medical Oncology in Toronto.

**Maria Mathews**, PhD, is Associate Professor of Health Policy/Health Care Delivery in the Division of Community Health & Humanities, Faculty of Medicine, Memorial University, Newfoundland. She has a PhD in Health Policy, Management and Evaluation from the University of Toronto and a Master's degree in Health Services Administration from the University of Alberta.

**Mina Mawani**, MHSc, is the Chief Development Officer at the Greater Toronto CivicAction Alliance (CivicAction), leading the organization's resource development and capacity-building strategies. Prior to joining CivicAction, Mina was CEO of the Aga Khan Council for Canada, and has also held key roles at the Ministry of Health and Long-Term Care, KPMG, and PricewaterhouseCoopers, working with the largest hospitals in Ontario. Mina has a talent for building consensus on tough decisions, and uses her business background and strong financial and analytical skills to ensure that a compelling vision is backed by a solid business plan.

**Elizabeth McCarthy**, RSW, MHSc CHE, has worked in the Ontario health care system for the past 25 years, most of them in hospital leadership positions. During a five-year period working as a consultant in a Ministry of Health and Long-Term Care regional office, she gained perspective on how local needs and interests are able to influence public health policy at a provincial level.

**Christopher W. McDougall** holds a BA and an MA in political science from McGill University, was a graduate student at the Institut de sciences politiques de Paris, and a visiting fellow at the Erasmus Mundus Master of Bioethics at the Università degli Studi di Padova. He is currently completing a doctorate in health policy and bioethics at the University of Toronto's IHPME. Christopher's research lies at the intersection of international law and relations, population health, and moral theory. His recent publications have focused on ethical and public-health arguments for improving infectious disease–control policy, multilevel health governance, and global health diplomacy and assistance. Christopher was also part of a three-year project at NCCHPP and the INSPQ to develop a wide array of tools and resources for the integration of moral reasoning into the everyday practice of Canadian public-health professionals.

**Major Brandy McKenna** is a Regular Force Military Health Care Administrator who has been serving with the Canadian Forces since 1996. Her numerous appointments have included administrative, operational, and clinical roles, both domestic and abroad. Her career highlight includes being deployed to the Role 3 Multinational Medical Unit (combat hospital) in Kandahar, Afghanistan, for a seven-month rotation (August 2007–March 2008) as the National Medical Liaison Officer/Administrative Officer. Having graduated from the Royal Military College of Canada (Kingston, Ontario) with an undergraduate degree in honours English (2000), she also completed a Health Management Certificate Program through Ryerson University, Toronto (2003), achieved her Certified Health Executive (CHE) certification through the Canadian College of Health Leaders (2004), and completed an MHSc in Health Administration through the University of Toronto (2011). Brandy is currently the Officer Commanding/Clinic Manager for 2 Field Ambulance Medical Clinic at Garrison Petawawa.

**Meghan McMahon** is a PhD student in the Institute of Health Policy, Management and Evaluation at the University of Toronto. Her research interests centre on health care financing and funding. She is also the Assistant Director of the CIHR Institute of Health Services and Policy Research.

**Wendy Medved** is a graduate of the MHSc Health Administration program in Health Policy, Management and Evaluation at the University of Toronto. She has a background in sociology, and has extensive research and project management experience, having conducted and coordinated numerous sociobehavioural, epidemiological, and clinical research studies on health-related issues. In 1994 she conducted a qualitative research study on the sociopsychological impact of in vitro fertilization treatment failure on childless women. She is currently a Policy Lead at the Health Council of Canada.

**Elaine Meertens** received her MHSc from the Health Administration program at the University of Toronto. A nurse with experience as a clinical manager, she is currently the Director, Cancer Planning and Regional Programs at Cancer Care Ontario.

**Paul Miller**, MD, MHSc, FRCPC, is a staff Emergency Physician at Hamilton Health Sciences Centre and Assistant Clinical Professor, Division of Emergency Medicine, Department of Medicine at McMaster University in Hamilton, Ontario. His academic interests include administrative medicine, systems improvement, and physician engagement.

**Gunita Mitera**, BSc, MRT(T), MBA, PhD candidate, is a Quality Initiatives Specialist at the Canadian Partnership Against Cancer in Toronto, Ontario. She previously worked as a Radiation Therapist at the Sunnybrook Odette Cancer Centre. Her research interests include health services research related to access to care, health policy, palliative care, and health technology assessment.

**Lucinda Montizambert** holds an MHSc (Health Promotion) from the University of Toronto and an MA in International Affairs from the Norman Patterson School of International Affairs at Carleton University. Lucinda currently works as a senior policy analyst at Status of Women Canada and is a member of the Society for International Development Board of Directors, Ottawa Gatineau, and chairs its Gender Working Group.

**Frances Morton-Chang**, MHSc, is currently a PhD candidate in Health Policy at the University of Toronto, where she pursues her keen interest in gerontology and health policy; her thesis examines the mix of resources required to maintain frail and/or cognitively impaired seniors (deemed eligible for LTC facility placement) safely in the community. Her work experience spans a variety of health sectors, including home care, acute care, long-term care, and charities, with a specialty in the area of dementia (particularly Alzheimer disease). She is also a sought-after consultant with Local Health Integration Networks, NGOs, and private and not-for-profit organizations, and a doting mother to two beautiful sons.

**Shaheena Mukhi**, MHSc, is a flex-time PhD candidate in health policy and works at the Canadian Institute for Health Information (CIHI). At CIHI, she is leading the development and implementation of the pan-Canadian Primary Health Care Voluntary Reporting System and comparative reports to improve access, availability, and use of primary health care information for quality improvement and health system evaluation and planning.

**Michèle Parent**, MSc, PhD, is an Aboriginal health scholar currently working as a consultant. She formerly taught at Nipissing University School of Nursing and the Faculty of Nursing, University of Regina. She is Métis and an active member of the Canadian College of Health Leaders.

**Allie Peckham** is a PhD student in the Institute of Health Policy Management and Evaluation at the University of Toronto. She graduated from the University of Toronto in January 2009 with a Master of Social Work. Prior to her studies at the University of Toronto, she completed her BA in Honours Gerontology with a Minor in Sociology at McMaster University. During her studies, she gained considerable experience in conducting both qualitative and quantitative research related to care for seniors and their informal caregivers in the home and community care sector.

**Yeesha Poon**, BSc, Phm, MBA, MSc, HTA, PhD candidate, worked as a Drug Advertising Reviewer at Advertising Standards Canada and is now Director of Market Access, responsible for drug formulary submissions across Canada, with Ferring, Inc.

**Caroline Rafferty**, MHSc, is a healthcare executive, graduate of the HPME program, and Registered Nurse. She has a broad range of work experiences within the public and private healthcare sectors. Caroline has worked in the development of public health policy that includes hospital funding, service integration, and EMR development. As a senior healthcare consultant, she has provided leadership for initiatives in a variety of healthcare sectors, nationally and internationally, to address cost, quality and access pressures. Currently, Caroline is focused on primary-care reform, where she continues to pursue her passion of public-policy implementation to improve access and system integration for the benefit of individuals and their families.

**Glen Randall** is Associate Professor in the Health Services Management area of the DeGroote School of Business and Member of the Centre for Health Economics and Policy Analysis at McMaster University. He holds a PhD in Health Policy, Management and Evaluation from the University of Toronto, as well as an MBA, MA, and BA from McMaster University. His research interests focus on the impact of health care policies on health professionals.

**Natalie (Wajs) Rashkovan**, MHSc, is currently working as a program and project manager for the University of Toronto Stroke Program (UTSP). The ability to exercise her research and project management skills over a broad range of health-related areas is what keeps her energized and loving her work.

**Melissa Rausch** is the manager of business development and special projects at SRT Med-Staff in Toronto. She received her MHSc in Health Administration from the University of Toronto.

**David Reeleder** graduated in 2006 with his PhD in Health Policy and Bioethics from the University of Toronto. After over 20 years with the Ontario Ministry of Health and Long-Term Care performing a variety of policy-related managerial portfolios, he currently operates as an independent healthcare consultant.

**Zahava R.S. Rosenberg-Yunger**, PhD, is currently a postdoctoral fellow at the Keenan Research Centre of the Li Ka Shing Knowledge Institute of St Michael's Hospital. She obtained her PhD from Health Policy, Management and Evaluation and the Collaborative Program in Bioethics at the University of Toronto. She completed an MA in Interdisciplinary

Studies at York University. Her research interests include health studies research, ethics, priority setting, health policy, and mixed methods designs.

**Eleanor Ross**, BScN, MScN, has been President of the professional associations in Ontario (RNAO) 1987–9 and Canada (CNA) 1994–6, and Vice-President of the International Council of Nurses (ICN) 2001–5. Her nursing practice has included teaching, research, clinical nurse practitioning, and administration. A number of awards and honours have been bestowed on her.

**Mark Rovere** is a Senior Policy Advisor in the Health System Strategy and Policy Division at the Ontario Ministry of Health and Long-Term Care. He was previously Associate Director (2010–12) and Senior Policy Analyst (2006–10) in the health policy research centre at the Fraser Institute. He holds an Honours Bachelor's degree and a Master's degree in Political Science from the University of Windsor, and is currently completing a PhD in Health Services Research (health policy) at the University of Toronto's Institute of Health Policy, Management and Evaluation (IHPME). He has authored and co-authored numerous studies, articles, and commentaries on a wide range of health and pharmaceutical policy–related issues.

**David Rudoler** is a doctoral candidate in the Institute of Health Policy, Management and Evaluation at the University of Toronto. Before pursuing his doctoral degree, he received a Master of Public Policy Administration and Law from York University. He also has experience working in a number of departments in the Ontario Public Service, including senior-level positions within the Ontario Ministry of Health and Long-Term Care.

**Somayeh Sadat**, PhD, University of Toronto, is a health care consultant experienced in population-based and clinical service analyses in support of health system planning, as well as process reengineering in support of quality improvement initiatives.

**Miriam Alton Scharf**, BScN, MHSc, had an extensive career in health care, working in community health, acute care teaching hospitals, and community-based organizations. In her management role in a multidisciplinary setting, she developed new programs and evaluated current programs focusing on goals and results-based management. Sadly, she passed away in June 2012.

**Brian Schwartz**, MD, is Associate Professor in the Department of Family and Community Medicine and the Dalla Lana School of Public Health at the University of Toronto, and currently serves as Chief, Emergency Preparedness and Executive Lead, Service Integration at Public Health Ontario. His academic interests are in health emergency management policy and practice, emergency medical services, and critical incident stress in health emergency responders. Dr. Schwartz is the recipient of awards of excellence from the Ontario Medical Association, the Ontario College of Family Physicians, and the National Association of Emergency Medical Services Physicians.

**Natasha Sharpe**, MBA, PhD, is President of Bridging Finance, Inc. Prior to joining Bridging Finance, Natasha was the Chief Credit Officer for Sun Life Financial's $110-billion global portfolio. Prior to that, Natasha spent over 10 years at the Bank of Montreal, where she led various teams in risk assessment and corporate finance. In 2010 Natasha was named as one of Canada's top 40 under 40. Natasha is a director of public, private, and nonprofit companies. She holds a PhD in health policy and a MBA from the University of Toronto.

**Shannon L. Sibbald**, PhD, is Adjunct Faculty in the School of Health Studies, Faculty of Health Sciences at the University of Western Ontario. She completed her master's and doctoral degrees though the Department of Health Policy, Management and Evaluation and the Collaborative Program in Bioethics at the University of Toronto. Her research interests include the management and translation of knowledge in various health settings (including primary, acute, and public health), health policy/health services research, and the ethics of resource allocation.

**Shahzad Siddiqui** is a Toronto-based lawyer. He is a graduate of the University of Toronto, where he designed an undergraduate program in health policy and did Master's-level courses with Dr Deber, before completing an LLB at Osgoode Hall Law School and an LLM at the University of Pennsylvania Law School. He has lived and worked in Zambia, England, Pakistan, China, Canada, and the United States.

**Louise Signal**, PhD, is a director of the Health Promotion and Policy Research Unit at the University of Otago, Wellington, New Zealand. She has over 20 years' experience in health research and practice, including as an advisor to the New Zealand Ministry of Health.

**Rena Singer-Gordon** graduated from the MHSc Health Promotion program at the University of Toronto in 1996. Currently, her company, Holistic Health Matters, specializes in bioenergetic healing solutions for body, mind, and soul. She lives in Thornhill, Ontario, with her husband, Stanley Gordon.

**Joe Slack** is a technical specialist in the Performance Measurement Department at University Health Network. He completed his MHSc in Health Administration at the University of Toronto and is a Certified Health Executive.

**Karen Spalding** is Director of the Graduate Program at the Daphne Cockwell School of Nursing, Ryerson University, Toronto, and a paediatric nurse, with a PhD focusing on health policy. The main focus of her research program is the role of government in health care, how it is shaped by the interests and actions of key political actors and professional organizations, and the consequences of health system changes for health care organizations, providers (nurses), consumers (parents and children), and governments themselves. She is currently co-investigator on several externally funded research studies, involving both quantitative and qualitative methods, of the delivery and organization of paediatric home care. As a nurse and health policy researcher, she is committed to ensuring that the new knowledge generated through her research is translated to key decision makers, consumers, providers, and government policymakers.

**Wendy Sutton** is a Toronto lawyer with an LLM in health law, and is a Vice Chair of the Workplace Safety and Insurance Appeals Tribunal. She was a member of the Interim Regulatory Council on Midwifery (Ontario) from 1989 to 1992 and President of the Toronto Birth Centre from 1990 to 2010. She is the co-author with Marilou McPhedran of *Preventing Sexual Abuse of Patients: A Legal Guide for Health Care Professionals* (2004).

**Phyllis Tanaka**, MSc (Nutritional Sciences), is a dietician and the Vice-President of Scientific & Regulatory Affairs for Food & Consumer

Products of Canada, an association that represents food and consumer goods manufacturers in Canada. She works specifically on policy and regulatory issues related to the nutrition-food-health paradigm. She is a member of Equal Voice, a non-profit organization with a mandate to change the political scene in Canada so that more women engage in and take political office at all levels of government. She resides in Toronto.

**Vera Ingrid Tarman**, MD, MSc, FCFP, CASAM, is currently the medical director of Renascent, and a staff consultant for the Salvation Army Homestead.

**Lee Tasker,** BS, PhD, received her BS in Kinesiology and Exercise Science (University of Waterloo) and her PhD in the interdisciplinary graduate program at the University of Calgary. Her research examined how the design of a motor vehicle accident insurance compensation system affects access to benefits for claimants who have sustained a traumatic brain injury, and how this, in turn, affects recovery, if at all. She is President of Lee Tasker Counselling Inc.

**Dan Tassie** graduated with a MScPl from the University of Toronto. He currently works as a research analyst at Ryerson University in Toronto.

**Fern Teplitsky** is an experienced educator, planner, and facilitator. She has a Bachelor's degree in Community Nursing and a Master's degree in Environmental Studies (Specialization in Policy and Planning for the Elderly in Ontario). For nine years, she was a Senior Health Planner with the Toronto District Health Council, where she specialized in planning issues related to seniors, community services, and long-term care facilities. Since 2003, she has operated her own consulting firm.

**Romy Joseph Thomas**, MBA, MHSc, CHE, is a Health Care Executive with special interest in health policy, organizational strategy, and operations. Romy's prior assignments include consulting and in the near past serving as COO of an academic health center in India. He has since moved to Toronto and now works for a health-service organization in capital planning.

**Sharon Vanin**, MHSc, works as Legal Counsel at Cancer Care Ontario. She is a graduate of Queen's University, Osgoode Hall Law School, and the University of Toronto.

**Kenneth Van Wyk**, MBA, is a practicing psychotherapist and the executive director of Christian Counselling Services. He is a PhD candidate at the Institute for Christian Studies in a conjoint program with the Free University of Amsterdam.

**Judy Verbeeten**, MD, MHSC, is a retired eye physician and surgeon who practiced in Toronto for 30 years.

**Jillian Watkins**, BASc, is a doctoral student in Health Policy, Management and Evaluation at the University of Toronto. Jillian's doctoral research focuses on the provision of home and community care services for marginalized seniors, specifically seniors who identify as lesbian, gay, bisexual, and transgender.

**Anne Wojtak**, MHSc, BSc, is the Senior Director of Performance Management and Accountability for the Toronto Central Community Care Access Centre. Her diverse portfolio includes corporate performance, procurement and contract management, strategic planning, risk management, research, and communications. She is an adjunct faculty member of the University of Toronto in the Health Policy, Management and Evaluation Program, where she is a guest lecturer on strategic planning and a tutor for Canada's Health System and Health Policy course.

**Rachel Wortzman**, MD, MPH, is a resident in the Department of Family and Community Medicine at the University of Toronto. Her professional interests include primary care reform, social determinants of health, and healthy public policy. Dr. Wortzman also received her MD and MPH from the University of Toronto.

**Betty Wu-Lawrence**, RN, BscN, MEd, PHCNP, is currently working as a public health nurse with Toronto Public Health. Among her many voluntary and community activities, she was an appointed as a council member for the College of Midwives of Ontario, 1993–6.

**Linda Gail Young** served as the Director of Personnel at Fort McMurray Region Hospital, Alberta, and as the Director of Human Resources and then as Vice-President, Human Resources at Surrey Memorial Hospital. After obtaining her MHSc (Health Administration) at the University of Toronto, she was Vice-President of Medical Operations for the Regina Health District. She passed away far too young and we miss her. Her husband, Dr Eric Young, wrote that she would have been delighted to hear that a second edition of the *Case Studies* book is being published, especially with her case study in it.

**Debra Zelisko** obtained her Master's degree in Audiology at Western University and has worked for over 20 years in hearing healthcare, in a variety of roles including clinical research, clinical practice, industry, as well as management. She is currently Vice President of Operations at Lifestyle Hearing Corporation. She is also completing her PhD in health policy at the University of Toronto.